A Physique Guide For Self Reliant Women

BODYMAGIC
A Great Body At Any Age

By Julie & Gary Walsh

Love to all the women that take control of their own body. A Precious Gift

BODYMAGIC - Books By The Same Authors.

A Man's Search For Meaning - *Identity Construction Of A Bodybuilder.*

Bodymagic - *Different For Girls*

Bodymagic - *A Beginners Guide To Training & Nutrition*

Bodymagic - *3 Legs & Abs Blasts*

Bodymagic - *3 Pecs & Lats Routines*

Bodymagic - *3 Upper Body Routines*

Bodymagic - *Fitness Facts*

Bodymagic - *Super-Gran Legs & Abs Routine*

Bodymagic - *Super-Gran Arms Routine*

Bodymagic - *A Physique Guide For Self Reliant Women*

Bodymagic - *A Physique Guide For Self Reliant Men*

Getting Better 1 - *Moving In The Right Direction* - *Ego Busting & Enlightenment In The Real World.*

Contents

Introduction

You can be whatever you want to be, though at times you may find that hard to believe. Life is too short to live through it being any less than the best that you can be. Imagine yourself in 1 year: how would you like to look and feel? Are you fit, strong, confident, proud and healthy? Are you the perfect role model for all of the people that know you? Are you working towards these goals right now or are they just wishes and hopes for the future? If your dreams seem far away or unrealistic you can bring them into your reality right now, in this very moment, by making a commitment to change the way you think and thus change your life. I wrote this book for you, to provide the simple guidelines that you need to coach and attain your dream body, health and fitness, becoming an ideal role model for everyone that knows you.

My job is to show you how you can have the body, fitness and health you crave for and become the star in your own life performance. I will tell you exactly what has worked for us. I will share our potent habits and you can choose which you can use in your life.

Your job is to make a commitment to yourself to undergo the coaching process, become your own coach and be ready to accept with an open mind any new ideas and the new you.

This commitment is the key you will need to unlock the energy that you need to achieve your goals. My experience in coaching and in life has shown me that everyone can take charge of their life and turn themselves around as long as they believe in themselves. Self belief gives you energy, awareness, focus and the confidence to take responsibility and that lies at the very heart of successful self-change. Use the simple workouts, strategies and habits outlined throughout this book to inspire and empower you to become your own fitness coach and make the changes you desire. Only you can really know yourself; only you will be there through your personal ups and downs. So find out exactly how you tick, what works for you and what doesn't, what keeps you positive and upbeat, what you do to turn your barricades into bridges and come out smiling. Your life is an amazing journey, so get enthusiastic about your future and generate some real excitement – you have everything to gain. Become your own biggest fan, because self belief is potent magic! Bodymagic.

Pay it Forward

Bad health habits are rife in our society today, as with the film of the same name, with this book we are paying forward any of our effective good habits or behaviour that might serve to help and influence others to reach optimum health, fitness and a body image to cheer. Our mistakes and successes can both equally serve as an influence. Allow our good memes to penetrate your mind and spread to your circle of influence. We will continue to spread the word but now pass these habits to you for you in turn to pass forward and in doing so influence significant others in your life, not with loud words but with your silent positive actions.

Keeping It Simple

Your body is the ultimate gift from Mother Nature, to transport your soul through this life and as such it should be offered much respect. Are you respecting your most precious gift? Can you pass on good habits and respect for your body and health to be a role model for your loved ones? We believe you can, we believe anybody can, you just have to desire the change and the influence will flow on naturally.

There has been much written about diet and fitness and as often happens with a popular subject it has become confused and often misleading. Each new expert contradicts the one before and each new diet promises but fails to deliver a "long term" solution to weight management and fitness.

This Book is different in as much as all we will do is inform you honestly what has worked and is still working for us and some of the habits that most definitely did not work.

We will not preach to you, but we also will not be telling you that you can reach your goals without making some drastic changes in both your habits and primarily the way you think about both, your own, and your family's lifestyle.

We are aware that we are fit and in shape because we resist being the same as everyone else in our habits. Initially you might think that you cannot make the changes needed. Then you may start to see the odd habit that you could, and are willing to shoe horn into your current lifestyle, this process then evolves until you have reached the point that suits you and makes you a role model. Wholesale change is never easy but a few changes here and there soon result in a lifestyle that suits your health, fitness and self image. Once you begin the evolution the new focus on what works for you brings change into your sights permanently and once you are open and receptive to change anything becomes possible.

We will not be entering in to long debates about which diet is better or which exercise programme is better. This is real life, we are going to give you the facts about the practical habits and behaviour that gives us results. What we eat, what we drink, how we exercise and generally how we win our "Energy In" (food & drink) "Energy Out" (any exercise/movement, just being alive) battle. Quite simply we will tell you based on a lifetime of trial and error, what has worked, and is still working for us and what doesn't work and never did.

So just to stress the point – this book will CUT THE C**P and give it to you straight. If you can take on board many of these habits you will make good progress. If you decide you can't make the changes, that is your choice and worth remembering here is that it all comes down to choices, we choose to live our lives in the bodies we see in the mirror and feel take us through life each day. Our aim is to keep it real so at least you will not be kidding yourself that there is a short term magic solution waiting to transform you overnight.

You will need the qualities of hard work and persistence in abundance but that is exactly what makes the end product so satisfying.

Do you not think if being fit, healthy and in great shape was easy we would all be that way and the value of being just so would diminish greatly?

It is the rare jewels that are hard to obtain and much sought after.

We hope this book will move you away from believing that there is a short term solution to your goals and stop the false hope given to you by the latest fitness gadgets manufacturer or diet guru that sells you the dream which all too often just adds to the nightmare.

Change the way you think!! Turn your thoughts on their heads. This honest voyage to fitness is a fantastic lifetime challenge and the journey is as much fun and gratifying as the results you will achieve. You can enjoy every challenge, savour every moment and actually make fitness a flow experience, your flow experience, or you can continue to fight it all the way, searching for the magic fix that never materialises but makes many people very rich at your expense. If something seems too good to be true, then it generally is!!!!

I say again – Change the way you think!! Change your false beliefs!! Begin today.

Good luck and enjoy.

Part 1 - Women's freedom

When it comes to the sporting body, are women free to choose who they are, what they do and how they think?

"It is generally accepted that the ideal body shape for women in Western cultures is very slim. In Western societies, slimness is a valued attribute for women, and is associated with attractiveness, self-control, social skill, occupational success, and youth" (Grogan, Evans, Hunt & Wright, 2004, p.49).

Whilst men take part in sports and whatever body shape manifests from the sport from Sumo wrestling and darts to bodybuilding, that sporting body is widely accepted and often revered throughout society. The female sporting body however is often ridiculed as being too muscular, unfeminine or masculine and "manly", often the female's sex is called into question. Males and females are both born with the same muscles however in most cases the female hormonal cocktail does not lend itself to developing muscle mass to the same extent as a male. Could it be argued that society holds women rigidly to the "ideal", and in many cases possibly prevents them from maximizing their true physical potential and gaining the benefits that an increase in lean muscle mass would bring them? The first section of this literature review will look at how deeply embedded dominant ideologies, not absolute truths, as is often the belief, shape the collective psyche of society with regards to women in sport. We will use the acceptance of netball as a female appropriate sport as evidence. The second section will provide evidence to show the health benefits of weight bearing resistance work that females may be missing through evasion of their true physical potential, together with constant dieting and an unhealthy fear of their own muscles. The next section will show how distorted images in the media may be the primary source for this unrest and lack of freedom women feel they have when it comes to body shape. Next we will look at how natural female bodybuilding may offer a model for women's freedom to choose their body. Finally we will turn to Ralph Waldo Emerson for his argument as to how women may begin to secure their freedom.

In order to find out why netball is the most popular female participant sport, as described below in sporting females, and whether it does have any real advantages in attracting female participants or not it is necessary to seek out relevant evidence to support this theory:

"As a non-contact game, played and controlled by women throughout its history, and linked to school and college contexts, netball has all the attributes of a feminine appropriate sport. It is the most widely played female sport in the country. (Hargreaves, 2001, p. 250).

This tells us that netball is considered feminine appropriate but how did this ideology come about. The games development will tell us more about how

Victorian values contributed to this situation over 100 years later. Here are some quotes from The International Journal of the History of Sport outlining these values for us:

> "Netball largely escaped the complaints about female muscularity, as it was not seen as contributing to muscle mass in the same way that other sports such as hockey and tennis were, it tended to be viewed as more graceful than powerful and therefore much more suitable for girls.........The discipline and restraint required of the netball player reflects the restraint required of feminine girls and women throughout the twentieth century. It is no surprise that nowadays the stereotype of the netballer is someone who is heterosexual and conventionally feminine. Contemporary uniforms, often made of clinging lycra with very short skirts, only reinforce these notions." (Treagus, 2005, p.101-102).

Looking at this it is hard to understand how such beliefs can stay with us to this day. Even to this day any female deciding against playing a female appropriate sport still faces being stereotyped as this quote shows:

> "Sports have been classified as masculine and feminine appropriate because of fiercely defended heterosexist traditions. Conventional femininity does not incorporate images of physical power and muscularity and female athletes who have such physiques have always stood the risk of being treated in a derogatory way. Women who play traditional male sports, such as cricket, football, rugby and basketball, face the greatest criticism and exposure to ridicule. The implications that athletes may be "pseudo-men", "unfeminine", "gay", "masculine", "mannish", "butch", "dykes", or lesbians put pressure on heterosexual sportswomen to play the "femininity game" and stigmatize homosexuality." (Hargreaves, 2001, p. 171).

The question remains though, could such ideology stand the test of time unless there were some truth in the idea that women have special traits that require purpose made sports to fit these needs and differences. Radical feminists argue that:

> "Radical feminists thus seek the creation of distinct and separate female cultures (e.g. sports based on sharing and cooperation, rather than patriarchal characteristics such as competition and aggression) that have the potential to provide more liberating and humane sporting experiences" (Malcolm, 2008, p.94).

Netball is one such sport and all indications are that netball is successful and the women involved with the sport do approach the experience in a unique way.

Can it be that there are biological differences in the sexes that mean some sports will have an advantage over others in providing the much needed experience? In discussing the biological and very real differences inherent in men and women neuropsychiatry's Louann Brizendine M.D., is less willing to speculate on psychological or sociological ideas, that have little to do with how the brain actually works. Though clearly a feminist, she warns that political correctness has no role in understanding behaviour. Yes, we may be able to alter our cultural attitudes or policies to make a better world, but first we must understand the facts about how brain biology - so different between men and women - shapes behaviour. Brizendine states:

> " Close social bonds actually alter the female brain in a highly positive way, so that any loss of those relationships triggers a hormonal change that strengthens the feelings of abandonment or loss. The intensity of female friendships therefore also has a biochemical basis." (Brizendine, 2007, p. 55).

Could this then point to actual biological reasons why "feminine appropriate" ideology within sport has been so enduring? Ideological theories aside netball just seems to fit the bill for many women at this time.

Now we move to see the problems faced by a sport widely considered as feminine inappropriate, female bodybuilding. In could be argued that female bodybuilding amplifies the body issues faced by sporty women in general.

> "Women experienced pressures from within the body building community defining the acceptable size and appearance of their bodies. They were engaged in a 'balancing act' where they were trying to attain a body that was muscular but not too muscular, and that maintained some aspects of traditional 'feminine' appearance. It is concluded that women who engage in Physique-level body building face complex layers of social pressure from within and outside the body building community" (Grogan et al, 2009, p. 49).

Women face health risks by trying to attain the ideal slim body revered by western society. Research was undertaken to assess bone mineral density in women.
> "The main aim of this study was therefore to investigate how physical activity together with performance in selected tests in adolescence and physical characteristics in adolescence and/or adulthood are related to adult

BMD in women. A second aim was to investigate whether performance in physical capacity tests for a specific body region in adolescence may be associated with adult BMD for this body region. Thus, physical performance tests were performed around the age of 16 years, coinciding with attainment of peak bone mass, and measurements of bone mass were performed at a second visit at the mean age of 36 years............ This supports earlier findings that activities started in late adolescence or young adulthood are not as effective in enhancing bone mass as activities started in earlier ages, i.e. around puberty. It also suggests that mechanical loading should be continued after puberty to maintain the increase in BMD gained from physical activity." (Barnekow-Bergkvist, Hedberg, Pettersson, Lorentzon, 2009, p.447).

This report shows that lifetime high impact and weight bearing activity started at adolescence, dramatically increases bone mineral density in later life, drastically decreasing the likelihood of osteoporosis. This is exactly the sort of exercise that women avoid in order to reach the ideal female form. Top of the list would be full body progressive resistance training, an extreme version of which, is bodybuilding. On this evidence it would appear that current ideologies could be harmful to women.

Here is another example of the damage perfect body ideologies can represent to young women athletes:

"A 15-year-old girl finishes a 1-hour dance rehearsal that prepares her for an upcoming recital. At the end of her practice, her dance instructor pulls her

aside to give her the usual critique and pointers. Instead of merely telling her to

work on her positioning, the instructor tells the dancer that before she will be

allowed to perform, she must lose 10 or more pounds. The instructor tells her that this weight loss will help her look like a "real" ballerina. In a track practice

across town, a 19-year-old woman talks with her teammates about the best way

to drop a few pounds before the next meet. Although her coach has never openly suggested weight loss, he has made it clear that the thinner the runner is, the faster she will be. Are these examples a clear representation of what today's female athletes face in terms of sports participation and body image? Does athletic involvement by young women put them at risk for eating disorders brought on by pressures to excel at their sports? Do some sports pose a greater threat than others to a woman's body image and eating behaviour? Over the past 20 years, female athletic participation has increased dramatically, and with this growth have come questions about the impact that athletic participation has on young girls and their sense of self" (Robinson & Ferraro, 2004, p. 115-128).

Both of these research projects build a good case for ideal female body concepts and ideologies being both physically and psychologically damaging to women of all ages.
There is some evidence however to show that a gradual acceptance of female muscularity is occurring and in some cases even sought after.

"The muscular physique for women was once largely unacceptable by many; however, in the wake of the current social trend, women's muscularity is not only accepted but has also become desired. Although in the past the ideal woman's body was slender, the present standards are much more specific, with the ideal physique being not only thin, but also muscular and toned. Despite this trend, societal norms seem to have an upper limit as to what amount of muscularity is acceptable for a woman to possess, resulting in women attempting to negotiate the correct amount of muscle and an intensification of the difficulty in trying to attain this ideal. Although there is still a continuum of body ideals, it has become increasingly clear that women do aspire to muscularity goals" (Mosewich, Vangool, Kowalski & McHugh, 2009, p.99).

Form this quote it would seem that although progress is being made women are still a long way from having the freedom to display a body without limitations. Where does the responsibility lay for keeping women locked into an idealised body image that is so damaging physically and psychologically? Two studies give an indication as to where the responsibility for promoting such idealised images may lay. The first quote here is based on research undertaken with young volleyball players, showing how their evaluations of body image were negative after looking at the perfect images depicted in non athletic poses, within a volleyball publication.

"Body image is heavily influenced by the social comparison process and involves evaluations of overall physical size and specific body parts—arms, abdomen, and thighs. Although the self evaluations of physical ability are predominantly positive, evaluations of body image are frequently negative and appear to be exacerbated by photographic poses that emphasize an athlete's aesthetic beauty rather than her athletic prowess" (Thomsen, Bower & Barnes, 2004, p. 266).

The next journal examined the eating habits of young women after viewing media images of the perfect female body.

"Among women with a discrepancy between perceptions of their actual body and the body their same-gender peers believe they ought to have, exposure to images alone and images plus congruent text led to a reduction in the amount eaten in front of female peers" (Harrison, Taylor & Marske, 2006, p. 507).

From this it would indicate that media manipulated images of how the perfect woman should look are the primary source for unrest, and the resulting lack of freedom that women experience when it comes to their physical appearance and ultimately their health.

There is no doubt that Western culture in the 21st century promotes unrealistic body ideals to women, and that nonconformity to these ideals leads to social disapproval.

In the book Body Image by Sarah Grogan (2008), she reviews much of the latest research on body image. In an extremely well cited and well researched text she argues that female bodybuilders provide a model of how women can resist mainstream cultural pressures to be slender providing they have the support from a sub cultural group, such as the bodybuilding community. They show that contesting the dominant slender ideologies can lead to feelings of empowerment and the construction of alternative body ideals. The fact that they are under pressure from the bodybuilding community to present as feminine should not take away from the fact that they have found a way to resist mainstream pressure to be slim, and to feel good about the look of their bodies (Grogan, 2008).

Ralph Waldo Emerson (1803-1882) - This gentleman may offer up a possible solution for prospective sporty women that are scared to take the plunge because of contemporary ideology, and sporty women detractors alike to consider. Both the aforementioned have lost an element of human freedom, to think what you like and to act how you like as long as it harms nobody. This is the path most of us take, happy to go along with society's program in exchange for a level of status and reasonable material circumstances, in essence to fit in. Though we all profess to be individual and breakaway from limitations, the reality is, comfort in conformity. In his 30 page essay called self reliance, Emerson called his philosophy idealism and sells the virtues of resisting conformity in order to find your true self. To follow your unique calling and resist being steered through a pre - programmed predictable life. If the thoughts and actions are predictable then so too will be the results. The only proper defence against numbing conformity due to the scripting of our lives by society is to find and walk the trail of uniqueness in both thought and action. In Self Reliance there are many calls to that end.

> "We but half express ourselves, and are ashamed of that divine idea which each of us represents.........What I must do is all that concerns me, not what the people think.....It is easy in the world to live after the world's opinion.... It is easy in solitude to live after our own...Nothing can bring you peace but yourself. Nothing can bring you peace but the triumph of principles" (Emerson 1841/2007, p. 20).

If we can apply this to our thoughts and actions then maybe we will become the unique individuals we are intended to be and recognise the same in others and applaud individuality and the right to be different in all people.

The literary evidence would indicate that a female appropriate sport may well be a way forward. However is that not then accepting the dominant male ideology that women should not be muscular or be allowed to develop to their true physical potential? The argument here is not whether women may enjoy netball but whether any woman or all women should have the unfettered freedom to enjoy sport and whatever body arises from that sport. So men have basically sanctioned and approved for women to play netball. Maybe it is time women are allowed to be bodybuilders, rugby players, weightlifters or whatever they choose without ideological condemnation of the resulting body.

Conclusion

Whilst much research has been undertaken in this field, much of the available data just repeats other studies. There would seem to be a tendency for the research to concentrate on the problems women face without really looking for possible solutions. Netball is a gender specific sport and can offer no real way forward as the women involved are finding comfort in conformity with societies acceptance that the sport and resulting physiques meet with its approval. An area for study and I believe an escape route for many women may be right in front of our noses. The term, or sport of bodybuilding conjures up images of extremely muscular, often chemically enhanced women. These images represent a major transformation for most women that makes them recoil with fear. The image conjured up is always the most extreme example of a muscular women that often the media has used to sensationalise the practice. Consequently since the conception of workout gyms in the 20th century women have avoided the free weights area and workouts that they believed would turn them into grotesque specimens or even worse make them look like men. When witnessing a competing female bodybuilder we see the extreme result of the corruption of what is in its purest, most natural form, the ideal physical solution for the female body. Now imagine women working out naturally without fear of morphing into a man, eating healthily and maximizing their natural physical potential without the fear that perpetuated myths and ideologies have imprinted on their minds. Maybe a future study on introducing and following a group of women into a world of bodybuilding without drugs and competition would prove very interesting and dare I suggest enlightening and empowering for everybody involved. I look forward to the day when gyms across the country are full of women doing their "thing" with strong tight feminine bodies, currently these spaces are men only clubs. No signs to bar the women just powerful ideologies, which are never absolute truths.

Another short study revealed that even within the gym culture the ideologies at work are powerful.

An investigation into the powerful ideologies that may be shaping how women at XXX gym exercise their bodies.

The argument for this case study is that women are deterred from taking part in any productive and healthful exercise and nutrition regimes at XXX gym, due to deeply embedded myths and ideologies. Although being dissatisfied with the way we look, and feeling fat can motivate us to exercise, it may also prevent us from engaging in exercise without limitations, due to concern about whether we have the right kind of body to fit in with a culture that promotes a slender ideal (Grogan, 2008).

In arguing that the ideal form which women aspire to is both psychologically and physically damaging, I will interview, observe and question, a small group of regular exercisers of XXX gym to find out why they exercise so differently from the males when we all have the same muscles. There is no physiological reason why males and females should experience exercise for their bodies in such drastically different ways.

Research Question -

In XXX gym, when it comes to the sporting body are females free to choose who they are, what they do and how they think?

Methodology

Questionnaires - 12 questions were used in order to discover how much control a group of exercising women at Gold's gym had over both their bodies and their workout philosophies.

<u>Case Study Questions</u>

Why do you exercise?

Are you satisfied with your body?

Do you believe your assessment of your own body is accurate?

How do you structure your workouts?

When you perform resistance training - Do you lift as heavy weights as possible?

Men and women in Gold's gym generally train in very different ways - Do you think males and females should exercise differently? Why?

What is your idea of the ideal female body?

If you had that ideal body - what will having that body bring you? Do you think it will change who you are, how you view yourself?

Do you think the ideal looking body would be the healthiest body for you?

Given your genetic potential - Do you believe your expectations are realistic as to the body you strive for?

Do you think it is ultimately you that has decided what is the ideal female body in your eyes?

When it comes to the female body, your body - Do you believe you are free to choose who you are, what you do and how you think?

Interviews - Another way to find out how women feel about their autonomy is by semi structured interviews. The same questions were used as a guideline for the interviews. The advantage of doing this rather than just asking women to fill out a questionnaire that asks specific questions is that the women are given the freedom to express how they feel, rather than just answering pre planned questions. This allows them to set their own agenda and address issues that are important to them, giving the technique more flexibility than questionnaire work.

Participant Observation - through personal involvement and as a gym member. I already have a good idea of their exercise habits. In this case the familiarity has allowed me to comfortably approach the girls as part of the scene, to discuss what is quite a sensitive topic. The cardiovascular equipment, treadmills, bikes etc at XXX overlook the gym area so I have been able to spend time whilst exercising also observing behaviour.

Field notes - Time has been limited but I have taken mental notes for the study. It would not be practical to stand and take notes physically. The practice would place me as alien in the environment and the women would be naturally suspicious.

Findings and Analysis

35 years ago, my first time in a workout weight lifting environment, no women present at all. The East Midlands weight lifting and bodybuilding club was not male only, that is just the way it panned out. Each and every gym I have attended since and there have been many, there have hardly ever been any women at all present in the lifting areas, and those that were, almost never lifted maximally. Both sexes possess the same muscle make up, why then do we behave so differently? Of the seven fit ladies I questioned, only two actually worked out intensely with no limitations, one a female bodybuilder and the other her daughter. One extremely petit lady Stacey said, "I am scared of becoming too bulky". Staff member, Lynn commented, "women will break their bones if they train like men". The ideal shape the majority of the women want is slim with big "boobs". In the 18 months I have attended XXX at least 5 times weekly, I have only seen two of the ladies in the serious workout area. This would start to explain why there are no other women in this area, if even the staff are afraid to lift in case they should suddenly sprout muscles overnight. It would seem that most are only mildly aware that the shape they want, is the shape powerful ideologies are leading them to desire. All of the women have connections within the fitness industry, most worked in the gym and yet the myths and ideologies were still effective in perhaps those that should know better or at least be aware of the facts. When asked if the ideal form would change their lives. "It would make me more confident", "I would be happy", " I would be more confident in every aspect of my life" and "if I thought I had the perfect body, I'd be so confident and naked all the time". What makes this all the more amazing is that each of these women would be the envy of most other women, they all exhibit slim bodies as required in society. Julie, a Mother of three and Grandmother twice over, is a female bodybuilder, she has impressive muscles including a very visible six pack that most young men would envy. When asked the question, when it comes to your body, do you believe you are free to chose who you are, what you do and how you think? Julie answered, "I would like to think so, but being more muscular than the normal female generates negative comments, looks and often rude remarks, there are plenty of compliments also, I wouldn't want to make you think it was all bad". Diane answered to the same question, "I think media, male opinion and comments decide women's opinion of the body for them. Kirsty believes wrongly of course that gym equipment is gender specific and that is determined by the women wanting to lost weight and men wanting to gain weight "different sexes use different equipment". This belief is in line with recent research outlining men wanting to become more muscular and women more slim

to meet body ideologies within society. Two weeks after the interviews and questionnaires I observed some of the girls workout sessions whilst I was working out. I wandered if there would be any change or modification in workout structure or behaviour due to our conversations and the fact that at least three of the girls expressed a desire to train differently once armed with some facts. I witnessed no change, light weights, high repetitions and exaggerated ranges of motion. The fact that the girls employed by XXX gym would all be considered ideal by society standards and that they held no previous knowledge with regards to exercise or nutrition could indicate that they were employed to facilitate the vastly male majority membership with ideal female forms to gaze upon and interact with. All of the girls working at XXX gym were also involved in promotional work.

Conclusion and Implications

In response to the research question - **In XXX gym, when it comes to the sporting body are females free to choose who they are, what they do and how they think?** I would argue that the females I questioned and interviewed are under the influence of extremely deeply embedded powerful ideologies that shape their workout and exercise behaviour. The implications of this is that females at XXX are being deprived of the basic ethical human right of obtaining any health benefits to be derived from correct and well informed exercise behaviour. At the same time the ideologically led behaviour can be both physically and psychologically damaging. I would also argue that this case study although studying a small group of females within a limited time scale at XXX could reflect issues amongst exercising females on a much larger scale.

Discussing the Effectiveness of Self Confidence and Coping Theories for Enhancing The Performance of a Mature National Level Female Bodybuilder.

There is a tendency to think of sport in relation to young people and totally disregard any more mature involvement in competitive sport. With the onset of improved medical care and knowledge on how to manage the body for life, sports men and women are now able to stay active in sports for much longer.

"A positive aging discourse emerged in the latter third of the 20th century in the related fields of gerontology and health care, exercise promotion and leisure. Positive aging discourses refer collectively to research, theories, images, or attitudes about celebrating later life as a period for enjoyment, good health, independence, vitality, exploration, challenge, productivity, creativity, growth, and development rather than solely focused upon decline, disengagement, and hopelessness. The literature includes multiple messages about autonomy for older people, alternative ways of viewing aging, advice on leisure and active living, the health benefits of physical activity, and exercise program development .... With the surfacing of these positive aging discourses, the associated health and fitness promotion movement, and the aging of populations, opportunities for sports participation in later life have increased. Thousands of people aged 60 years and over compete in and train for physically strenuous individual or team sports such as track and field athletics, cycling, swimming, long-distance running, triathlons, tennis, squash, field hockey, ice hockey, soccer, and basketball at Masters and Veterans tournaments. The rising leisure trend of older competitive athletes across many western countries presents an intriguing context for exploring how older people negotiate multiple understandings of aging and physical activity when they talk about their experiences in sport and when they actually compete" (Dionigi, 2006).

Using bodybuilding as an example, the over 40's category for men is now recognised as the category with the most consistently high standards. The overall champion at the recent British championships was indeed the over 40's winner also. There is now an over 50's category. In some countries these two categories have been raised to over 45 and over 55, in recognition that many athletes are just reaching their peak at 40 years of age. So with this in mind, a discussion on self confidence and coping strategies using the unique experiences of a competitive, mature, woman bodybuilder (49), also a mother and grandmother, is more relevant than ever as we increasingly see older athletes competing in sport at some level. The first section will focus on outlining and painting a picture of some of the problems women face that could and possibly should have an effect on their self confidence.   The following section then discusses current theory with contemporary research examples and how relevant is that theory when applied to a mature woman bodybuilder? How does she cope? Finally and in conclusion what implications may be drawn from the discussion?

Female Bodybuilding a Unique Sport.

> "It is generally accepted that the ideal body shape for women in Western cultures is very slim. In Western societies, slimness is a valued attribute for women, and is associated with attractiveness, self-control, social skill, occupational success, and youth" (Grogan, Evans, Hunt & Wright, 2004, p.49).

The female sporting body is often ridiculed as being too muscular, unfeminine or masculine and "manly", often the female's sex is called into question. Males and females are both born with the same muscles however in most cases the female hormonal cocktail does not lend itself to developing muscle mass to the same extent as a male. A woman choosing bodybuilding as her sport has many important choices to make, often changing her body permanently to one that falls way outside society norms. Here is how participants in a study perceived muscular women.

> "Participants perceived hyper muscular women, as compared
>
> to the average woman, as having more masculine and fewer feminine interests, less likely to be good mothers, and less intelligent, less socially popular, and less attractive"(Forbes, Adams-Curtis, Holmgren & White, 2004, p.487).

Female bodybuilders find themselves with no secure place even within the bodybuilding subculture.

"Women experienced pressures from within the body building community defining the acceptable size and appearance of their bodies. They were engaged in a 'balancing act' where they were trying to attain a body that was muscular but not too muscular, and that maintained some aspects of traditional 'feminine' appearance. It is concluded that women who engage in Physique-level body building face complex layers of social pressure from within and outside the body building community" (Grogan et al, 2004, p. 49).

How does a woman remain a self confident individual when her sport, which is her actual physical being is vilified from within and without. What coping strategies does she implement mostly inadvertently to continue her sport with passion and spirit?

"Often commentators and critics have marginalized and demeaned female bodybuilders by describing them as grotesque freaks, he–shes, and worse" (Forbes, Adams-Curtis, Holmgren & White, 2004, p.488).

Bodybuilding also entails most of the physical performance taking place day to day in the gym, where confidence needs to be high. A hostile male dominated area. There are times during the season when a bodybuilder looks for personal records and visible physical improvement every single time they are in the gym as a sign they are on target with their diets, supplements and training programmes. Self confidence is vital. The show aspect, happening for some maybe only once a year for a matter of minutes then displays the results of the past months performances in the gym, combined with the result of specific nutritional habits added to the rather severe, some would say acetic contest preparation. Confidence and success in the gym carries a bodybuilder on the crest of a wave all the way to show time. A bodybuilder particularly a woman walks around carrying her sport with her every day in a society that mostly likes to show it's disapproval for anything they do not fully understand. It could be argued that a woman with muscles falls into this category. With this difficult situation in mind how effective are the sport confidence and self efficacy strategies for enhancing performance?

Self confidence

The results of the cited study below revealed that self confidence was strongly related to sport performance, more strongly related than cognitive anxiety. The study also reported that self confidence has a greater impact on men than it does on women. As to why this would be, the study indicates in the discussion that there may be a sex threshold for self confidence relating to sports performance. Further study in this direction is needed and more studies including women were also suggested (Woodman & Hardy, 2003). Knowing that self confidence is vital to sports performance, Bandura's theory of self efficacy should be critically assessed in relation to our mature athlete.

> "Self efficacy refers to situation-specific self confidence, as opposed to global self confidence. It is the performer's perception of her competence to succeed in a given task at a given time..........self efficacy will predict actual performance if necessary skills and incentives are present" (Hardy, Jones & Gould, 1996, p.46).

The next study took place on women training for self defence, not only did the women's self efficacy improve on self defence skills but also across many other domains, such as self defence abilities, sports competencies and coping skills.

> "Trained participants also experienced a significant increase in more global aspects of personality, including perceptions of physical self-efficacy and assertiveness......... trained participants experienced a boost in multiple domains of self-efficacy not directly tapped by the intervention (Weitlauf, Cervone, Smith & Wright, 2001, p.1683).

It would appear that an overall boost in self efficacy and global self confidence both inside the discipline and outside had taken place. It could be argued that drawing a parallel between self defence training and women's bodybuilding would not stretch the imagination too much. Both disciplines deal with strength and power and controlled aggression. Our bodybuilder has become more confident in the gym and most definitely her confidence has improved in many other situations. However, the attention attracted by a woman bodybuilder when preparing for a competition, once or twice per year, a condition so far away from a society norm could be argued to actually make her feel more uncomfortable during that period. At the same time her efficacy within the gym amongst her peers and around the subculture would be imagined to be high. This would make an interesting research project for the future. The four factors that determine self efficacy are listed as performance accomplishments, vicarious experience, verbal persuasion and emotional arousal (Hardy, Jones & Gould, 1996). Our bodybuilder competes with good success at national level. Are these significant factors in her success? Performance accomplishments - always respected as an extremely hard trainer, stronger than many men on various lifts, not having any women peers to compare herself against, overall performances are always a positive experience. Many watch her workout in apparent awe, which could just be because it is unusual to see woman reaching her strength potential. One could most definitely argue for performance being a positive factor. Vicarious experience - difficult, as stated before there are no women bodybuilders present except on competition day. Inside the comparisons are invariably with men, however outside there are other competitors and women bodybuilders available to view online in contests and training and this is definitely a process our woman undergoes. Several women have gained considerable money and fame from bodybuilding, with personal appearances, guest posing spots etc, so it could be argued that this is a factor also. Verbal persuasion - this arguably is the factor most responsible for our woman's success. Bodybuilders are an extremely supportive group and the men and women alike support our woman totally. The encouragement is constant and unsolicited. Win or lose. Finally to emotional arousal and yes one has to be aroused for both training and competitive performance, this however is an accepted constant, part of being a bodybuilder, if there were no emotional arousal to either performance, then one might argue why would one choose a bodybuilding lifestyle? Also bodybuilders use stimulants such as caffeine before performances to provide a guaranteed level of arousal every time. In the next study nine sources of confidence were identified: Preparation, performance accomplishments, coaching, innate factors, social support, experience, competitive advantage, self-awareness, and trust. Six types of sport confidence were also identified: skill execution, achievement, physical factors, psychological factors, superiority to opposition, and tactical awareness. This study appears to be taking current theories and taking a giant leap forward (Hays, Maynard, Thomas, & Bawden, 2007). There are also differences in how gender is related to sources of confidence. Females placed much emphasis on personal performance whilst males derived confidence from winning. In 1998 it was proposed that athletes rely on additional sources of confidence that are influenced by social, organizational, and demographic factors. Consequently, the revamped model of sport confidence proposed by Vealey in 1998 identified the sources of confidence that were specifically relevant to athletes. We will discuss them and how they may be relevant to our female bodybuilding example. The sources are, mastery, demonstration, physical & mental preparation, self presentation, social support, vicarious experiences, trust in coaches, environmental comfort and situation favourableness (Hays, Maynard, Thomas, & Bawden, 2007). How do these sources that have not already been discussed apply to our athlete? Mastery in this example comes as a result of constant physical and mental rehearsal of the poses that are compulsory and the free posing round which is performed to music of the competitors choice. This rehearsal becomes part of the bodybuilders daily routine which is fine tuned and adapted according to any perceived weaknesses or additional knowledge gained. For example a new pose that may suit better than an existing pose may be suggested by the coach or respected peers. Advances in training methods and nutrition practises may also become a factor. The process is ever changing and constantly searching for relevant and well researched new knowledge to gain an edge. Our bodybuilder happens to be married to her coach, so the trust as with the attention she receives is 100%. A personal trainer on call 24 hours a day. This is also a major source of the social support needed and the environmental comfort of having your coach training, eating and sleeping alongside you. The demonstration and self presentation sources of confidence, gain as the show draws closer. The reason for this is that all being well with the training, nutrition and of course health a bodybuilders physique improves as contest day approaches, confidence improves along with the physique improvements. A bodybuilder training pre contest will be receiving copious amounts of positive feedback from within the sub culture and that boosts performance in the gym. It is widely accepted that the best training period is in the months prior to a contest. Improvements in both strength and appearance happen on a daily basis. Mental practise is applied by our bodybuilder having the posing music on her portable music device and rehearsing the routine over and over in her head whilst at work. That just leaves situational favourableness, something that makes the bodybuilder believe it is her day. This is interesting because with the preparation of posing, nutrition, training and then on the day, tanning and suit choice, there is little that a bodybuilder can do to affect the result. The confidence and feeling that the situation is in her favour can only come from perfect preparation and the belief that that will be enough on that day to sway the judge's opinion in her favour. On the day of the show, once the other players disrobe, a fair assessment of final position can be arrived at. Maybe then more than any other time does the support team need to be positive and focused. However the bodybuilder being in the best shape of her life will be confident. A bodybuilder in this situation but failing to win, then evaluates her performance as to whether it was enjoyable and whether further improvement can be made for future performances. Unlike many sports a bodybuilder visibly carries her efforts with her and often this is reward enough.

"Results of the present study seemed to suggest that males focused more on successful competition outcomes, whereas the majority of female athletes

identified good personal performances as a source of their confidence. These findings are in accordance with research that has identified different antecedents predict self-confidence in males and females............. The results of the present study certainly raise awareness of possible gender differences in the goal orientation of those competing on the World Class stage" (Hays, Maynard, Thomas, & Bawden, 2007, p.450).

With this quote in mind, our bodybuilder upon placing 2nd or 3rd will always want to talk about performance and preparation over victory or lack of it. Endlessly looking at and comparing pictures and video clips to search for areas of obvious improvement. Never has her placing resulted in her not enjoying her experiences. Upon being asked if she was angry that she hadn't won a contest that maybe she should have, she replied - "No, not really because I think I looked really good". The fact that the judges may have got it wrong, a fact she has no control over did not bother her at all. This leads nicely into some current theory on motivation that works on the level of improving self confidence and coping and can be applied on site with ease. They are cognitive approaches. Cognitive approaches concentrate on specific aspects of how we think. Weiner's model of attribution is based on two factors:

1. Whether the responsibility lies with the individual(internal) or situation(external).

2. Whether the attribution is stable over time or will vary from one situation to another.

How we attribute success and failure is related to self esteem and affects performance.

Self serving bias dictates it is more likely that success will be attributed to ability and failure to task difficulty. Inconsistency is attributed to luck or effort, the self serving bias means success is attributed to effort and failure to luck.   Martin Seligman (1975) discovered that when early negative experiences and consistent failure have occurred then the learning is such that there is no point in continuing to make efforts. As a result any form of adversity is faced with an attitude of learned helplessness. Learned helplessness can develop at any time and even elite athletes can lose motivation upon meeting with successive failures (Jarvis, 2010). Both Weiner's attribution theory and learned helplessness benefit from reattribution training, a practical solution. If young athletes can learn to become helpless or attribute failure to permanent, pervasive and internal circumstances then the opposite must be true and exposure to success and viewing adversity as temporary, specific and external can help them develop a more optimistic approach to adversity and so increase intrinsic motivation. In Learned Optimism, 2006, Seligman recommends a simple **A**dversity, **B**elief, **C**onsequences, **D**isputation, **E**nergisation approach to cognitive therapy. A is the adversity. B is athlete belief or attribution about A. C is the consequences of that often illogical belief. D is disputing the logic behind and at the root of B and finally E is realigning with the new belief (Seligman, 2006). The appeal of such a simple cognitive approach would be obvious in dealing with athletes of all ages. The reaction to adversity could become part of the coaching philosophy and would quite easily be passed on to athletes informally on a situation to situation basis. Reattribution performed informally in the field would appeal in situations where it is not practical to sit in one to one situations, there would also be a much better chance of the attitude becoming part of the culture for the athlete as with our bodybuilder. It is important for the athlete to feel in control. In the following journal it was shown that lack of control was enough to create helplessness. With this in mind it could then be argued that increased athlete autonomy would also assist in the reattribution process, another valid argument for embedding reattribution talk and thought into the sporting athlete's culture. (Gernigon, Thill & Fleurance, 1999).

An inability to cope with the stressors in sport may result in withdrawal from the sport or a drop in sports performance. Problem focused coping includes planning, setting goals and seeking information. Each of these elements are a built in part of our bodybuilders day to day lifestyle and contest preparation, up to the most minute detail regarding nutrition, training and posing practice. Emotion focused coping includes support, relaxation and wishful thinking. Our bodybuilder uses meditation and visualisation again as a built in part of her day to day bodybuilding lifestlye, attempting successfully to utilise a holistic approach to an extremely demanding lifestyle (Nicholls & Polman, 2007).

It could be argued that for our mature bodybuilder a more stable lifestyle and family background makes a significant contribution to how she copes with her sport. One could not leave a discussion about a mature athlete without briefly consulting Maslow's hierarchy of needs which would indicate our athlete's current levels as being esteem and self actualisation and part of those processes being her sport, the lower levels have long been secured in her life. It could be argued that Maslow becomes more relevant when discussing mature athletes.

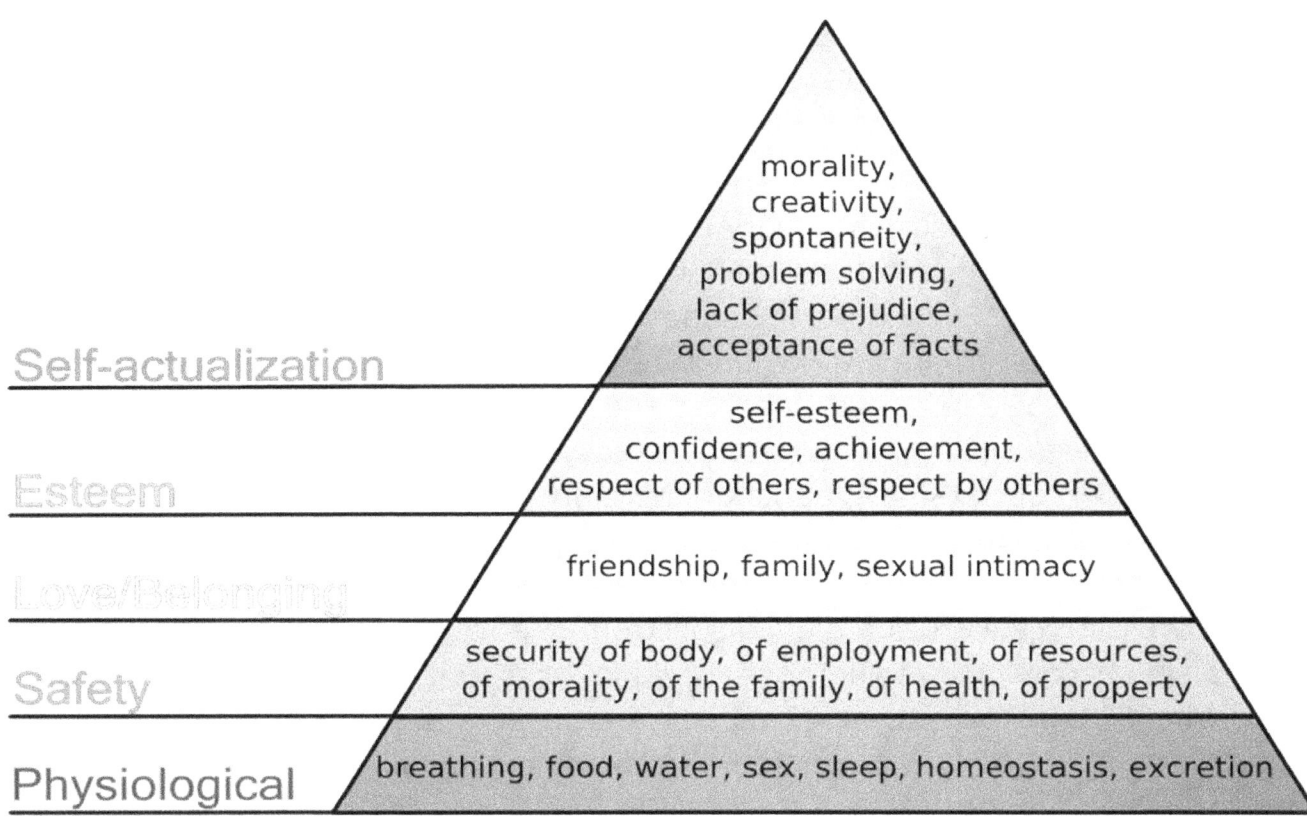

Figure 1. Maslow's hierarchy of needs

"Maslow's hierarchy implies that human growth is associated with adult maturity, a decrease in the prepotency of "lower" motives and an increase in the prepotency of "higher" motives. These hypotheses were evaluated with data from 1,712 participants who had been tested with the Reiss Profile, which is a standardized assessment of a comprehensive range of enduring (trait) strivings. The results provided some support for Maslow's general idea of human growth: The lower motives (such as eating and exercise) were stronger for younger versus older adults, whereas the higher motives (such as honour and idealism) were stronger for older versus younger adults. The results demonstrated a new method for studying some of the issues raised by Maslow" (Reiss & Havercamp, 2005, p.41).

Could it then be the case for security being a contributing factor in sporting confidence also. We have all seen sports men and women perform badly when their much publicised personal lives are less than secure. It can be seen clearly that traits highlighted in the pyramid - confidence, self esteem, problem solving and an acceptance of facts would all be major assets when discussing confidence and coping. Maybe there are some lessons to be learned for younger athletes and coaches regarding athlete maturity and stability. Can maturity be coached?

Conclusion

In conclusion, the current theory and studies explain well a mature female bodybuilder's confidence issues. Both the self confidence theory and coping theories discussed play a role in enhancing her performance both in the gym and on contest days. There are no doubt differences in sources of confidence and coping applicable to both gender and age, and there would need to be more studies carried out using mature and mixed gender participants. Findings were applied to our example, although there are some quite unique issues in bodybuilding the theory could transfer to many other sportswomen and men, in other sports. There seems to be an emphasis on youth when dealing with sporting issues. Both genders and the full spectrum of ages need to be researched as athletes become increasingly active within sport well into their golden years. Retirement from top level sport happens later in life and sports now invariably run masters tournaments and events.

"CHOICES"

The Ethical Dilemmas Facing Women Bodybuilders and how a Holistic Approach to a Bodybuilding Lifestyle could be the Answer.

"Often commentators and critics have marginalized and   demeaned female bodybuilders by describing them as grotesque freaks, he–shes, and worse" ("(Forbes, Adams-Curtis, Holmgren & White, 2004, p.488).

Why would a woman choose such a sport, how might she make the choice to build her body and how might she justify the bodybuilding lifestyle under such prejudice? In part one we will briefly outline some of the problems women face. Next we will look at how a woman might arrive at her lifestyle choice. Following we will look at how she may cope with the hostile aggressive environment of a hard core gym and the arena and retain life balance whilst doing the right thing. Finally a look at the question of the attainment of body perfection.

No Place For a Lady?

> "It is generally accepted that the ideal body shape for women in Western cultures is very slim. In Western societies, slimness is a valued attribute for women, and is associated with attractiveness, self-control, social skill, occupational success, and youth" (Grogan, Evans, Hunt & Wright, 2004, p.49).

The female sporting body is often ridiculed as being too muscular, unfeminine or masculine and "manly", often the female's sex is called into question. Males and females are both born with the same muscles however in most cases the female hormonal cocktail does not lend itself to developing muscle mass to the same extent as a male. A woman choosing bodybuilding as her sport has many important choices to make, often changing her body permanently to one that falls way outside society norms. Here is how participants in a study perceived muscular women.

> "Participants perceived hyper muscular women, as compared to the average woman, as having more masculine and fewer feminine interests, less likely to be good mothers, and less intelligent, less socially popular, and less attractive"(Forbes, Adams-Curtis, Holmgren & White, 2004, p.487).

It could be argued that bodybuilding is a selfish, self centred, aggressive and narcissistic sport at best, dominated by males and producing more body image issues than any other sport (e.g. Grogan, 2008; Pope, Philips & Olivardia, 2002). The body is central and nothing else matters. Women bodybuilders find themselves with no secure place even within the bodybuilding subculture.

> "Women experienced pressures from within the body building community defining the acceptable size and appearance of their bodies. They were engaged in a 'balancing act' where they were trying to attain a body that was muscular but not too muscular, and that maintained some aspects of traditional 'feminine' appearance. It is concluded that women who engage in Physique-level body building face complex layers of social pressure from within and outside the body building community" (Grogan et al, 2004, p. 49).

As can be seen from the three quotes, this is indeed a lifestyle decision of gigantic proportions for any woman to make. Just recently the United Kingdom Bodybuilding & Fitness Federation has decided to withdraw its women's physique category leaving dozens of women members with muscles and nowhere to compete. Bodybuilding is a sport of extremes, extreme diets, extreme training, extreme discipline, often extreme drug use and generally an extreme lifestyle. As is fitting the sport has a seedier side and true to form that is also more extreme than you will find in any other sport (e.g. Hotten, 2005; Klein, 1993; Arnold, 2008). A sport with no boundaries. Our woman bodybuilder must see all that is wrong in the sport and the way the sport consumes many that enter the fray. How then may a woman happily make a choice to move so far from society norms to a sport that as yet doesn't really have any clear direction for women and how upon making such a choice could this lifestyle provide happiness and peace of mind throughout her life? How should she live and how can she do the right thing now and continually into the future?

All Things Considered

In making her choice, she will initially look to the wisdom of existentialists such as Kierkegaard, Nietzsche, Heidegger and Jean Paul Sartre. Existentialists view freedom as both our greatest blessing and our biggest burden. Existentialists maintain that with her freedom to make choices our woman must know that she is 100% responsible for the result(Wartenberg, 2008; Harwood, 2010; Barrett, 1958; Cox, 2009). In their eyes failing to make choice would be an act of bad faith. In many cases awareness of this responsibility would inject fear into the decision making process. The result for our woman is a sense of empowerment and clarity. There is no confusion, she will weigh her options carefully, make a decision and accept full responsibility for better or worse.

> "The existentialists encourage people to develop their uniqueness, their own special qualities. This means that the answers people develop to the fundamental questions about how to live their lives are ones that they have to work out as individuals" (Wartenberg, 2008, p.5).

Ralph Waldo Emerson may be able to help with this choice, offering sporty women such as our bodybuilder that are scared to take the plunge because of contemporary ideology another route to consider. The aforementioned have lost an element of human freedom. That is to think what you like and to act how you like as long as it harms nobody. This is the path most of us take, happy to go along with society's program in exchange for a level of status and reasonable material circumstances, in essence to fit in. Though we all profess to be individual and breakaway from limitations, the reality is comfort in conformity. In his 30 page essay called self reliance, Emerson called his philosophy idealism and sells the virtues of resisting conformity in order to find your true self. To follow your unique calling and resist being steered through a pre - programmed predictable life. If the thoughts and actions are predictable then so too will be the results. The only proper defence against numbing conformity due to the scripting of our lives by society is to find and walk the trail of uniqueness in both thought and action. In Self Reliance there are many calls to that end.

> "We but half express ourselves, and are ashamed of that divine idea which each of us represents.........What I must do is all that concerns me, not what the people think.....It is easy in the world to live after the world's opinion.... It is easy in solitude to live after our own...Nothing can bring you peace but yourself. Nothing can bring you peace but the triumph of principles" (Emerson 1841/2007, p. 20).

By conforming our woman would be powerless to help in implementing any change within her sport. Michel Foucault maintains that power and knowledge within the field is the only way to resist oppressive regimes(Markula & Pringle, 2006). In the case of our bodybuilder this is not by being rebellious but rather by acting holistically and raising the profile of women's sport and in this case bodybuilding. Her goal should she choose to compete would be to act as an active ambassador for all that is good in women's bodybuilding, thus influencing any detractors to rethink their judgements, a role that maybe all sports women should become aware of. In continuing to find help with this decision and calling on Kantian ethics, the categorical imperative asks 'What if everyone did this'(Cox, 2010)? This question answered would seem to be no bad thing, in the unlikely event that all women began to explore their physical potential and ignore current ideal female body concepts and ideologies, which are both physically and psychologically damaging to women of all ages. This would appear to be a decent thing. Aristotle's virtue theory suggests finding the golden mean of your virtues in order to strike a balance in your life, this is exactly our woman's aim if choosing to enter the sport(Harwood, 2010). Can she find the golden mean, can she live a good life with meaning and above all can she make a difference(Cox, 2010)? Much of this decision making process is determined by others, particularly the negative aspects.

> "Each person constantly confronts the existence of other people, not simply as objects in his world, but as subjects who see him and judge him and reduce him to an object in their world. To be an object in the world of the Other, to be for the Other, to be in danger of being belittled by the Other, this is the meaning of being-for-others"(Cox, 2009).

Our woman must take into consideration that she has no control of what others think of her but must know that they will have thoughts, judgements and opinions, some good, some bad, but all generally based on very little knowledge. This dramatic statement from the Sartre play "No Exit", maybe a bit harsh but shows how others are viewed by an Existentialist for effect.

> "So this is hell. I'd never have believed it. You remember all we were told about the torture-chambers, the fire and brimstone, the burning marl. Old wives' tales! There's no need for red hot pokers. Hell is - other people" (Wartenberg, 2008, p.47).

Now there is already much for our prospective woman bodybuilder to consider before making her decision on whether she can live a moral life as a competitive bodybuilder. To end this section she needs to take counsel on happiness and peace of mind, left to the end as other issues may affect the outcome of her achieving her ultimate goal which is happiness for herself and for any person involved in her life. Utilitarian's would advise our woman that it is the consequence of her actions measured and evaluated in happiness versus pain that should direct her choice. The greatest aggregate well being for all involved being the right choice (Furrow, 2005, p.44). Utilitarian John Stuart Mill, was the first to distinguish between higher and lower pleasures, higher pleasures being more valuable and rewarding than lower pleasures (Mill, 2001). In this instance lower pleasures may be the pleasure felt in the body during a workout or that gained by seeing your peak conditioning before it fades again. As mentioned before bodybuilding is a sport of extremes and the extreme conditioning needed for competition is often offset by a bodybuilders off season condition which is fat and bloated and causes them to cover up making them miserable (Klein, 1993). Our woman has already mastered the art of happily staying in shape or close to contest shape year around and with her mindful approach to training and life in general including meditation. She views her body as a working ever changing sculpture, a gift that she lovingly and creatively values. Experience has taught her that purpose and meaning are more fulfilling than the pleasures gained from materialism and any hedonistic pursuits. She will be happy and knows she will receive the full support of her friends and loved ones. She looks forward to the new adventure.

Mindful in the Mayhem
For any person never having entered a hard core gym, they can be intimidating

places, even more so for a lone female (Klein, 1993). Cursing seems to be compulsory and the topics of conversation are those reserved for men only clubs. For our woman to be part of this environment but not affected by it, either by judging it, or becoming influenced by it, she has developed the idea of Buddhist mindfulness to use whilst working out. Mindfulness focuses her on her workouts, conscious breathing on cardio and being "in the moment" on her exercises, feeling the muscle, the weights and the sensations whilst blocking out the white noise that makes a gym an extremely turbulent place. Add to this a smile for other members and help whenever needed and she has managed to become part of the scene without compromising her moral standards. Conscious breathing techniques and mindfulness are featured in books written by Vietnamese Buddhist Monk Thich Nhat Hahn in 2008 & 2009 entitled Happiness and The Miracle of Mindfulness respectively. These techniques help our woman achieve balance in an extremely turbulent society.

A Question of Perfection

Bodybuilding as a sport whether competitive or not tends to subscribe to the idea that more is better. Our society seems to follow the same route. This prompts the question, Is there any peace of mind in "more is better"? The endless quest for perfection can be seen everywhere in bodybuilding circles. Perfection is a concept that has no clearly defined lines in any context so how can it be achieved? Betrand Russell even argued that any object is seen differently by each and every person viewing it. If you look at a chair, the angle you look, the light, your eyesight and all of your internal thoughts and memories affect what you are seeing, and what you see changes by the millisecond (Russell, 1912). If you apply this to perfection, any person for a brief moment will see perfection in what they see according to all of the above, and their personal perception and preferences as to what perfection is. Why would any person strive to achieve such an impossible outcome? Perfection may be judged at any time by any person without all the striving. There is far more peace of mind in not trying to achieve the impossible. Therefore it could be argued that for peace of mind being able to see perfection all about you is best. That would mean ignoring any other image of perfection you are being sold by any person or institution in society, as just plain immoral.

Conclusion

The sport of women's bodybuilding has many detractors and indeed it could be argued that is much wrong with the sport. This essay has attempted to show that with the correct approach participants don't have to sacrifice their right behaviour in order to be part of a sporting sub-culture, and if enough individuals can show correct moral behaviour from within the sport then change is possible as the sum of the parts increases. A woman can be a bodybuilder happily and live a balanced life with meaning.

Part 2 - Handy Habits & Tips

Some Handy Habits and Personal Philosophies That have served Us Well for Gaining & Maintaining the Motivation That Can Also Help Lead You to Your Success.

Influence

Parents affect their children's outlook in life so much. Some bad habits are so ingrained in families that the children don't stand a chance of getting fit. Are we letting our indifference to health and fitness affect those around us, particularly the ones we love? This role really is so important. We all influence our nearest and dearest silently all the time with our memes, this is not a role we can decide we don't want. Memes are the mimicked behaviour, the transferring of ideas, beliefs and attitudes to others and it all takes place mentally and silently. Memes pass from mind to mind via hundreds of thousands of imitations, they are not necessarily good or bad; they simply spread easily. Memes impact our behaviour throughout our lives and can influence our habits if we don't realise and change those ingrained beliefs that are not serving us well. Are we sending out the right messages? Could our children, friends, parents or neighbours be setting us the right example? Are we setting them the right example? Do we take our position as role models seriously? Do we even realise that we are all role models? Just because we are older does that mean we cannot learn from our children? We have a lifetime of bad and some good habits just waiting to be passed on to our friends, children and even neighbours. When is the right time to take our role model status seriously? Does the fact that the results are not immediately obvious like they would be with bad behaviour or poor manners mean that we ignore our responsibilities? Whether we realise the consequences of the example we set or not, there are, and will always be people that love us and look to us for a lead in life. We influence others and that is a fact. We all make mistakes and none of us are perfect but there has to be a time when we look to set or follow examples of others with habits that will set up our families for generations by actually changing the activity culture. Are we teaching our kids by example, to eat, drink and sit around doing nothing or play computer games? Is our fear of exercise influencing our children, significant others or any person that spends time in our company on a regular basis? Do you think walking is for people that don't have cars or can't drive? We can all make good or better health and fitness habits part of our culture permanently by starting the ball rolling with small changes here and now.

If you are overweight, unfit and sedentary and every social occasion for you involves food and drink, if your idea of relaxing is watching television or playing computer games, then you are following an example that could lead to a miserable life and an early grave. You are also setting this behaviour as normal and making it part of your culture to be handed down to future generations via your memes. In effect this behaviour has become part of your legacy. I know this may sound harsh but that is the whole point, our lifestyles are killing us and we do nothing but joke about it until it is too late. Obesity is no laughing matter. Heart attacks are not funny. Bad habits lead to misery sooner or later is that what we want for ourselves and for our families? To stress this even more our influence and roles as mentors is preordained whether we like it or not that is how society habits are reinforced. And no longer can our ingrained habits be dismissed as not harming anyone but ourselves that is simply not true and just plain irresponsible. Overnight with these discoveries we have become aware that we are even more responsible and closer bonded to all of humanity. Just for a second as you sit there ask yourself this question. Discounting your wise words and we all have plenty of them, what messages are you sending out with your lifestyle and your behaviour? Do you live a do as I say not as I do existence?. Are you 100% happy that your message is the one you mean to deliver? Julie and I know that we have much to work on i our lives, but we also thrive in the knowledge that how we behave and our lifestyle can and does make a real difference to people one way or the other. This awareness give real meaning to our lives that may otherwise have gone unnoticed. This influence is less about loud words than good deeds, habits and behaviours that will silently flow from mind to mind and become learned behaviours. A point worth considering here also is that while we are thinking about our influence on others we ourselves are constantly under attack by mind viruses both good, bad and indifferent.. Not to panic but be mindful of what you expose yourself to in the way of negative and sensationalised bad news, violence and advertising. These mediums can weaken even the strongest resolve. On the flip side be receptive to good news, nature and all things positive and you will set yourself up to lead by example. You can ensure you are back in control and not being brainwashed and conditioned by an often complaining and selfish society or businesses wanting you to use their unhealthy products for the sole purpose of increasing their profits.

Inner Fitness

For many years self help exercise books have been produced, full of facts, most of them are very accurate in the information they provide, although most of them are not providing anything more than a short term fix. With all of this expert advice available, still human beings are collectively becoming more obese and less fit. We are failing as a species to grasp the concept of how to look after our amazing, nature gifted bodies. On countless occasions I have started to write my book and each and every time have not been able to convince myself that we are offering or contributing any new ideas or wisdom that will really help anybody that may be struggling with their fitness and all that relates to that fitness, such as self esteem, confidence, depression etc. As I sit here at my computer, I know that there is little we do not know about exercise and nutrition programmes after 35 years being totally addicted to the subject and a former gym owners and personal trainers for over 20 years. Clients would drive for miles for our expertise and bed side manner. We knew we could motivate people to great levels of fitness when we were with them, however to guarantee long term success we needed to be able to teach them how to do that for themselves and in order to do that we had to understand exactly what it was we were teaching. We knew every exercise and principle and could teach those with consummate ease. This knowledge and experience however does not offer the key to fitness for all people. We knew the answer to why Julie and I in our forties and fifties had no problem maintaining top levels of fitness was more complex than that but never really managed to put our fingers on exactly what separated us from other people when it came to success in that area of our lives. We knew that there are no special exercises or machines that can bring about dramatic results, we knew that the answer was actually inside of each of us and the key was, and still is, our motivation. Psychologists Sigmund Freud, Alfred Adler and Abraham Maslow would all have different theories on what motivates us from sex, power and life meaning respectively and maybe they are all right but how does that work in the real world. The key for the rest of us is to find a model in the real world that works and follow that example as best we can with our lifestyles. So task number one is to find a positive model and look at their habits and refine ours accordingly. We are often asked what our secret is, well the nearest we can come to a secret is to reveal our habits and maybe the secret is revealed as the sum of all of our habits. The secret is inside of us and not in equipment or special diets. We in turn can then become that positive role model for our nearest and dearest and the ball starts to roll. With this book we hope to become your model for fitness success and share our very typical human story of ups and downs. We have seen many books being presented by seemingly perfect fitness professionals, never eating junk food and never missing exercise sessions. We really believe that aspiring to emulate this perfection will never bring any person peace of mind and that improvement, not perfection should be the target of any and all fitness regimes. More is better will never bring any peace of mind and that includes with your fitness and body image.

One thing we need to make very clear is that the success we have experienced with our fitness and physiques had only until recently purely been in that area of my life, it has taken 35 years to realise that if we approach the rest of our lives with a similar philosophy, we could have as much joy throughout our lives.

Our lives had become a hopeless mess, the simple act of changing the way we approached that same life, miraculously remedied the 20th and 21st century disease that had ailed us and probably has infected many of you reading this book.

We had reached a desperate stage in our lives, that looking back and with our new outlook does seem very surreal, but I know many others must face the same creeping society disease and may appreciate the views of a family that has come back from the brink. How? Simply by looking at and thinking about life differently. This sounds so simple now but maybe at the time we were just perfectly primed to accept a solution that was within us all the time. We are now sure that the answer to every problem we ever come up against is not in drugs, sex or material possessions, but rather sitting quietly inside of us waiting to be consulted.

Now both in mid life and at long last taking responsibility for our own lives and happiness, no longer searching for happiness outside of ourselves, we feel ready to share some of the habits that have enabled us to maintain excellent fitness and physiques and spread over enriching the rest of our lives. I can now write this book without feeling like it is just another revamped exercise manual. We have learned some very hard lessons in our lives and these habits have not been easy to arrive at, we have lived our lives the hard way and with that said would not change one single day of it. We are the people we are today because of our life experiences. The most exciting part for us is that we are learning about life and our roles till the day we die and still we will never be close to having all of the answers.

Our habits, and we are very much a work in progress, encompass the welfare of mind, body and soul as we have discovered this symbiotic relationship is essential to both success and happiness. We look at our habits in a number of life areas that we feel are vital to a balanced existence. Looking back, we realised that every book we had read and every goal we had set in the past had been fitness and physique orientated, our lives had no balance, and we needed to use our physical success as a model for the rest of our lives. We had control over our fitness and physique and were a great team, however every other facet of our lives was totally out of control. Our businesses and there have been many had all succeeded and then failed, our relationship and at times our lives were on the rocks and we firmly believe if it weren't for the fact that we were training partners, we would not have survived, the gym seemed to be an area of neutrality, our Switzerland. What was so different in the gym to any other area of our lives? Look at other areas of your life, you will see aspects of your life that you are successful in and yet have no control over your fitness or physiques, instantly you will have the start of a model to base your exercise and fitness needs on. As it turns out it seemed that the only difference was the way we thought about and subsequently applied ourselves to that area of our lives compared to, at that time, all others. We had a victim mentality in every other area of our lives except our fitness, where we were in control and confident. In fitness and physique we were and will always be self reliant, in the rest of our lives we were conforming to unsuitable ideals, constantly chasing happiness in its guise of more is better. Looking back, where is the peace of mind in forever having the philosophy of more is better? Continuing to look back, and that is not something we like to do these days, we both agree that Julie was always ready to embrace the changes but unknowingly needed to have me there by her side, my influence had to change for both of our sakes, not to mention our three fantastic children.

We had lost two friends through suicide in the space of 12 months, we were following that same destructive path. Massively stuck in a rut of despair and only seeing a downhill life path, on the recommendation of a very special friend and maybe in desperation I began to read a few self help books. I cannot explain why as at that time I never sat still long enough to read books, just magazines, and would say that I have always been the world's biggest cynic, believing that people that write these books are doing it for the money only. Being an analytical person, I started to see much logic in the books I began reading and it was obvious that I needed to change the way I thought, take responsibility for my life and maybe I could turn things around. I believe the technical name for this process is cognitive therapy and bibliotherapy is therapy via reading books that help lift depression and generally improve one's state of mind. Julie and I would have long discussions about the books I was reading and I would even read to her while we lay in bed. I know, sounds like a thrill a minute, but really it was. We hadn't been able to see the fantastic life that was right in front of our eyes. We had very little to change, we had all that we needed in our extraordinary lives. I am now an avid reader, I cannot believe I spent so many years avoiding books; maybe they reminded me of school. I even have a shelf of books that are waiting to be read; as I type there are 16 new books on that shelf. My body tingles at the thought of all of that new reading. I think I am a bookaholic or should that be biblioholic? I no longer need a magazine full of glossy pictures and idle gossip to spark my interest.

The following pages include some of the habits and philosophies we have developed in different areas of our lives, we have much to work on in certain areas but now thankfully we are heading in the right direction with extreme optimism. We have no fear and look forward to an incredible experience. We hope you will be able to take whatever you find useful to adapt for use in your own lives and ultimately arrive with a balance that brings you happiness and contentment. Many of these changes we credit with saving our marriage and we can honestly say they have been life changing for us and any person whose life is aligned to ours. We are in love with life and the possibilities once more.

Different for Girls

Should the way women exercise be radically different to the way men exercise? In our opinion there should be no such thing as gender appropriate exercise as there are no relevant differences that would affect exercise and results from exercise. we feel that gender appropriate training only serves to slow down or negate the potential results available to both genders. I am going to generalise for a second and I apologise if the following generalisation does not fit with you. Boys like lifting heavy weights and girls see mainly cardio as the way to reach their goals. Goals which most often are aimed at achieving a society ideal body portrayed in the media. Often these goals are unrealistic for the individual. Both genders use every justification in the book to avoid the basic fact that for whatever reason they enjoy one more than the other. The facts are that we all have the same muscle and cardio-respiratory system. The only real difference is that women do not have the capacity to build the massive muscles which they are so worried about sprouting all over their bodies and the obvious genetic potentialities we all have. Incidentally I have never known muscles to appear on anyone suddenly and unexpectedly just because they lift weights and with muscle there is a definite use it or lose it situation which comes into play. I honestly prefer weights as does Julie because that is how we are able to sculpt our bodies and obtain the more rewarding quantifiable results. For Julie and I we even feel that it helps to work out with members of the opposite sex and whenever possible over the last 30 years that is what we have done. There is rarely any domination and we compete on how hard that we both train not on how much weight we can lift. The combination is perfect our strengths and weaknesses complement each other very well. Julie keeps me honest on the cardio. There are no special gender based exercises only those you have been lead to believe are that way for various commercial reasons based purely on myth. So come on girls get in that weights room and tear it up a little. Maybe teach the guys how to behave and understand that there are no men only areas in the 21st century.

"At no point do I claim any special mastery over how to live life, but I am committed to finding a formula through experience that could assure a person some success". - **Benjamin Franklin.**

Perfection

Perfection or the ideal, whose idea exactly is the perfection human beings strive so hard to attain. Well without apportioning any blame the ideologies and images which portray perfection to us need to be unattainable, that way we all continue to spend our money on achieving the impossible. The media and associated industries need us to be dissatisfied. Let us take a look at perfection in a different way. If man had a hand in designing nature which he often does with his landscaped gardens, all would be symmetry, straight lines, ordered colours and uniformity in appeal. Try to imagine a single tree designed by man and then a forest of those trees with accompanying flora and man designed wild life. Have you got that image? Now think of the rain forest with all of the seemingly random shapes, colours, sizes, the amazing waterfalls and diverse wildlife. Which is more perfect to you? Without doubt, Mother Nature can never be surpassed even when man has the plans and blueprint she still remains unsurpassed. So, this would indicate that man's idea of perfection is never as perfect as A Mother Nature original. Then maybe we would come to the conclusion that man's idea of perfection is always a pale imitation of the original. Now for a moment, holding the image of a man made forest with identical symmetrical trees in nice neat rows, picture a main street in any town or city. Now imagine, the ideal body image for men and women portrayed in the media for this era, visualise everyone has finally achieved this look. Each and every man, woman and child identical. Is that perfection? Now imagine the same scene our creators way, all of us different, unique and happy that way. We can all be fit and strong but just the way we are shaped is our creators perfection. We are created whole and perfect, then we tend to abuse that creation with poor nutrition habits and no exercise. We each have a genetic potential, that is perfect and fits our world as does every piece of the rainforest jigsaw. The vision of perfection sold to us by the media is simply false and unrealistic. Perfection is surely reaching Mother Nature's genetic potential for our unique self, through exercise, nutrition, peace of mind and good habits. We are already perfect creations but often we mess up that gift with poor and misguided lifestyle habits. Love who you are and be the best version possible of you, not a media creation. Next time you are wishing for that media created perfection, think, of the rainforest or any of Mother Nature's creations of which you are one and find your inspiration. Then find joy in the knowledge that the creator got it right and you can never be improved upon. Work every muscle in your body as nature intended, they are part of your body for a reason, to be used. Don't store fuel (fat) you are unlikely to have any future need for that stored fuel. Get moving, get happy and laugh at societies idea of what is ideal. Embrace your natural shape, exude confidence, love your wrinkles and hair, see aging as the amazing time of life that it really is. Above all appreciate the whole of the human race as potentially perfect just the way they were created. Never lose sight of your perfection.

> "We but half express ourselves, and are ashamed of that divine idea which each of us represents.........What I must do is all that concerns me, not what the people think.....It is easy in the world to live after the world's opinion.... It is easy in solitude to live after our own...Nothing can bring you peace but yourself. Nothing can bring you peace but the triumph of principles" (Emerson 1841/2007, p. 20).

If we can apply this to our thoughts and actions then maybe we will become the unique individuals we are intended to be and recognize the same in others and applaud individuality and the right to be different in all people.

Be Your Own Coach

In delivering this book and information to you we are obviously expecting you to become your own coach. We are able to carry on our fitness lifestlye because we are coaches and we have an awareness of what is needed and we take full responsibility for our own progress. This responsibility or ownership coupled with the learning and subsequent improvements are what make fitness so enjoyable and are key motivating factors. In simple terms the buck stops here.

Motivation

There are many theories on motivation and a general understanding and acceptance of what may motivate you is helpful if you are to be coaching yourself. Many of these theories do seem to be at least somewhat age and sex related but that is no hard and fast rule and there are always exceptions. I also believe that motivational factors are different for each individual and also may change at different stages in any person's life. It is important to accept what motivates you and to accommodate that drive in your programme selection. We are all driven primarily for the need for food but I think we can discount that as our motivation in this instance, unless you starve all day and then leave your dinner at the end of an assault course. Maybe not that practical and there is bound to be a McDonalds somewhere on the course. An actor asks what their motivation is before they perform so let us see if we can narrow down exactly what your motivation for changing your body and fitness may be.

Sigmund Freud theorises that we are driven by our repressed sexual urges. Alfred Adler states that we are driven by the search for power to make up for what we believe we are lacking, so inferiority, inadequacy and insecurity determine the strength of our drive and ultimate goals. He uses Napoleon as an example of an inferiority complex. He was highly motivated because of his lack of stature. Erik Erikson believed that identity crises are essential for us to form ourselves and that we are driven by forming those identities. The last 2 psychologists I will mention here are Viktor Frankl, who believed that man's search for meaning is ultimately what drives him. And finally to Abraham Maslow whose hierarchy of needs shows that we have an order of needs that begins with food, water, shelter and safety and goes up through the higher values of self esteem to ultimately becoming self realised and driven by values and life meaning. I think it is fair to say that we are complex organisms and all the above are true to some degree in most of us.

Young men are generally the most obvious in what drives them and they are training either to excel in sport or just to be bigger, stronger and more attractive to any prospective mates, thus conforming to a society ideal portrayed in magazines and television. The bigger and stronger image is for other guys mostly to strengthen their identities in the pack. This drive quite easily leads into the middle years in men as well particularly if they are in amongst the young guys at the gym. Sadly muscular size is overly revered in society but that is just the way it is. So if you are a guy and your motivation is to get bigger and stronger that is great just remember that fat is not the way to go. Gyms are full of size monsters that are just plain overweight. Cardio, leg work, good eating habits and stretching need to be included in your workouts. Nobody is fooled by Mr upper body except Mr upper body. Quality above quantity is the way to go, it may take longer but will be well worth the wait.

For men the society acceptance threshold for being overweight is higher than for women. An overweight guy is "a big bloke" and totally accepted up to an invisible limit, where he becomes fat. For women that limit is much lower and society is less forgiving of overweight women.

For young women it is not important to be strong and powerful and in fact a woman with muscle could be frowned upon, again there seems to be a line not to be crossed. For a while that line was determined by Madonna's stringy, yet muscley arms. Madonna though is quickly replaced by the next must have celebrity body just like the latest model of a car or mobile phone catches the desire of consumers in a capitalist society. Generally young women are motivated by reaching a weight or dress size acceptable to both society and themselves. You could then say that forming an identity that is shaped by the media is the driving force for women's fitness and that the painfully thin photo-shopped role models are the gold standard. These motivations lead to women wrongly avoiding weight training in favour of attempting to burn off as many calories as possible with cardio and men not seeing the need to do cardio and spending all their time getting big, yes, and fat. For women this motivation is quite consistent throughout the years.

As men age they start to reach an unacceptable level of both fitness and fatness and health concerns may arise. Confronted with the middle years, they decide to do something about it. This stage being bigger and more powerful is not as important, often married with kids and settled the need to attract a mate is less of a drive. This is often where the drive is to improve the quality of fitness and subsequently the quality of life, the time for more meaning and where being free of health problems becomes much more important, something as a youngster we tend to take for granted. This stage is very similar with women of the same age, a realisation that improved health through nutrition and fitness not only makes you look better but improves your moods and the quality of your life, all factors that produce excellent motivation. Have you found your motivation amongst the sex, power, meaning or identity in here anywhere? Desire is the key to motivation but it is taking action to meet your desires that produces results.

Motivated people have a dream, show passion and enthusiasm, work with a practical and flexible plan and never ever give up. Motivation is the driving force that makes you gleefully hop out of bed in the morning, full of yourself and happy to be alive. When you are motivated, life is full of magic, and when you are not motivated you need to get there and quick. Motivated people are passionate and positively full of themselves, their enthusiasm and excitement is contagious and they attract people to them. Do whatever it takes to stay motivated, dream, fantasise and imagine the unique body and fitness that the future you will earn and turn into reality, very soon.

Our Motivation

Now, true to the theme of the book and to keep it simple. What honestly motivates us to keep training after more than 30 years of intense gym work?

Gary – For me, I started because I had a low self image, I was thin and sporty but very shy, in many ways despite my physical changes I still have an unrealistically low self image. Also motivated by what can be achieved potentially, the dream. A friend once said that " I constantly needed smoke blowing up my arse", which means I needed and searched for other peoples acceptance and admiration. Although not as bad as I use to be I would say the same still applies. I am working on not needing others acceptance and convincing myself that it really doesn't matter. Nowadays I exercise because I love it, it makes perfect sense and I am in my element with it. I love the way it makes me feel, I love the way it makes me look. I love the challenge that Father time has set for us in seeing how long we can make our bodies last, and how it feels like home. I am comfortable with all things fitness. I have come a long way with fitness as part of my life and to me it is inconceivable that it would be any other way. Fitness is part of me and who I am, fitness has always been a positive constant in my life. Another very motivating factor is being in control of your body as opposed to losing control to the many temptations life has to offer.

Julie – Initially Julie was motivated by me and worked out because I did, she says she became aware of how her body was changing and could change more as she went along and that further motivated her. The compliments she received were a big plus and having her body bounce back after having children because of her hard work and great attitude helped. To this day, for Julie, how she looks and feels is the deciding factor in continuing to workout and she says it has made her a much more positive person in general. Not using excuses or whinging about anything that takes effort to achieve is a reward not easily seen, she often smiles when she hears how others negatively talk themselves out of anything involving any effort or use childbirth as an excuse for being out of shape. To Julie they are depriving themselves of one of lives pleasures by constantly believing their own false excuses. Being a fit healthy and positive hardbody that believes physically the sky is the limit when it comes to improvement is motivation enough for Julie. Julie also adds that competing in bodybuilding shows is also good motivation, a motivation she came to late in life. Julie entered her first show aged 48 and a grandmother. She won.

FIT HAPPENS !!

Habits

Widely regarded as the Father of modern psychology, William James noted in his book The principles of psychology in 1890, "when we look at creatures from an outward point of view, one of the things that strikes us is that they are bundles of habits". James also noted that while the actions of most animals are automatic, and relatively limited and simple, because of our wide variety of desires and wants, humans have to consciously form new habits if we are to achieve certain results. The problem is that creating new, good habits requires work and application. James wrote that the key to good habits is to act decisively on the resolutions you make. You are the sum total of your habits and influences. In changing bad habits you don't suffer, you reap the benefits. A friend of mine got into jogging to reduce his expanding waistline, but disciplined himself to start everyday at the same time. While good habits are hard to develop, they become easy to adhere to; in contrast, bad habits come slowly and easily but are hard to live with. A good guide is the people in your circle of influence and who influence you and that you spend your time with. If you want to stop smoking, quit drinking and start getting up early, you will not achieve it by spending your nights in bars. You acquire habits by choices - choose good habits and they make you. Choose bad habits and they break you. Our character, fundamentally, is a composite of our habits. Habits are influential factors in our lives. Because they are consistent, often conscious patterns, they constantly, daily, express our character and produce our effectiveness or ineffectiveness. Bad habits wait on us forever. They don't ever go away. They will always be there, just around the corner, lurking and looking for an opening. If you're addicted to food or alcohol or cigarettes or even the wrong person in your life, if you've got a bad habit of any kind, I don't think it just disappears. If you stop setting goals for the future, if you start living in the moment again, that's when those bad habits will push their way back into your life.

To develop a habit in our lives we need all three of the following **Wisdom/Knowledge** (what to do and why), **Mastery/Skill** (how to do) and **Desire** (The motivation). My job with this book is to provide you with Wisdom of what to do and why to do it in order to reach your dream you. Also my job is to provide you with the wisdom of how to do it, although mastery of the practical skills of actually doing it are down to you and your self coaching.

To form a good habit you must be convinced that it is desirable. When your desire for the change is greater than your desire to continue with the old habit, you are already on the road to success. Now finish this sentence.

I am motivated by a desire to

_____
_____
_____
_____

In other words what is your motivation for developing new habits for coaching yourself to change?

This is all very well but what is the one habit that we have formed that helps more than any other in changing your lifestyle? We discuss this habit to form habits next.

Our Most Helpful Habit Forming Habit

Ironically you will need to form a new habit to help you break and form other new habits. This is the single best habit we have ever formed. This habit can take on every new habit you have ever wanted to form and give you a day to day analysis as to how you are doing.

My journal is a black and red notebook with affirmations stuck all over the front, this innocent looking notebook is the best habit you could ever form. You could even keep your journal on your pc, I actually do both now but personally I think the whole idea of handwriting it adds to the feeling of intimacy. You could even make it a blog but then you have to watch what you say and you really need to be able to confide in your journal without fear of recriminations from any direction but the self. Handwrite it and just take my word for that being the cosiest way to keep a journal, just curled up comfortably in the corner with a cup of tea.

Your first entry will be "JOURNAL WATCH DAY 1 – today I started to write a journal for the first time ever, I am not sure how I will do but apparently if I can keep it up for about 30 days it will have become a habit". After this you will chit chat to yourself about this and that maybe even ad an "EXERCISE WATCH DAY 1 – today I have decided to form the habit of exercising in some way shape or form each and every day. I began by joining the local gym. I was nervous at first and am nervous about going back tomorrow for my induction, I guess this feeling is normal." You will get more and more into using your journal, I even use it as a springboard to mailing people I am close to but do not see regularly for whatever reason. It's just like talking to a very close friend. You can dream, fantasise and just generally let off steam.

I have given up drinking alcohol. I have formed the habits of meditation and visualisation in the same way.

Here are some progressive days of my "meditation watch" that may be of interest to you as to how I deal with the ups and downs of forming any new habit. These are actual journal entries, written seconds after meditation.

Meditation Watch day 1 – Settled in for 15 minutes, putting on some nature sounds – went Ok, set my phone for 15 minutes and used AH! as my mantra. So it went, deep breath in through the nose hold for 4 secs and then AAAAAAH! out of the mouth. I did struggle to quiet my mind but rhythm developed and I felt good afterwards, a little spaced out. I caught myself thinking a few times but I suppose with practise I can focus on breathing and how the AH! feels resonating in my head. A quick summary; I felt a bit daft but I am a believer and I definitely felt spaced out for want of a more accurate description. Had a giggle when I pictured myself.

Meditation Watch day 2 – Jacob joined me for my meditation today, I could learn a lot about relaxation from him. Found my mind wandering again but did relax once I found my breathing rhythm, struggle to settle in to the rhythm at first. I think maybe I am trying to hard with the breathing, so I changed the way I thought about it and it seemed to work. Jacob stayed asleep on my lap the whole time.

Meditation Watch day 3 – 20 minutes today, set my phone again, yesterday was good, today I struggled to settle, no rhythm and Jacob even decided to leave after a couple of minutes. Oh well, 2 steps forward and 1 step back. My mind is very active today, I have had many ideas for my writing appear in the last 24 hours. It occurs to me that I finished off some chocolate early this morning something I eat very rarely, it had been left in the fridge by my Mum, that poor meditation is probably confirming what I already know about how chocolate affects moods adversely by upsetting homeostasis.

Meditation Watch day 8 – I decide that timing a meditation is probably counterproductive so I don't set the timer and I leave off the sounds of nature. Goes well, I still need to quiet my chatterbox, but I think I am improving.

Meditation Watch day 9 – Best yet, this time I have a dream, a vision in my head and my mind seems to approve greatly and I have the best meditation yet. I will try to combine my meditating with visualisation in the future.

Meditation Watch day 14 – I followed a guided meditation that I have downloaded today, it felt very good, something to stop my mind wandering so much.

Meditation Watch day 17 – Up later today, struggled to get up, feeling plug pulled. I sat in my dressing gown and had a cup of tea before showering, that is rare. Eventually showered and settled down to meditate, went really well, lasted at least an hour and I felt so much better when I had finished.

Meditation Watch day 19 – We have visitors so I stayed in bed to meditate this morning with Julie next to me, different surroundings and a new test for my concentration. At one time I almost gave up. I didn't and that just strengthened my resolve. Strange phenomena to report; in my deepest moments I became aware maybe 2 or 3 times that I pulled myself away from a thought or a state, not sure what, but could not see anything clearly. I can only describe it as a deep awareness of a new state of mind but I am clueless as to what? Where? Who? Why? or How? Interesting though as I was very aware of pulling away and trying to instantly remember or see the thought but it had gone.

Meditation Watch day 21 – The evolution continues, I have split my meditations up to suit me. I have one for body, gratitude, prosperity and sanctuary. Generally going well.

Meditation Watch day 29 – I lay in bed meditating today, I complete 2 guided meditations. Absolutely could not concentrate at all, I did persevere but my focus was poor, this was not one of the great meditations, Buddha has nothing to worry about, not that he worries at all.

Meditation Watch day 30 – Didn't meditate this morning. My aim is to do it before I sleep tonight. 30 days is a crucial time in forming new habits, I need to be vigilant and not let the meditation habit slip this time around. I have been grumpy and restless all day. Later I force myself to meditate, the change in mood and feelings is remarkable. I shower and the new less grumpy Gary settles down for the night with Julie. I can't let a habit so beneficial slip this time.

Meditation Watch day 31 – I am up early and shower and settle down to meditate, it goes great and I think even though I only missed one morning that it had made a difference to my day. I won't let this habit slip.

I hope this illustrates how any new habit involves a lot of persistence and just how easy it is to give up at any given time when any day doesn't live up to your expectations. With the journal it gives you the chance to each day look at any adversity you come across logically before you let a knee jerk reaction spoil your ultimate purpose. I have learned from experience that I can't flood myself with many new habits at once as the need for some focus is essential. Initially I had a whole host of new habits listed but ended up confused and spreading my mental resources too thin. I find if I work on one or two related behaviour changes at the most it is easier to focus throughout the day. Once they become habit, I still use the journal to check up on myself, I suppose you would call them secondary habit watches. Currently my main habit change is to become a better listener. Julie sees me type this and says "that will take at least 30 years let alone 30 days". I listen to what she says, shrug and all she has done is bolster my resolve to succeed and improve my listening in one sentence. What a team, Oh! Yes and she is great at finding memory sticks that I frequently lose as well.

I do feel that humour is essential to life but also to your journal and never take yourself too seriously. To illustrate I have taken an insert from my journal; "Upper body today, we are snapping pictures for the book once more. Julie and Shaunie are performing, it occurs to me that 2 trained chimpanzees would be more useful but that is probably being unfair to the chimps. We finish and skip the shower as Shaunie is late for college, I stink but we need to get off quickly, even though agreeing with me the girls don't follow suit and despite my sacrifice we are late anyway. When we arrive home I download the pictures and video clips and it turns out the chimps did worse than I thought. None of the clips are any use as the camera was the wrong way around. Never mind, there is no urgency, if we take enough we will eventually get what we need, I hope!!! The chimps spend the rest of the night searching for Shaunies lost keys. I seriously think I may get them swing bars installed in the garden but they may annoy the neighbour's cat. I hope Shaunie and Julie return to me soon, but somehow I doubt it. The evening goes by smoothly as is normal. Yes! I love them both as much as ever and I find it all really funny and that includes my reaction to their keystone cop routines, they are just having fun, and when Holly joins them it seems to get worse. The other day all three and Smudge & Jacob were crammed into the bathroom discussing who owned which toothbrush and why somebody had to retrieve a toothbrush from the waste bin.

I wouldn't trade it for anything. These moments are what go to make up life as I love it.

To summarise habits–

1. Don't try to set too many new habits at once.
2. Whilst in the phase of forming a new habit or breaking an old one, keep a close eye on your day to day progress for 30 days, after that, review the habit for as long as you wish.
3. Form the habit of using a journal, it will be the best habit you have ever formed. You will only need to spend about 15 minutes on your journal if you feel time is an issue but I guarantee once you form the habit you will want to spend more time talking to yourself about yourself and all that is happening in your life. Use some humour "don't take yourself to seriously" and have some fun with it.
4. Expect zig zag progress to forming new and breaking old habits, new habit forming hardly ever works in a straight line to success. Negative feedback allows you to re-adjust and reach your ultimate target.

Self Discipline

Forming new better habits leads us to one of the most important habits you will need to develop in order to succeed. Self discipline is often ignored as one of the key reasons for success in improving your health and fitness and achieving your dream body. In cartoons you often see a character with a demon on one shoulder and an angel on the other stressing over a decision that has to be made. Both can offer you a convincing reason to follow their lead. The physically easier route is always to follow your demon. He will tell you not to workout today, you are tired, you have done enough, you don't need to train legs, you deserve doughnuts and chips and this once won't hurt. He will follow up with suggesting you watch the television or have a nap or do what your friends are doing, as long as they are not doing anything healthy or strenuous, he will tell you there is no time or you have other things that are more important. You will make a great team because the deltoid demon will tell you whatever it is you need to hear to justify not working out or eating badly. You will believe that this only happens to you and fit people don't have the demons, well you are so wrong and the demons have fooled us on numerous occasions in the past. When he does fool you the trick is to bounce back more committed than before and learn to ignore the little beast, don't let one demon encounter put you off for life. You learn that once you get moving and ignore him you gain the energy you need and an empowering feeling of triumph because you have disciplined yourself to follow your dreams against what seemed like insurmountable demon odds. All joking aside though the fact is that without recognising you will need self discipline you will never reach your goals. Saying, " I didn't feel like it today" and any reasons used to excuse yourself from your chosen path become a habit just the same as any other repeated action, each time it seems to become harder and take longer to get back on track. Any gym computer will show you that once members lower their exercise consistency they soon stop exercising completely, the same will apply if you are exercising away from a gym environment. And, trust me on this one, there will never be a time when you regret ignoring your friendly deltoid demon and follow your dreams. Get up and get moving and he vanishes and you will start to feel energetic and human again. The top of the list of natural mood enhancers is exercise. When your motivation is waning, it could be that your workout needs changing because you are just bored with the old one and have reached a sticking point in your progress. Nobody says you have to do the same thing all the time, recognise the fact that the more you learn the more flexibility you will have within your programmes to motivate you. Most of all recognise and accept that you will often not feel like doing what you need to do, you will need self discipline. Don't rely on others this is "SELF" Discipline. Most often the last thing you feel like doing is the thing you need to do most. "Change the way you think and the things you think about will change". We love that idea and it is so effective, all you need is the awareness that your thoughts are in charge, to make it happen for you. Be consistent in your habits, keep that daily journal and you will succeed or have to explain to yourself why not, trust me it is easier and far more rewarding to just do it.

To Summarise Self Discipline :

A habit you need to develop and develop is exactly how it will happen, self discipline is like a muscle and the more you exercise it the stronger it will become.

Expect self discipline to take that good old zig zag route again with each perceived failure or as we know it with each episode of feedback you will get back on the fast track towards improving yourself discipline.

Don't forget to give yourself a break and don't beat yourself up if you have lapses. Don't take yourself too seriously. Self discipline will happen just like any other habit, and you will never be perfect, so don't even try as there is never any peace of mind in striving for perfection.

Setting Goals

I have mixed feelings about goal setting as I feel, and have seen something as simple as a person weighing themselves turn them from a positive and motivated individual into a self confessed failure in front of my eyes. Nothing deflates certain personalities quicker than perceived failure. In our eyes this is not even an issue, in health and fitness as life there are no failures and it is not a competition. Perceived failures are just part of the process to success in reaching your goals. At worst we all have to navigate around obstacles we know as failures at best they are your guiding lights to progress and success. We suggest you take the latter view, why look at it any other way?

So the big question is – **How do we set goals that do not turn out to be counterproductive?**

Julie and I sat for hours chatting about goal setting and how we approach this in our training. We have nothing detailed and specific written down. So our first question to answer was - do we have goals? We both decided that we do. Ok! Next question – where do we now keep our goals? Well we both keep our goals in our journals, when we see something we need to work on we log the fact that it is a priority and watch it for 30 days and then just informally after that to ensure the new habit doesn't slip too far. You may wish to detail your goals more thoroughly, but we believe that is when you set yourself up for disappointment, constantly number crunching to check your success and missing the big picture. We both decided that we keep a very positive body image embedded deep in our subconscious minds, put there from years of seeing the finished article as we daydreamed, this is undoubtedly the safest and best place for your goals but being honest this has happened for us totally by accident and through force of some very good habits. Although I do use creative visualisation now, we arrived at this level of fitness and physique by unwittingly using the skills I now deliberately employ in other areas of my life.

I asked Julie what her desire was for her body and her fitness and how she saw herself in her perfect scene. She pointed out that she always saw certain areas of her body as better than they are now. For example, her legs and glutes are less likely to carry any fat in what she holds in her mind. She said that in all honesty the fitness for her was the fantastic by-product of attaining the body, if you get the body the fitness just comes along with it, a two for one. That would indicate that Julie is motivated by the need for an identity based on her body. She stated that her real physique is always a tad behind the subconscious Julie. I asked if this meant that she was dis-satisfied with how she is now, she answered that she does have her moments like any person does but she is very happy with her body 99% of the time. We theorise that the subconscious image of us is where we are aiming to be and is just enough of an improvement on reality in our eyes to keep us both motivated. In summary Julie is satisfied but more than happy to welcome positive changes to her physique. This attitude lends itself to a relaxed approach to any goals and avoids constant disappointment for falling short.

Self Image - For any goal to be realistic and attainable one must have an accurate self image and yet most of us do not see ourselves accurately at all. This inaccurate evaluation of ourselves is always lower and limits our potential. In psycho cybernetics by Maxwell Maltz he likens it to having two boxes one small one inside a much larger one. The small box represents our image of our self and our capabilities, the larger box represents our fantastic potential. The void between these two boxes needs to be filled by improving our self image with that all important self belief and ridding ourselves of self imposed limitations. As an example of how we limit ourselves again taken from psycho cybernetics. A person that has a fat self image convinces themselves that they have a sweet tooth and cannot resist rubbish food, they can't find the time to exercise and nothing they do works. This becomes their reality, you cannot escape self image but you can change that image. If you feel that you really need work in this area to improve self image, I heartily recommend the above book- Psycho Cybernetics by Maxwell

Maltz and there are others that I will list at the end. Anything is possible if you believe in yourself.

Ok, now with self image as a work in progress or perfectly Ok we will look at how this information can best help us set goals that will inspire us with minimum effort. The results we want can be facilitated by setting goals whether we write them down or have them all stored in our onboard computer, so for us it is our handwritten journal and our minds. We need goals for every aspect of our fitness related behaviour particularly as in many cases we are setting out to form new habits.

Our habits ensure we achieve our goals each day. To give an idea of what I mean I will break down a typical day for me. None of this list is written down as it is habitual behaviour but nevertheless has to be completed for our deltoid angel to rest peacefully, having vanquished her deltoid devil adversary for another day. Should we at any time consider that we are falling below our own expectations on any of these, we hand the goal over to our journal to once again reinforce the habit. Any new goals get the journal treatment from the word go.

Our HEALTH AND FITNESS goals for the day –

- A little and often feeding schedule including moderate protein and carbs with healthy fats. Any current eating plan could fit here, zero carb days etc.
- To walk the dogs for at least 30 minutes
- To go to the gym and workout whatever has been planned. This get to the gym goal has goals within the goal. There are also goals in the workout to achieve, for instance 30 minutes cardio at a set heart rate level, or a perceived exertion level of very hard, and a workout to complete to our satisfaction. The feeling post workout has to be one of having given a good honest account of ourselves. We never leave the gym thinking "that'll do" or "next time". Workouts have to be challenging. I cannot remember ever leaving the gym without completing the work out.
- The feeding "little and often" carries on with our shake post workout and then throughout the day till bedtime, don't worry we do eat some proper food for dinner. Your feeding schedule is the key to your results and is determined by your size and activity levels and your goals of either fat loss or muscle gain.

For me the day starts at about 4am with a shower and a meal replacement protein shake before I settle down to meditate for up to an hour, I then write my informal journal. I get to work on my current project for my first stint of the day until about 9am. I have another shake at about 8am as I work. My goals for feeding are to take on board moderate to high protein and moderate carbs throughout the day either from solid food or more conveniently liquid form, being heavier my requirements are greater than Julies. At 9am we both take Jacob & Smudge over the park for a long run lasting about an hour. We have fortified porridge when we get back. I do a little more work and then we get set to leave for training at about 11am. We pack our bags to include shakes for immediately after training and water. Upon arriving at the gym (a major goal), arriving is where most people fall down, we set about our first workout goal and today for me it is completing a tough but satisfying 20 minutes on the cross trainer. I have always found cardio is where I need to make a special effort as it is where I will justify slacking off. I never slack off these days and complete a hard 20 minutes alternating between high and low levels. After cardio I stretch, I perform 8/10 stretches, each for 30 seconds, another goal achieved. My next goal is an upper body workout. I perform 10 upper body exercises in a set order very intensely with good technique and the exercises have to pass my inbuilt "hard work" test, another goal completed. I shower drink my shake and return home. I know when I need to feed next at all times, this avoids me ever eating out of control or missing valuable feeds. Progress hinges on training, sleeping and feeding. All three need to be planned and in your goals, if not automatically then logged in your journal until they are ingrained in your behaviour.

For anybody thinking that my schedule is suited to this, maybe you are right at the present time but for the last 35 years whatever job I have been doing, wherever I have been and even working abroad I have always managed to design a schedule to keep up my fitness needs. Planning is the key, if you rush out of the house each morning without a plan for your nutrition and exercise needs, you will fail. YOU are responsible, nobody else, so save your excuses and just get on with it. Once it becomes habitual you will wonder what you were worried about. Maybe one of your main goals will be to plan and prepare each days feeding schedule for your success. I have used shakes in the past because I just think it is convenient and measurable nutrition. In each shake I get X amount of protein carbs etc and if you can measure something you can adjust the levels either way upon evaluation of your progress. We rarely leave home without a shake onboard and there are lots of healthy fast food options like Brazil nuts, dried fruits and all sorts of bars and drinks now on the market. Porridge is quite nice even when cold in a sealed container, just match your taste buds up to your imagination and find your healthy nutritious solution. This is just one of many skills you will need to master as your own coach. I will leave the feeding schedule for the moment. We will discuss nutrition options later and I will give you some valuable sources to obtain your healthy convenience foods.

Remember that goal setting doesn't mean that you are stuck with those goals. You can change your goals as often as you want and feel it is needed. Also it does not mean that you become emotionally addicted to achieving them. Goals should help you flow and give you a clear focus and direction to direct your energy toward. Goals are there to help and support not hinder you in your true purpose. They are not taken too heavily or seriously but at the same time you must give them enough weight and importance so they are of real value to you. Start with simple obvious things and you change and develop them as you go along.

Ultimately goals are set to help you form new habits and get rid of some of your existing ones. These new habits need to hold the promise of improving the quality of your life experience otherwise there will be little motivation to reach your goals or change our existing habits.

I will now outline the Habits we credit with our fitness success to assist you with the goal setting process. This is how we do it.

1. We plan to exercise every day. This leaves us room to manoeuvre and missing a session doesn't become failure as five or six workouts a week is still something to be proud of. Aiming high always give you a good average workouts per week. We witness trainers that aim for 2/3 session per week and quite regularly miss them and yet when asked they say " I work out 3 times per week", firmly believing that they really do 3 workouts per week. Goal 1 – aim high with your workout regularity. Aim to get some exercise everyday and you will always achieve a good average. Any less than 3 times per week is really not enough anyway and you should be doing something on a daily basis. It is wise to get out of the habit of thinking everyday exercise is too much, it is not, our bodies are created to move so give them what they need everyday not just a few days per week. Walk, run, play sport or get to the gym but every day is your aim, it doesn't have to be super intense every day, intensity interspersed with more moderate days like taking a long walk is perfect. Get yourself moving

and away from the temptation of boredom or low energy eating. The number one way to energise your body is to exercise. A long walk with Jacob and Smudge is often as well as other exercise in our day, if we have nothing planned that walk can be just a little or a lot longer

2. We plan to eat little and often, always knowing what and when our next feed will be. Protein shakes are food. Anything with a calorie content is food whether you eat it or drink it. We never have a constant supply of crap foods in the house, no alcohol either, if you are serious about getting and staying in shape you need to avoid the temptations so don't buy them. You will be setting an example for all of your loved ones, if it's not good for you then it's not good for them and why would you want to be introducing them to habits they will struggle to change when they inevitably need to.

3. We always do balanced workouts that over the week include – Cardio, weights for every muscle group and stretching.

4. We always work hard, not going through the motions. It is not enough just to turn up you have to train intensely. The last set on all resistance exercise is done to failure which means we couldn't do another rep if our live depended on it.

5. **If I were to recommend one habit as the most important to your successful progress in fitness and most other aspects of life this would be it!!** Keep a journal, this is a good way to discipline yourself to keep your habits as it is difficult to kid yourself. I cannot praise the process enough. There is no fun in writing up failures each day but there is much satisfaction is seeing your progress and success and looking back on your feelings, it allows you the opportunity to re-align your goals each and every day. The journal also allows you to spot a problem before it becomes much of a problem at all. Sitting and writing about your dreams and expectations is good also. This can include anything and doesn't have to just be about your health and fitness. If you have a bad day it is good to talk to yourself about it in your journal and turn it around for the next day. You journal can be a day to day assessment of your whole life.

6. Meditation and visualisation are both part of our lives, most of our goals are held in our heads. Visualising your ideal scene is great when meditating and the relaxation felt in your often tight body from workouts is very therapeutic. See it, believe it and know you will surely get there in the end.

7. This may surprise you but one of our goals has been to avoid getting into the habit of watching too much television. We find this habit

addictive and energy sapping and very powerful. How many times do you find yourself watching other peoples crap lives unfolding before your eyes and passing for entertainment? Or sit looking for absolutely anything to watch rather than move your backside? We feel that apart from the odd exception television depicts the worse side of human nature and never energises but rather saps the energy from your body and to cap it all for some reason we all sit and eat while we do nothing. For us that is a bit of a negative double Whammy! and a habit we have to fight to avoid but the effort is well worth the gains. Our main living room no longer has a television in it, we have it housed in a small room adjacent. We mainly watch selective sporting events and often they are recorded so we can make it fit our schedule as opposed to letting the devil box in the corner dictate our lives, not to mention the position of our furniture. Just as a side to this, our conversations and family moments are much more rewarding without being distracted by the television on in the background all the time. I recommend you try it, you will not miss it until you are bored and then you should get the message and find something better to do. Each of us at some time does have the odd programme we like to watch but that doesn't now entail any person in the room having to watch it and becoming hypnotised as well. As you can see, I am quite a critic of the negative effects that television and computer games have on our overall fitness, energy levels, social skills and activity habits. DOH! Sorry about that it is just one of my hot buttons, I have been sucked in once too often. At one time I had watched so many re-runs of friends that I began quoting the wisdom of Phoebe, Joey, Chandler, Rachael, Ross and Monica at the most indiscriminate moments, now that is sad and most definitely time to take stock of your meme library. I guess the fact that I have just mentioned them all by name shows I am some way from a total cure.

To summarise goals –

Your goals will ultimately be achieved by setting your new habits and breaking destructive habits. If you change nothing then nothing will change.

Self belief is of paramount importance. Visualise what you want and do not accept no for an answer. Anything is possible.

Use your journal to focus daily on your progress, thoughts and plans.

Once you are focused do not become goal obsessed, relax and let it all happen perfectly.

Know and accept that you will not reach your goals without having to deal with some negative feedback, your progress line will be a zig zag, never straight.

Approach each moment of adversity with an optimistic view and move onwards and leave it behind. It really doesn't matter. Never dwell on small matters.

Develop "the happy little place in your head" where you can go when you need your motivation bolstered. Make it your planned reality. It will happen if you want it with emotion, passion and then let it go.

Try to make meditation a part of your daily routine, a time to relax and put all that is happening into perspective.

Know that the way you think is the key, all you ever have to change is inside of yourself, if you are having bad feelings, your negative thoughts are causing them. Look inside, never outside.

Last but not least, have some fun and never take yourself too seriously.

Take all of this on board and it is not a matter of how but rather WHEN you will succeed.

Coaching Yourself

Now before you start to self coach you need to vanquish a vision from your mind. That vision is the one of the personal trainer pushing the client really hard and being mean and way too hard, ruthless and unreasonable. I also need you to forget all that has gone before this moment. Your coaching philosophy will focus on your potential and future possibilities and not on any past mistakes. You are going to need to get to know yourself maybe more than you ever have before and this area of knowing yourself in fitness will spread throughout your entire life and begin to influence all that know you in a silent and extremely positive way. In succeeding in your challenge, and you can't fail as failure is only feedback you will change the memes you emit forever and pay forward your new healthier attitude to future generations.

There are certain qualities that a good coach needs and as you are about to become a coach you will need similar attributes. You may find you already have most of these in abundance so don't be phased by the long list.

> **Responsibility, Reliability and Dependability** – You are responsible for your life and fitness, just you and nobody else, if you are blaming any person or situation for any shortcomings or adversity you need to stop that habit now and take full responsibility for yourself now. You also need to be reliable and dependable. You need to be somebody you can rely on. If you can't depend on yourself then who can you depend on? Never let yourself down.

> **Calm, Persevering and Patient** – Persevering with your aims and goals is a must for success, remember that zig zag progress line we spoke about. However you must be calm and patient and not running around like a headless chicken. The perseverance you need to display is a calm, patient, grim determination to get where you want to be, you need to know you will get there and simply relax.

> **Honest, Detached and Objective** – This can be quite difficult as often we see ourselves not at all as we are. I will assume here that you have a good self image and are really rather fond of yourself, if not then you should be as you are perfect as you were created. Step back and take a good long look at yourself, take into account your feelings also. Try to block out any unwanted feedback from well meaning and not so well meaning others. This is about the body you live in not the body others think you should live in. Your body is the ultimate gift for living your life in and housing your soul what do you need to do to honour that precious gift so you are satisfied? That is so simple in theory but not quite so easy in practice, step back and

be very considered. Be as honest as possible, detached and objective and you will be on the right track to flow to exactly where you want to be.

- **Understanding, Kind and Supportive** - When you motivated to achieve a goal it is easy to be impatient with people around you that have no such motivation and may even be inadvertently sabotaging your efforts. Remember that was you just yesterday and understand their lack of understanding, eventually they will surprise you. Should you come across others that are in a similar boat to you or have a goal that you do not understand, accept that you do not need to understand and be kind and offer your support, that support will return to you. We are all too keen to jump in and offer our opinions and judgements. Offer the same understanding, kindness and support to yourself when you are beating yourself up. Give yourself a break.
- **Interested, Keen and Curious** - Keep your interest in yourself high, stay keen and curious, read and learn. Avoid settling in a rut. Change is good.
- **Attentive and A Good Listener** - Listen to others, much of what you learn and also dis-guard will come from being a good listener
- **Intuitive, Sensitive and Observant** - Learn to listen to your instincts when it comes to training. Often your initial reaction will be accurate. Listen to your body. Just BE.
- **Aware, Self aware, Mindful and Well Informed** - Be mindful, when you are training, focus on the moment. You will never be aware if your inner chatterbox is constantly taking your attention. This is good advice for all of your moments. Live in the now, not the future or the past. The past is over and the future does not exist only as an illusion in your head. NOW. Avoid gossips and negative people. The saying "misery loves company" is very true. Don't let others share the grumps with you. The grumps are contagious, don't let them grab you. Look out for the Mrs Grumpy opening line "the weather is crap today" or similar, then on to the rest of her poor life that is actually pretty great. Golden Rule - No point in complaining about something you can never change. I have a friend who spends all of her time talking about her lack, however she is away on holiday every second she gets, at least once a month. Her life really does not lack for much at all. Moaning has become a habit for her. Try this: say to yourself how amazing the weather is, recognise the awesome power of mother nature every day. I guarantee it is as easy as changing the thought. Swapping an old habit of complaining with a new one of appreciating. This works for everything. When someone complains to you about the weather or anything else allow yourself a smile. That is being mindful, aware and in the moment. Regain control.

➢ **Self Discipline, Self Motivation and Self Confidence** - Just do it. I know, you've heard it all before but that is what self discipline is. Set yourself your weekly, monthly or yearly workout schedules and see the benefit in reaching your high standards. Have pride in your ability to adhere to your schedule and stay motivated. Self Confidence will follow. Self discipline is a must, don't look elsewhere. Motivation will increase along with your total involvement in your goals and formation of new habits. There will be days when motivation is low and you are not very disciplined, accept that fact and stay on track. Remember that the path to your goal is never straight and zig zag your way to success.

➢ **Open Minded and Receptive** - Last of all in this section, always listen with an open mind. There will be times when the answer to your current sticking point or problem is right in front of you. A open mind will allow you to see the solution. A closed mind will keep you stuck in that dreaded rut. Remember in looking for a solution, the answer is never to do the same thing you have always done. That will continue to give you the same results. You will never achieve a different outcome by doing the same thing. A new approach will give you a different outcome. Always keep an open mind.

Mind Body & Soul

The Secret to your Success is inside of you – Change the way you Think

Habits – *The building blocks of change. Change is only real if it has become habitual. The same applies for both constructive and destructive habits, learn to recognise them honestly.*

Many of these habits and this behaviour may seem quite obvious but it is often the attention to detail that makes for success. Attention to doing lots of small things right can add up to a very effective programme of exercise and nutritional habits and a resulting very nice big thing. Having solutions at your finger tips to any problems or questions that may arise helps to avoid barriers to your progress, turning them into bridges to enable you to flow through each and every day regardless. The more chances you give to excuse yourself from exercise and healthy eating, the less likely you are to succeed. As you read through you might like to highlight any ideas that may dovetail into your lifestyle with relative ease. All of the ideas will take effort until they become habit and then, like us, you will just do them automatically, effort free. We have included some habits that purely allow harmony with other gym users and are mostly common sense.

Work on Developing Stronger Fitter Attitude First - The tools for creating your perfect health, fitness and body surround you but without the right attitude and behavioral changes they are just about useless. The best fitness centre's and equipment will serve no purpose without a well developed positive attitude driving your progress. Looking for short cuts will only waste your time, total fitness and a body you are proud of requires habits for life. Habits that need to be neatly slipped into your busy life to further enhance your experience. You will not need to find many hours per day, quality not quantity is the way to go. The reason most people fail in reaching their fitness goals is that they have unrealistic expectations, often fed to them by industry professionals, over selling the dream. The first truth you have to deal with is that your fitness and physique goals will take hard work for the rest of your life. The good news is as you begin to see the changes in fitness and physique you start to enjoy the hard work and discipline that it is costing you. The main point to remember from this is that the time you spend in the gym will only be fruitful if the time you spend away from the gym recovering, sleeping and feeding is close to perfect. You will need to cover all the bases and your success is guaranteed, time to turn all your barricades into bridges.

Develop an Optimistic Style – When all is going smoothly it is relatively easy to adhere to your exercise and nutrition plans, it is only when you are faced with adversity that you will determine your path. Each setback is a fork in the road and your ability to deal with yourself realistically is a key to your success. One missed session or one junk food moment doesn't mean you are a failure and everything has to go back to normal because you can't do it. Your new habits will eventually become your new norms. This process is an evolution and your target is to improve on existing habits. When facing adversity, accept that you are human, be realistic about what has happened, putting it all into perspective and then carry on. One slip up, or many, doesn't define your achievements; keep your eye on your ultimate intention. Two steps forward and one step backward is far more common progress to this sort of evolution anyway and as the habits become ingrained in your behaviour there will be less variation. Author Martin Seligman covers this subject very well in his book Learned Optimism. A very enlightening read.

Take Responsibility for Your Fitness and Physique - The real truth here is that there is only one person responsible for you fitness and physique. That person is you. If you want to be successful, you have to take 100% responsibility for everything in your life.

This is generally a gradual process and it is important not to be impatient with yourself.

In fact most of us have been conditioned to blame something other than ourselves for our poor levels of fitness. We blame our kids, bosses, husbands, friends and life in general for not having the time. We blame childbirth if our physiques are less than our ideal. We even blame our parents for dealing us a crap genetic hand. We are masters at justifying our failures. It is time to stop looking outside of yourself for the answers to why you haven't created the fitness and body you want, as it is you that creates the quality of fitness and the body you choose to live your life in.

You – no one else!

To achieve major success in fitness and body sculpting – to achieve those things that are most important to you – you must assume 100% responsibility for your health and body. Nothing less will do.

Clutching at Straws – If a gadget or special diet promises fast results, appreciate that if it seems to be good to be true then it probably is. The diet and

fitness industry is full of promises, made to desperate people wanting a quick fix. If it was that easy, surely we would all be super fit and lean. We are not. You can't get fit and you don't burn fuel (fat is stored fuel) if you don't move. On the other hand if you are looking to build bigger stronger muscles you must overload your muscles, meaning you have to work and all the pills and potions in the world will not help without that commitment to progressively more physical work. Look at it this way; if your car sits in the garage does it need any fuel? No, and the same is true of us, if we don't move we don't need much fuel and yet at those times of minimal activity we usually spend more of our time taking on totally unnecessary fuel.

Give Up All Of Your Excuses - Being 100% responsible for YOU means you have to give up all your excuses, all your victim stories and all the reasons why you can't and why you haven't up till now, and all your blaming of outside circumstances. You have to give them all up forever. You have always had the power to make it different, to get it right, and to produce the desired result. You chose not to exercise that power. Who knows why? It doesn't matter. The past is past. All that matters is from this point forward you choose to act as if you are 100% responsible for your fitness and physique. What do I need to do different next time to get the results I want? How can I tailor my life to reach my goals? In the course of a week I have lots of women and men approach me or Julie about fitness and their physiques and without fail every single one of them without prompting makes excuses or justifications with regards to their own bodies or fitness. They may think the excuses are for me but really they are excusing themselves for not living up to their own expectations. Women assume Julie has never given birth or that we have no job or family to keep us busy. These assumptions are all designed as excuses to themselves for how they feel about their bodies. We are all guilty of this, STOP IT NOW! No more excuses. The platform for success is to love yourself now and every day.

Fail to Plan, Plan to fail - Develop the habit of planning your daily feeds and exercise, prepare your food and meal timing. Don't allow yourself the excuse of blaming the local shops or dining places for having no healthy options, take responsibility. Protein shakes, nuts and dried fruit all make handy nutritious snacks. We love Brazil nuts, apricots and dates. Plan it from shopping list to mouth.

The Bodies We Live In Today Are The Result Of Choices We Made Yesterday - You only have control over three things in your life – the thoughts you think, the images you visualize and the actions you take. How you

use these three things determines everything you experience. If you are not happy with your results you have to change your responses. Change your negative thoughts to Positive thoughts. Change what you daydream about, visualize what you want. Change your habits. Change what you read. Change your friends. Change how you think and everything will begin to slot into place as if by magic.

Skipping is great but as an exercise not when it comes to Meals

- Once you have planned your feeding schedule, don't skip feeds, thinking you will gain, you will not and eventually you will feel the urge to eat out of control, stick to your plan.

If You Do What You Have Always Done, You'll Keep Getting The Same Results You've Always Got

- No matter how comfortable you are with the way you have always attained your body and fitness if it doesn't really give you the results you need, CHANGE IT! Continuing the same behavior and expecting different results. That just won't happen. If what you are doing currently would produce a better body and improved fitness, the improvements would have already shown up! If you want something different, you are going to have to do something different.

Get Moving

- Up your daily activity, walk more often. Remember walking or running the same distance uses the same amount of calories and when you are wandering around you won't feel the need to boredom eat. Use the stairs, park further away, walk, walk. Look upon your ability to move as the blessing it is, not a chore.

Give Up Blaming

- You will never become successful as long as you continue to blame something or someone for your lack of progress, if you are going to improve, you have to acknowledge it is you that thinks the thoughts, makes the choices and took the actions that got you to where you are now. It was you!

Give Up Complaining

- In order to complain about something, you have to believe that something better exists. We always complain to someone that can't make a difference. Changing might be uncomfortable, difficult or confusing. And so, to avoid risking any of those experiences, you stay put and complain about it. Either accept that you are making the choice to stay where you are, take responsibility for your choice, and stop complaining or take the risk of creating your body and fitness exactly the way you want it. Put up or shut up!

All in Moderation - Very cliché' but with nutrition anything in healthy food groups in moderation is a good rule.

Train smart and long workout sessions are not smart - Currently our gym workout schedule is 20 minutes intense cardiovascular and 45 minute weight sessions every other day with optional cardio on the other days. Total time at the gym time is approximately 90 minutes including shower time till bright eyed and bushy tailed, ready to take on the world. Keep the sessions short and productive. You are more likely to find the time if you don't have to find so much of it.

Fitness and Body Shaping Becomes Easier - To be successful, face the facts squarely, do the uncomfortable and take steps to create your desired outcome, it will become comfortable much quicker than you realise. Don't wait for disasters and then blame something or someone for your problems, push forward with a positive attitude. Once you start to respond and act quickly fitness becomes easier. You start to improve both internally and externally. Old talk like "Nothing ever seems to work for me" is replaced with "I feel great; I am in control; I can make things happen." Uncomfortable is just fear, feel the fear and do it anyway. Opportunities are waiting for you, he or she that dares wins. Download a simple beginner workout now and start soon. If you are making excuses as you read this, STOP and just do it. I promise you will never regret the day you ignored your fears and changed your life.

It's Simple But That Doesn't Make It Easy - The bottom line is that you are creating your fitness and the body you live in the way it is. The current YOU is a result of all your past thoughts and actions. You control your current thoughts and present feelings. You are in charge of what you say and do. You also control what goes into your mind – the fitness books you read, the diet experts that you listen to. Every action is under your control. To be fitter and to attain your ideal body all you have to do is act in ways that produce more of what you want.

It requires concentrated awareness, dedicated discipline and a willingness to take risks and experiment. You have to be willing to pay attention to what you are doing and to the results you are producing. Ask anyone you know for feedback. "Is what I am doing working?" Ask your trusted trainers or yourself as you become more expert. "Could I be doing it better? Is there something more I should be doing that I am not? Is there something I am doing that I should stop? How do you see me limiting myself? Don't be afraid to ask. The truth is the truth.

You are better off knowing the truth than not knowing it. And once you know you can do something about it. You need feedback. One word of caution here! Beware that the people you ask have no motive for hampering your progress. Jealousy can be very damaging, a worried spouse or friend feeling left behind. Also don't listen to the self appointed gym member and fitness experts unless they have a CV that enhances their credibility, you know the guys and gals every gym has at least one. You need CUT THE CRAP constructive feedback.

This book is full of proven success principles and techniques you can immediately put into practice in your fitness and nutrition schedules. You will have to suspend judgment, take a leap of faith, act as if they work and try them out. Only then will you have firsthand experience about their effectiveness for your body and fitness. You won't know they work until you give them a try. No one else can do this for you. Only you can do it. The formula is simple do more of what is working and less of what isn't, and try new behaviors to see if they produce better results. Start slowly, give your body and mind the chance to adapt to the physical and lifestyle changes, build up methodically to where you want to be.

Can't make the gym? Just get active and have fun - Activity
sessions are great, we walk our dogs over the local park at least once every day, twice if we have the time. For me this is also a great time for listening to motivational audio books or great music on my iPod. What a productive use of time and a great way to actively relax. The dogs are not essential to this activity.

Add some variety - There are many ways to achieve your fitness goals,
varying your plan of attack and changing your routine can freshen everything up. Far more important is to remain consistent and intense in your workouts. As your knowledge increases so do your options. Never be afraid to mix it up a little or a lot.

Results Don't Lie - The easiest way to find out what is or isn't working is to
check the results you are producing. You are either maintaining your ideal bodyweight or you are not. You are both fitter and stronger or you are not. It's that simple. Results don't lie! Don't kid yourself. Be ruthlessly honest with yourself. Are you eating sensibly? Are you training well? Do you need to increase your training intensity or change your eating or drinking habits to reach your goals, be realistic in your appraisal of yourself. Above all else, BE HAPPY!

Decide What You Want - You have to decide what you want to do. What
do you want to accomplish? Where do you want to be? What does your success

look like to you? Be as clear and as detailed as possible whilst remaining realistic. This is not about what other people want you to do or how they want you to look. This is about pleasing yourself and nobody else. Plan to be the best version of yourself and everything else will fall into place. At this stage it isn't important to know how you are going to get there. Just be clear on where it is you are going and what you will look like and how you will feel. Be clear, then relax and enjoy each and every day as your new positive life unfolds.

Don't get sidetracked - The local gym expert and every gym has many is always well meaning and helpful, however there are no magic exercises and his way is not the only way, stick to your plan and change when you are ready.

Being in control - Learn to plan your own workouts and basic nutrition. I will outline how in the chapter entitled "Planning your own workouts". If you learn only one thing from this book, make it this skill. I want to teach you to become self sufficient.

Don't settle for Less Than You Want - If you want to get the most out of fitness and body you will have to stop saying "I don't know; I don't care; it doesn't matter to me. When you are confronted with a choice, no matter how small or insignificant, act as if you have a preference. Not being clear about what you want and making other people's needs and desires more important than your own is simply a habit. Break the habit by practicing the opposite habit. The best version of you is better for everyone in your life.

"The greater danger for most of us is not that we aim to high and we miss it, but that it is too low and we reach it."

Michelangelo

Aim High – Have Bigger Visions - Big dreams attract big results. Never limit yourself. It doesn't take any more energy to create a big dream than it does to create a little one. Have fun.

Don't Let Anyone Talk You Out Of Your Vision - There are people that will try to talk you out of your vision. They will tell you are crazy and it can't be done. There will be those who will laugh at you and try to bring you down to their level. Don't let them. Show them, not with loud words but rather with deeds. Influence them by being the best you can be, you will need no words, no preaching, just be yourself and watch your positive influence grow.

See your world from a different angle - At a convenient time enjoy a "leave the car at home" weekend, you will be surprised how much fun it can be and shocked to see that you can survive a whole weekend without the car. Don't weaken, if you have to shop or go visiting, or take the kids to the park, the aim is to increase your activity and get a whole new slower paced view of your world.

Look good, feel good - Buy yourself exercise apparel that is both comfortable and that suits you, the chance of enjoying your experience is vastly improved if you feel good about yourself. The gym can be a great place to express yourself, look around and smile at the characters in your gym, leave the judgement to others. You can really have fun with this. It really doesn't matter, so don't take yourself too seriously.

Compliments where they are due – Being complimented always makes us feel good. We are all too quick to criticise others, try the opposite for a change and see how good it also makes you feel. If you see another person doing well, tell them, we all need to know our efforts are not in vain.

Visualize You with Your Ideal Fitness and Body - Put on some relaxing music and see yourself and your life with perfect health and fitness and the body you will have. How is it different from now? How is your confidence? How are your relationships? How about your wardrobe and social life? Exactly how has your success affected your lifestyle? Close your eyes and go to the future. Are you full of vitality? Are you strong and flexible? Do you enjoy exercise and eat well? How long do you live to? Are you open, ecstatic and in a state of joy all day long? If you want, write it all down. Every day review your vision. Share your vision with a good friend whom you can trust to be positive and supportive. You will find that when you share your vision, some people will want to help you make it happen. Others will introduce you to friends and resources that can help you. You'll also find that when you share your vision it becomes clearer and feels more real and attainable. And most importantly, every time you share your vision, you strengthen your own subconscious belief that you can achieve it. **Believe it's possible**. For a more in depth explanation of "Creative Visualization", explore the book by the same name by Shakti Gawain.

"You can be anything you want to be, if only you believe with sufficient conviction and act in accordance with your faith; for whatever your mind can conceive and believe, it can achieve".

Napoleon Hill – *Best- selling author of Think and Grow Rich*

Believe In Yourself - Sooner or later those who win are those who think they can. Most people fail not because they lack the skills or aptitude to reach their goal but simply because they don't believe they can reach it. Look at setbacks as new opportunities, learn from them and just keep on rolling. Believe, and win. Look yourself in the eye in a mirror and forcefully tell yourself what you are going to do. Whatever your dream is, look at yourself and declare you are going to achieve it, no matter what the price. Believing in you is a choice. It is an attitude developed over time. The past is past, you must choose to believe you can achieve anything you set your mind to – anything at all – because, in fact, you can. It might help you to know that the latest research now shows that with enough positive self talk and positive visualization combined with the proper training, coaching, and practices, anyone can learn to do almost anything. With the right attitude you have already succeeded.

As in life balance is the aim - Work your weaknesses as much if not more than your strengths. Balanced fitness should have good flexibility, aerobic fitness and symmetrical strength over the whole of the body.

Create a special environment for yourself – Make the gym a place you enjoy. Speak to as many people at the gym as possible without letting the contact interfere with you workouts. Listen more than you talk. The one place you will not be considered rude if you train in between conversation is the gym. The skill to be mastered is to remain focused on an intense workout whilst retaining a sociable approachable demeanour. Remember, people, not plush fixtures create your ultimate experience.

No More Saying "I Can't" – You Can and You Will! - As you are going to be successful you need to stop saying "I can't" and all similarly related words such as "I wish I were able to." Your brain is designed to solve any problem and reach any goal that you give it. The words you think and say actually affect your body. You are born with a feeling of invincibility but little by little it is conditioned out of you by the mostly accidental emotional and physical abuse that you receive from your family, friends and teachers until you no longer believe you can. Remove "I can't" from your vocabulary. Maybe add "No limits" or "I intend" to your thoughts and speech. No more what ifs.

What Others Think About You Is None Of Your Business – If having others believing in you and your dream was a requirement for success,

most of us would never achieve anything. You need to base your decisions about what you want to do on your goals and desires – not the judgments of your parents, friends, spouse, children or co-workers. Quit worrying about what other people think and follow your heart. I always try to avoid negative talking people, just by choosing not to listen. I try to change the conversation to a more positive subject and if that fails I accept it and move on. Negativity can be remarkably contagious; I intend to avoid that social disease as much as possible.

A saying springs to mind, not sure where I heard it but I know I used to care too much about what others thought of me, consider the following.

"When you're 18, you worry about what everybody is thinking about you; when you're 40, you don't care what anybody thinks of you; when you're 60, you realise that nobody's been thinking about you at all."

Surprise, surprise! Most of the time, nobody's thinking about you at all. They are too busy worrying about their own lives, and if they are thinking about you at all, they are wandering what you are thinking about them. So don't worry about them, think about yourself and more ideas to help you achieve your body and fitness goals.

Never judge - Never stereotype any gym member, the scariest looking person is always the nicest person in the world. Gym intensity can be misunderstood as general hostility, it is not. In our experience, all people we have spoken to in gyms are "smashing chaps" once the barriers are down. Never be afraid to speak first. I find the attitude I portray tends to reflect back.

Be prepared for success - Always have your post workout feed in your bag with you. This is a very important meal, along with breakfast it is the most important feed of the day. A 30 gram protein and 60 gram carbs shake, recovery begins immediately upon finishing. There are specialist products on the market. We always use a high quality meal replacement shake for the added vitamin and mineral profile and antioxidants.

Goal Setting - Once you know your fitness and body purpose, determine your vision and truly clarify your needs and desires you have to convert them into measurable goals and objectives and be certain you will achieve them. Whatever goal you give your mind it will work day and night to achieve. Goals need to be realistic, specific and measurable such as I will weigh 140lb's by 10am on September 20th. Nice and clear. I must stress being realistic and don't see reaching your goal as the end but just the start of your amazing transformation,

just a small step towards your vision, your dream YOU. Write your goals down and read them three times each day, close your eyes and picture them as if they were already accomplished. Take a minute to feel what you would feel if you had already accomplished each goal. This will increase your mind's desire, closing the gap between reality and your vision, bringing it ever closer. Carry your most important goal with you written as gratitude for achieving it. *"I am so happy weighing 140lb's."* Live the result. Set more than one goal and set them for all aspects of your life, make it interesting and create a positive aura all around yourself, for the whole of your life picture.   Success in one area always creates success throughout your life. Create a goals book, an A4 size pad. A page for each goal and use pictures, words, phrases, depict each goal as having already been achieved, and when new goals arise simply add them to your book. Look at your book regularly. Alternatively, we have five notice boards up on our wall with the following headings – **Health and Self** – **Lifestyle** – **Love** – **Money** – **Career and Wisdom**; they are all full of cut out pictures, photographs and words connecting us to our dreams. I have heard them called dream boards, vision boards but whatever you wish to call them, they are fun and make us feel good and when you feel good anything is possible. To summaries have all your ultimate dreams and desires in your book or on your board and then set your goals accordingly to reach the desired result.

Comfort Zones

Comfort Zones -Most people go through life holding on to negative images about themselves. They stay in a comfort zone of their own making. They maintain inaccurate beliefs about reality or harbour guilt and self doubt. When they try to achieve their goals, those negative images and pre-programmed comfort zones always cancel out their good intentions no matter how hard they try. A good example of this is how fitness centres or gyms are often depicted as bad places full of shallow people, fitness fanatics and posers by people that are uncomfortable at the thought of being in such places. The same people then enlist likeminded people to agree with them thus separating themselves from the place or mere idea about the place they are so uncomfortable with. This is just an expression of a fear. The answer is to let go of limiting beliefs and change your self image. Think of your comfort zone as a prison – a largely self-created prison. It consists of the collection of cant's, must's, must not's and other totally unfounded beliefs formed from all the negative thoughts and decisions you have accumulated and reinforced during your lifetime. As an example, I wish I had a crisp five pound note for every time I showed a nervous newcomer around a gym as they echoed these fears only to see them a few days later in a new comfort zone, the dreaded gym and scary people they had feared so much only days earlier were now their new friends for life.

Should you train with a partner or not? - Exercise with somebody
with similar drive to yourself, I am lucky enough to be able to exercise with Julie
or my youngest daughter Shaunie. We have fun but always maintain the focus of
why we have made the effort to be at the gym. For me it is the chance to work
my body to somewhere close to full potential, maybe I would compare the
experience to getting the chance to take your car around a race track after
dawdling around at 30 mph the rest of the time. The feeling of really opening up
your physical prowess is very invigorating. For this you need to either train on
your own or have a reliable and influential training partner that motivates you, a
relationship that works both ways. A partner's strength or fitness level is
immaterial as you are not competing with them; however a happy positive attitude
is always a bonus. There will be days when your partner pulls you through and
vice versa. For me, I have found that Julie's strengths of cardio fitness and great
legs have been my weakness in the past so for me we are a training match made
in heaven. Julie and Shaunie always challenge me with their positive outlook and
their shrug of the shoulders attitude to adversity. The great sense of fun they
bring to the gym is an added bonus in what can be an overly serious environment.

Make Permanent Changes - By thinking the same thoughts, maintaining
the same beliefs, speaking the same words and doing the same things you are re-
creating the same experience over and over. To change this cycle, you must
instead focus on thinking, talking and writing about the reality you want to create,
not the current reality you are experiencing. An example would be your food
shopping list, if you are taking in too many calories currently and you continue to
buy the same foods, big surprise nothing will change. Learn about some lower
calorie foods that you could enjoy and substitute them for other high calorie
options. I have some nutritional recommendations later for you to try. Some
small changes to your diet can add up to large calorie savings over time.
Remember, any changes have to be sustained for life so make sure you can live
with them. This is not about losing loads of body fat and then gaining it again,
this is about a fitter, healthier more gorgeous you for life. Another good change is
that in addition to an exercise programme you can increase the amount of walking
you do each day, these small changes have an accumulative affect over time and
again add up to some impressive calorific savings over time. 1 mile a week adds
up to 52 miles each year, two marathons. That is not only very impressive but
very wise, take it further, imagine 1 mile extra each day, 365 miles a year, now
that is 14 marathons. Wow! By now you are seeing that some small changes can
lead to some very impressive results. The tip here is to realise that it works the
other way as well and a small chocolate bar or glass of wine each day can undo all

of that hard work. Our daily walks with Jacob & Smudge are a highlight of our day and not considered hard work at all.

The significant problems we face cannot be solved by the same level of thinking that created them

Albert Einstein

Smile - Always maintain your sense of humour. Don't take yourself too seriously.

Balance - Keep a sense of perspective, fitness is to be part of your life, not rule your life. Workouts need to be efficient and not too long. Don't spend too long, you will be back very soon.

Keep your workout flow – It will happen, you will get engrossed in a conversation and your workout will suffer just don't let it become one of your new habits. Avoid being the trainer that lets the occasional set of exercise ruin a perfectly good conversation, remember your goals and what you need to do in order to achieve them.

Disciplined in your approach - Make your workouts structured and measurable, give them order and timing.

Work at your level – At times, particularly with a partner this can be hard. Keep your exercise form and technique consistently of a high standard; never sacrifice good form for extra weight. I guarantee you will see this happening all around you, stay strict with yourself. If your ego takes over and the weight you are lifting and what other people think of you is paramount in your thoughts your progress will halt or you will get injured. Train smart. You are not a weightlifter; you are training with weights to attain a goal. Trust me on this one, when you forget about what you are lifting and just train hard, increased strength will be a by product of your good habits.

H_2O - Always ensure you drink plenty of water throughout the day and during your sessions. Most of us are aware of this but still very few of us drink enough.

A tidy gym is a happy gym - Please develop good housekeeping whilst at the gym, always put your weights away and be aware of hazards on the floor, such as weights other users have neglected to put back.

In Learning to Plan Your Own Workout You Are Taking the First Steps to Self Reliance

Achieving total fitness is all very well if you copy a workout and eating plan to the letter it can produce limited short term results. However much like the saying with regards to famine that if you give a man fish he will eat for one day but if you teach him how to fish he will eat for life, becoming self reliant for your fitness needs will give you the tools to maintain and motivate yourself to succeed for as long as you desire. Our aim is to avoid the dreaded yo-yoing exercise and diet scenario, where one exercises and diets to perfection for a period of time to achieve a goal, but never forming any permanent long term sensible habits and then returns to bad habits and the fitness and weight come and go accordingly, only each time the bad habits seem to have a worse effect. The worse part of this is that we always blame ourselves for failing because the miracle diet and exercise schedule delivered weight loss and fitness as promised. That is only partly true, the miracle schedule failed to take in to account the crucial factor that any changes have to be permanent and any Spartan schedule will only ever be possible short term. Exercise and fitness has to become habit and fit into your lifestyle on a permanent basis, normally this means slower progress but permanent change. Look back for a moment and reflect on fad diets and exercise videos by celebrities for fast money every year, promising the earth but rarely delivering. How many of those celebrities or new ones, as celebrity status is often delicate, return the next year with another new answer for you? How many of us fall for it again, because it has a new name and is based on new science and we have over eaten during the holiday period? How often do we see pictures of our new celebrity fitness heroes in magazines soon afterwards, having yo-yoed out of shape? Another few questions for you – How many of the aforementioned do you think are photos that have been enhanced for the look of absolute perfection set before you as an example, is that realistically attainable? Am I being unfairly cynical or just realistic?   Could it be that we need to choose our own influences as opposed to having them thrust at us by the media? The Tortoise approach and not the Hare, slow and steady wins the race. Consistent good habits over a period of time will always be favourable to the all or nothing approach. In this instance knowledge is the power for us to balance our fitness and life at our own unique pace.

There are many ways to formulate exercise plans and many ways to achieve results. We in no way claim that our way is the only way but we do claim that for us this has worked and is an excellent practical strategy for any person looking to manage their own fitness levels for life in a more balanced way.

Progressive Fitness – We will structure our programmes in such a way that we will arrive at 4 different levels depending on current fitness levels, the time you have available and the commitment you choose to make to your fitness. We recommend that you walk before you can run; it is always wise to progress through the levels when you begin. Your own perception of your fitness may not be accurate.

Use it or lose it – Fitness is very much a use it or lose it scenario, whilst we are young we may maintain a reasonable level of fitness just running about but as we age fitness levels decline rapidly if we do not have an active schedule to maintain these levels. For this reason if you have an enforced lay off even for as little as a week or so it is wise to drop the workout level down a little to build up again. This also helps if at any time you cannot meet your fitness commitment, you can just do the beginners circuit programme which will offer a pleasant change and give you balance until you can commit more time once again.

Variety – Even though the workouts will offer much variety within each level, you may just decide that you would like to use the approach of another level for the odd session. We often do this and it re energises us and the change proves to be a great motivator. When you are used to heavy body part training a full body circuit approach can be quite a fun challenge and vice versa. Keep an open mind.

Starting Exercise Weights – You will find initially that your starting weights will be all over the place until you get to know your strength on each exercise. The tip here to avoid injury is to always start light.

Understanding – There may be words we use that you are unfamiliar with, we will attempt to explain these as we go along. The exercise names may seem like a foreign language until you have used them for a while. For any gym based workouts members of your gym staff will show you any exercise you are unsure of. Below are a few explanations of common terms.

Rep (etition) – Is the term used for one single completed example of an exercise, so for example if you did a single press up that would be one rep (etition).

Sets – Is the term given to a grouping of reps. Again an example would be if you completed 20 abdominal crunches on the floor that would be 1 set of 20 reps. If you then waited for 1 minute and completed another set that would be a total of 2 sets of 20 reps. **Stretching sets** – We have a slightly different approach for stretching one static stretch held for 30 seconds constitutes 1 set.

Rest between sets – It is important that when doing multiple sets that your rest time in-between each set is consistent for each set. The rest can vary from 0 for circuit workouts up to 30 sec, a minute or longer for absolute strength workouts. Most of our workouts will either be circuit (0 rest) or 45 seconds for multiple set workouts. This is why when socialising in the gym you stay focused on your schedule as your workout can become long and disjointed and lose much of its effectiveness. A stopwatch can be useful when you first start working out until that rest time becomes ingrained in your subconscious behaviour.

Body part terms – Lats (back) - Pecs (Chest) – Delts/Traps (Shoulders) – Tri's (Triceps) – Bi's (Biceps) – Quads/Hams/Calves (Legs). You may find other gym users use slightly differing terms but will find your way with these.

PART 3 - Diet & Training

GETTING STARTED

Progressive Fitness – We will structure our programmes in such a way that we will arrive at 4 different levels depending on current fitness levels, the time you have available and the commitment you choose to make to your fitness. We recommend that you walk before you can run; it is always wise to progress through the levels when you begin. Your own perception of your fitness may not be accurate.

Use it or lose it – Fitness is very much a use it or lose it scenario, whilst we are young we may maintain a reasonable level of fitness just running about but as we age fitness levels decline rapidly if we do not have an active schedule to maintain these levels. For this reason if you have an enforced lay off even for as little as a week or so it is wise to drop the workout level down a little to build up again. This also helps if at any time you cannot meet your fitness commitment, you can just do the beginners circuit programme which will offer a pleasant change and give you balance until you can commit more time once again.

Variety – Even though the workouts will offer much variety within each level, you may just decide that you would like to use the approach of another level for the odd session. We often do this and it re energises us and the change proves to be a great motivator. When you are used to heavy body part training a full body circuit approach can be quite a fun challenge and vice versa. Keep an open mind.

Starting Exercise Weights – You will find initially that your starting weights will be all over the place until you get to know your strength on each exercise. The tip here to avoid injury is to always start light.

Understanding – There may be words we use that you are

unfamiliar with, we will attempt to explain these as we go along. The exercise names may seem like a foreign language until you have used them for a while. For any gym based workouts members of your gym staff will show you any exercise you are unsure of. Below are a few explanations of common terms.

Rep (etition) – Is the term used for one single completed

example of an exercise, so for example if you did a single press up that would be one rep (etition).

Sets – Is the term given to a grouping of reps. Again an example

would be if you completed 20 abdominal crunches on the floor that would be 1 set of 20 reps. If you then waited for 1 minute and completed another set that would be a total of 2 sets of 20 reps.
Stretching sets – We have a slightly different approach for stretching one static stretch held for 30 seconds constitutes 1 set.

Rest between sets – It is important that when doing

multiple sets that your rest time in-between each set is consistent for each set. The rest can vary from 0 for circuit workouts up to 30 sec, a minute or longer for absolute strength workouts. Most of our workouts will either be circuit (0 rest) or 45 seconds for multiple set workouts. This is why when socialising in the gym you stay focused on your schedule as your workout can become long and disjointed and lose much of its effectiveness. A stopwatch can be useful when you first start working out until that rest time becomes ingrained in your subconscious behaviour.

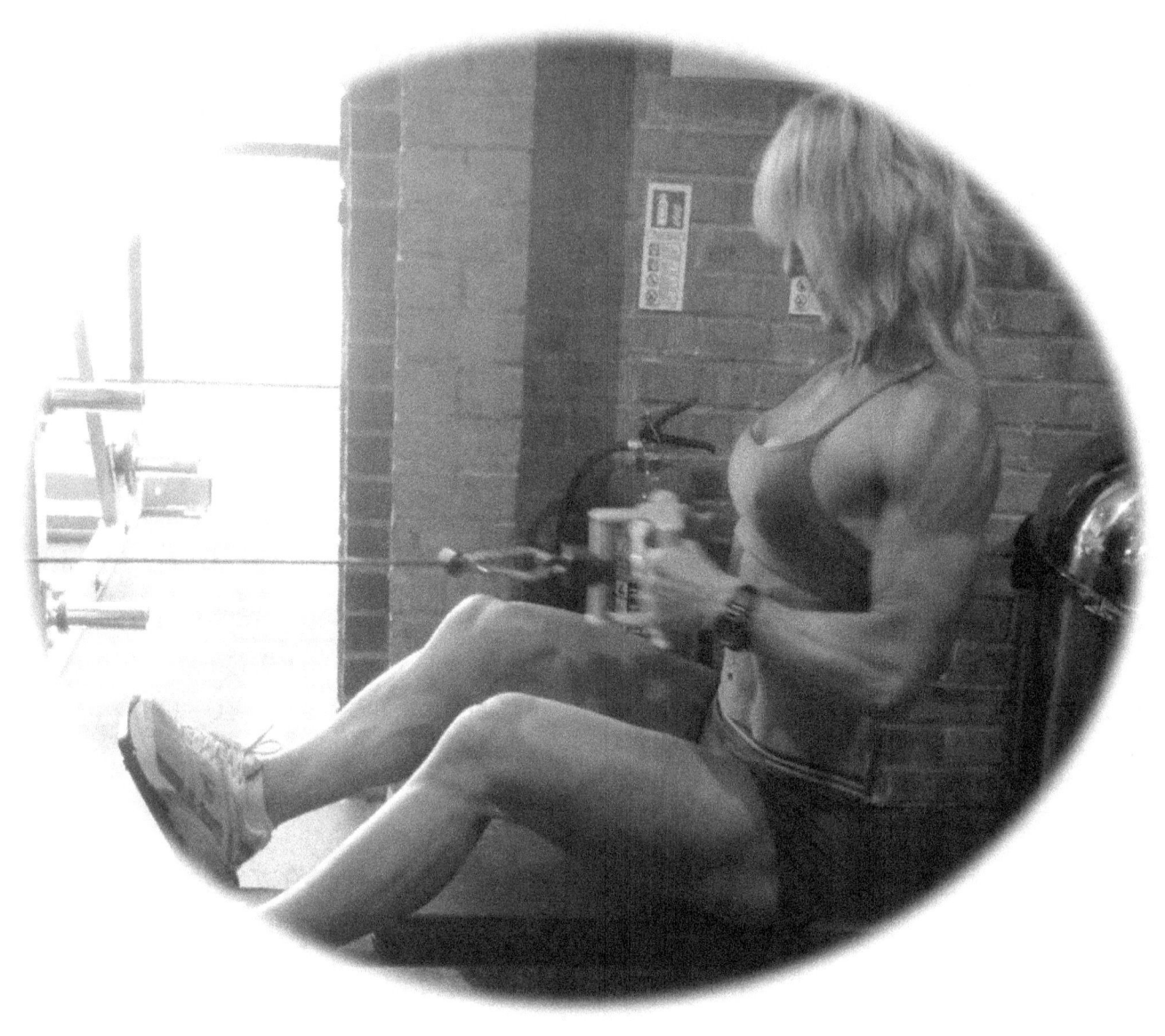

BEGINNER TO FIT

Getting started

Getting started - Elsewhere on this site you will find a gallery of exercises for you to use. They are under the headings of the various body parts, with sections for cardio-vascular and stretching. You can substitute what you have access to at your gym. For the examples we will fill in the exercises and you can just use ours to get started before moving on to formulating your own well structured workouts. All exercises correspond to those found in our gallery and in most gyms. The stretches are lettered accordingly. Our example is gym based but there are plenty of other alternatives, just match your choices to the resources you have readily available.

Full Body - Circuit to attain a good level of full body fitness.

Cardio - 5/10 mins rowing

1. **Lats - Reverse Grip Pulldowns**
2. **Legs - Dumb-bell Straddle Squats**
3. **Pecs - Incline Dumb-bell Press**
4. **Legs - Bodyweight Lunges**
5. **Delts - Dumb-bell Lateral Raises**
6. **Legs - Dumb-bell Step Ups**
7. **Triceps - Pulley Pushdowns**
8. **Abs - Basic Crunches**
9. **Biceps - Dumb-bell Curls**

Cardio Finish 5 mins cycle

Stretch for the whole body.

Week 1 = 1 circuit with 5 mins cardio (exercises I-IX) for three alternating days, ideally Mon, Wed & Fri. We are aiming for sets of 15 repetitions

Week 2 = 10 mins cardio - Complete the exercise circuit (1-9) twice.

Week 3 = 15 mins cardio - Complete the exercise circuit (1-9) three times.

Week 4 - Changing from circuits to multiple sets workout = 15 mins cardio – Now we change the way we do the exercises. Complete 3 sets of each in order 1-9 with 30 sec rest in-between each set. The first set should be the same weight you have been using for your circuit, aiming to increase the weight each set whilst keeping immaculate form. Now we allow the reps to drop to between 15 and 8 in order to workout with heavier but manageable weights. If you are able to get 15 reps comfortably the weight is too light and if you cannot get 8 reps the weight is too heavy. A normal rep range whilst increasing the weight may look like this - Set 1 = 15reps, Set 2 = 12reps, Set 3 = 8reps. For week 4 we only need 2 workouts with at least 2 days in-between. Any additional workouts will be cardio only, 30 mins minimum and stretch. You will notice that we are now doing different exercises each session to work the muscle from different angles. Any exercise can be replaced with any from the same section of our gallery or any you may know already. There are plenty of additional workouts on our site for you to attempt at any time. This ability to change will be a major factor to your continued motivation. Many trainers do the same workout for years, others change on a regular basis. Change works for variety, convenience and just to freshen things up.

Week 4,5 & 6.......Full Body - Multiple Sets Workout .... 3 sets of 8-15 reps / 30 sec rest between sets. Twice per week, 2 days rest from weights in-between.

Complete 1 x 30 minute cardio and stretch session on any other day with this programme. For the following example, Wednesday or a Saturday morning would be good days for your stretch and cardio.

Workout 1 (Monday)

Cardio - Cross Trainer - 20 minutes intervals

1. **Lats - Reverse Grip Pulldowns - 1 warm up + 3 x 12 reps**
2. **Legs - Dumb-bell Straddle Squats - 1 warm up + 3 x 12 reps**
3. **Pecs - Incline Dumb-bell Press - 1 warm up + 3 x 12 reps**
4. **Legs - Bodyweight Lunges -1 warm up + 3 x 12 reps**
5. **Delts - Dumb-bell Lateral Raises -1 warm up + 3 x 12 reps**
6. **Legs - Dumb-bell Step Ups - 1 warm up + 3 x 12 reps**
7. **Triceps - Pulley Pushdowns - 1 warm up + 3 x 12 reps**
8. **Abs - Basic Crunches - 1 warm up + 3 x 20 reps**
9. **Biceps - Dumb-bell Curls - 1 warm up + 3 x 12 reps**

   Assorted Stretches

   Cardio - Treadmill for 5 minutes cool down

Workout 2 (Thursday)

Cardio - Bike - 20 minutes intervals

1. **Lats - Seated Pulley Rows - 1 warm up + 3 x 12 reps**
2. **Legs - Dumb-bell Lunges - 1 warm up + 3 x 12 reps**

3. **Pecs - Incline Dumb-bell Flyes - 1 warm up + 3 x 12 reps**
4. **Legs - Leg Extensions -1 warm up + 3 x 12 reps**
5. **Delts - Delt Press Machine -1 warm up + 3 x 12 reps**
6. **Legs - Lying Leg Curls - 1 warm up + 3 x 12 reps**
7. **Triceps - Incline Dumb-bell Triceps Ext - 1 warm up + 3 x 12 reps**
8. **Abs - Knee Tucks - 1 warm up + 3 x 20 reps**
9. **Biceps - barbell Curls - 1 warm up + 3 x 12 reps**

Assorted Stretches

Cardio - Treadmill for 5 minutes cool down

For many of you variations of any of these two workouts will be all you will ever need. **A full body circuit** is a very efficient way to achieve and maintain a very good level of fitness, Three times per week added to good nutrition and a more active lifestyle generally and you will have an admirable level of total fitness. **A full body multiple sets** workout will allow you to build more strength than the circuit workout but at the expense of some endurance. Simply by adding one extra intense cardio workout and ensuring you work hard on your pre workout cardio will balance that loss very well.   Periodically changing from one of these to the other will allow you to achieve a good level of both fitness and physique you need and give you the variety to motivate you. That of course, is assuming you are working very hard when you are in the gym.

We are often asked if only training once per week on a full body workout would give any improvements? Well the honest answer is yes, any activity is better than no activity at all. If the workout is added to an active lifestyle, maybe even including other forms of less intense exercise it can work very well. However if that is all the exercise you are doing and you are sedentary the rest of the time, all you will be doing is maintaining some fitness at best, and that is unlikely to be enough to motivate you to continue with your program as we are all motivated by seeing a degree of improvement from our efforts. As the saying goes "you reap what you sow". Ideally a minimum of three good intense exercise sessions every week added to your other good activity habits would be optimum.

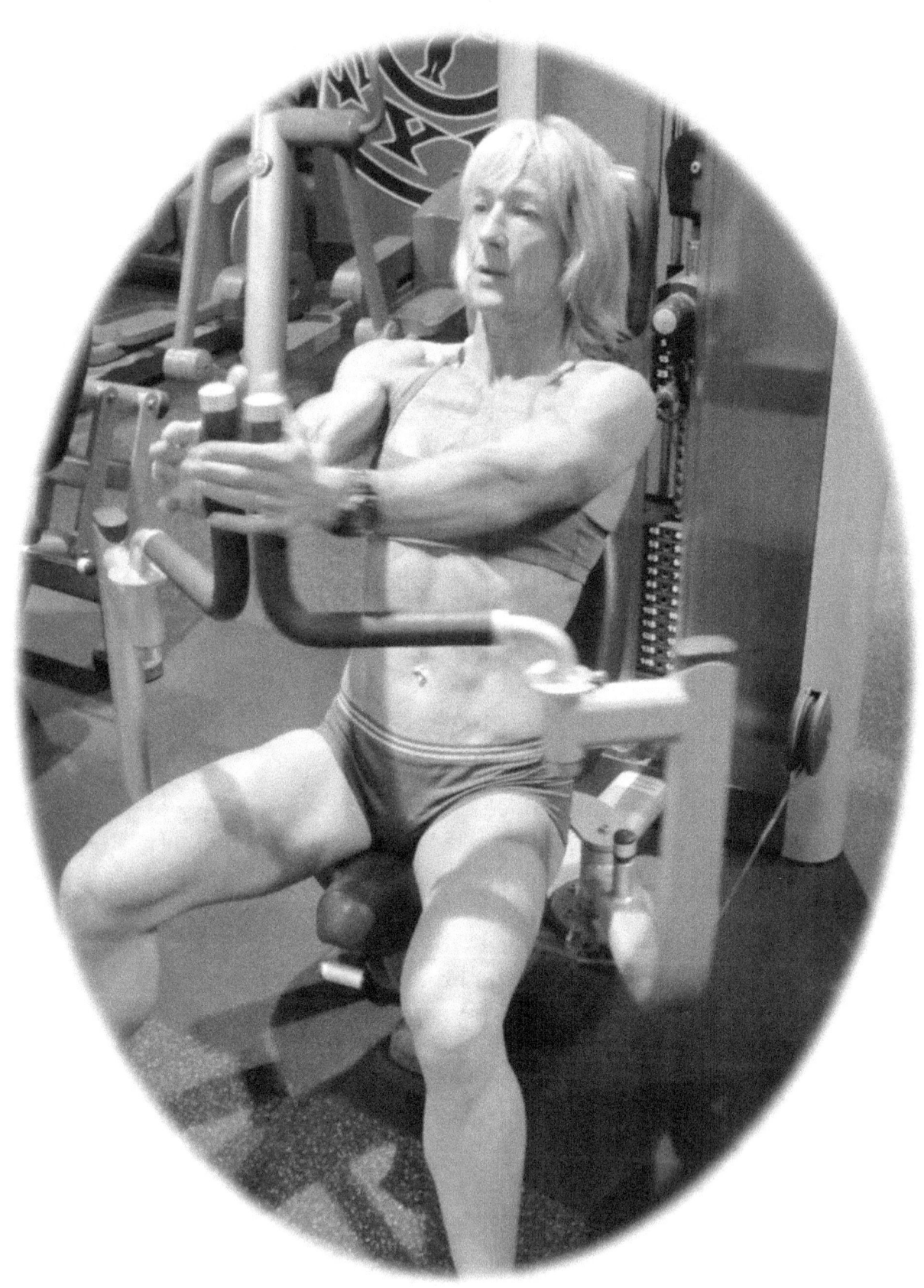

THE NEXT STEP

Split Routines – A Split routine is the name given to workouts where you train your body parts separately over a number of sessions, this enables you to concentrate all of your energy on just one or two areas of your body each session. Many people that do split routines use the opportunity to do more of what they enjoy, their strengths, and less of what they should be working on, their weaknesses. This is why you see men with big arms and spaghetti legs. Legs are hard work and you can cover them up so why work them because nobody will notice. WRONG! The important thing about any schedule is to maintain balance between the body parts. The reasons for this is that progress over all will be much easier, injuries will be less and let's be honest a body lacking symmetry doesn't look great does it? A good rule is to prioritise your weaknesses, that way you will even up your body and enjoy training all of your body not just some of it whilst hiding the rest. The first routine we will look at is a straight forward upper and lower split. When choosing split workouts it is important to understand that the investment in time does take a substantial jump. They are however very rewarding and actually become essential once you reach a level of fitness that dictates the next logical step has to be increased intensity. The upper body and lower body split is the workout that we use most of the time it enables us to train intensely with adequate rest for each body part. We alternate weight training days always doing at least 20 minutes intense cardio at the start of each session. We then have the option of cardio, stretch and abs days in-between our weight sessions. A typical 8 days for us for us would look like this.

1. 20 minutes intense cardio - **Lower Body 1**
2. **Off** – day after heavy legs often taken off for recovery, although light cardio and stretch session is always a good idea.
3. 20 minutes intense cardio – **Upper Body 1**
4. Optional - Between 30 & 60 minutes cardio, stretch and Abs
5. 20 minutes intense cardio – Light, higher rep, **Lower Body 2**.
6. Optional - Between 30 & 60 minutes cardio, stretch and Abs
7. 20 minutes intense cardio – **Upper Body 2.**
8. Optional - Between 30 & 60 minutes cardio, stretch and Abs.

We love this routine because it has much flexibility and variety and if we need to take additional days off we can miss the odd cardio and abs day without impacting our progress or fitness at all. It can also be shuffled around if our schedule dictates we can't make certain days, for instance it would be ok to do upper body one day and lower the very next day on the odd occasion. The workout can be every day of the week or every other day of the week, as the intense cardio on weights days can be enough if your work it hard. We guarantee if you take this workout on, there will be periods when you are motivated and train each and every day and other times when alternate days are just fine. The body's natural rhythms just seem to work this way. Periods of high energy and motivation interspersed with periods of less energy and motivation both moods are accommodated with this, our favourite workout.   On the following pages we have our last eight days workouts. These are intended as outline plans for you. You can insert your own exercises and do different cardio variations. If extra days off are needed, the cardio days are optional and we will occasionally drop one or two of those. As you can see this set up is very flexible and can be adjusted to suit any particular time restraints that you may come up against.

1. Lower Body 1

Cardio - Cross Trainer 20 minutes intervals

1. **Barbell Squats - 4 sets 15/8 reps - upping weight each set.**
2. **Lunges - 3 sets 15/8 reps - upping weight each set.**
3. **Leg Press - 3 sets 15/8 reps - upping weight each set.**
4. **Toe Press - 3 sets 15/20 reps - upping weight each set.**
5. **Leg Extensions - 3 sets 12/15 reps - upping weight each set.**
6. **Lying Leg Curls - 3 sets 12/15 reps - upping weight each set.**

Assorted Stretches

Cardio - Treadmill for 5 minutes cool down

2. Light Cardio & Stretch – Active recovery session – An active recovery session is often programmed the day after a particularly hard work out to promote recovery. The idea is to get nutrient rich blood into the recovering area to speed the recovery process. We also find these sessions loosen up what can be very tight leg muscles. A Heavy leg workout as you learn to train intensely is a very taxing workout. The cardio should be about 30 minutes at a moderate intensity and then stretch until your body regains an acceptable level of mobility. We find that downloading and playing some relaxing music on our i pods makes this a thoroughly enjoyable session and we leave the gym feeling much better than when we arrived.

Active recovery can be used any time you feel the need and would naturally fall on your cardio days on this programme.

3. Upper Body 1

Cardio - Cycle 20 minutes intervals

1. **Seated Pulley Rows - 3 sets 12 reps - upping weight each set.**
2. **Chest Flye Machine - 3 sets 12 reps - upping weight each set.**
3. **Machine Pulldowns - 3 sets 12 reps - upping weight each set.**
4. **Incline Dumb-bell Press - 3 sets 12 reps - upping weight each set.**
5. **Upright Rows - 3 sets 12 reps - upping weight each set.**
6. **Triceps Pushdowns - 3 sets 12 reps - upping weight each set.**
7. **Barbell Curls - 3 sets 12 reps - upping weight each set.**
8. **Triceps Machine - 3 sets 12 reps - upping weight each set.**
9. **Machine Preacher Curls - 3 sets 12 reps - upping weight each set.**

Assorted Stretches

Cardio - Treadmill for 5 minutes cool down

4. Cardio, Stretch & Abs

1. **Cardio - Stepper - 10/20 mins intervals**
2. **Cardio - Rower - 10/20 mins intervals**
3. **Cardio - Bike - 10/20 mins intervals**
4. **Abs Machine - 3 sets 15/20 reps**
5. **Pelvic Tilts - 3 sets 15/20 reps**
6. **Crunches - 3 sets 15/20 reps**

Assorted Stretches

Cardio - Treadmill for 5 minutes cool down

The intention with the cardio is to perform at least 30 minutes intensely. If you are feeling good you can carry on up to about 60 minutes. You can perform your cardio on as many pieces of equipment as you wish but please ensure that you hurry between pieces as we need to keep your heart rate elevated. The key is to keep moving.

5. Lower Body 2

Cardio - Cross Trainer 20 minutes intervals

1. **Leg Ext & Leg Press Superset - 3 sets 12 reps - upping weight each set.**

2. Toe Press - 3 sets 15/20 reps - upping weight each set.
3. Hack Squats - 3 sets 12 reps - upping weight each set.
4. Seated Calf Raise - 3 sets 15/20 reps - upping weight each set.
5. Leg Extensions - 3 sets 12/15 reps - upping weight each set.
6. Lying Leg Curls - 3 sets 12/15 reps - upping weight each set.

Assorted Stretches

Cardio - Treadmill for 5 minutes cool down

Supersets – Two exercises grouped together with minimal rest in-between them. Worked as one exercise. You will normally find you are able to use less weight with superset training than with straight sets. The intensity is greater as there is more work in less time.

6. Cardio, Stretch & Abs

1. **Cardio - Cycle 5 minutes**
2. **Cycle Crunches 3 sets 15/20 reps**
3. **Cardio - Cross Trainer 5 minutes**
4. **Leg Lowers 3 sets 15/20 reps**
5. **Cardio - Treadmill 5 minutes**
6. **Angled Knee Tucks 3 sets 15/20 reps**
7. **Cardio - Stepper 5 minutes**

Assorted Stretches

Cardio - Treadmill for 5 minutes cool down

This session gives you the opportunity to perform short intense 5 min bursts on cardio with your abdominal exercises alternated in-between. This offers some variation in routines to keep your motivation up.

7. Upper Body 2 – Supersets.

Cardio - 20 minutes Cycle - intervals

1. **Chest Flyes & Press Ups - 3 sets 12 reps**
2. **Straight Arm Pulldowns & Reverse Grip Pulldowns - 3 sets 12 reps**
3. **Dumb-bell Lateral Raises & Machine Delt Presses - 3 sets 12 reps**
4. **Barbell Curls & Triceps Pushdowns - 3 sets 12 reps**

Assorted Stretches

Cardio - Cycle for 5 minutes cool down

Supersets– Can be performed for the same body part or opposing body parts. They are great for saving time and generally improving your fitness because your heart and lungs are worked much harder than with regular sets routines.

8. Cardio, Stretch & Abs

1. **Cardio - Cycle 10/20 minutes intervals**
2. **Cycle Crunches 3 sets 15/20 reps**
3. **Cardio - Cross Trainer 10/20 minute intervals**
4. **Leg Lowers 3 sets 15/20 reps**
5. **Cardio - Treadmill 10/20 minute intervals**
6. **Angled Knee Tucks 3 sets 15/20 reps**
7. **Cardio - Stepper 10/20 minutes intervals**

Assorted Stretches

Cardio - Treadmill for 5 minutes cool down

VARIETY RULES OK - AN ALTERNATIVE PLAN
Diet & Training
How to Tailor Your Diet to Fit Your Training Needs. What Works for Us.

You are what you eat. The most important part of any body boosting programme is the diet.

There has been a big pause for thought between writing the rest of this book and taking on this section without repeating all you have heard before. Without any doubt finding the motivation to exercise is comparatively easy compared to adhering to nutritional practises that will help rather than hinder your progress. We discussed how we approach our diet and decided that we are usually either on one of two regimes, a muscle gain or on a fat loss diet. We are either trying to gain muscle with minimal fat gain or trying to lose fat with minimal muscle loss. Each diet serving to maintain low fat levels and a good healthy percentage of lean tissue. It did occur to us that we also need to offer ourselves and our readers something in the middle that can do both, but compromises a little in both lean muscle held, and overall bodyfat levels. We proceeded to test the diet on ourselves and as I write we are on what we feel may be an optimum diet for both high muscle and low fat levels. A diet flexible enough to be adjusted for either result, more muscle or less fat and also a diet that allows for the flash in the pan mentality that we have found amongst clients over the last 20 years. Julie is currently preparing for her next show, so it is fair to say the "optimum diet" will need to be up to the task.

There is nothing really new in the diet world and we have adapted and experimented with other diets and mixed them with what we believe is a little common sense for active people, to arrive at our current practises. True to the philosophy of this book, all the practises here have been used by us, we have no outside interest in nutrition companies, any sources we mention are used purely as paying customers. We are trained in nutrition management however we are not nutritionists, if you have any peculiar dietary needs you will need to research whether the diets are ok for you.

The way the exercise dovetails with this diet is important so there will be a total plan of exercise and diet to follow. I will publish the programme and the nutrition exactly as we plan to follow through from now until show time in June.

BodyBoosting Optimum Diet & Follow on Training Programmes. Parts 1 - 3.

We will deal with the training programmes first. Currently we are on a maintenance training programme, I call it that but if any gains come our way or any fat is lost that is all good. There are two tough full body programmes and are completed alternately every four days (ish) 3 sets of each exercise 8/12 reps flat out - as follows:

PART 1 - Goal = Maintenance - Duration 2 months

Day 1 Full Body Maintain Programme "A" Carb-Boost Day

Day 2 Carb-Boost Day

Day 3 Zero-Carb Day

Day 4 Zero-Carb Day

Day 5 Full Body Maintain Programme "B" Carb-Boost Day

Day 6 Carb-Boost Day

Day 7 Zero-Carb Day

Day 8 Zero-Carb Day

Day 9 Full Body Maintain Programme "A" Carb-Boost Day

Day 10 Carb-Boost Day

Day 11 Zero-Carb Day

Day 12 Zero-Carb Day

Day 13 Full Body Maintain Programme "B" Carb-Boost Day

And so on ....

Full Body Programme "A"

1. 5 minutes cardio warm up
2. Pelvic Tilts and Decline Sit up's super set.
3. Seated Calf Raises
4. Parallel Grip Pulldowns
5. Leg Extensions
6. Chest Flyes (any)
7. Lying Leg Curls
8. Upright Rows
9. Triceps Pushdowns
10. Barbell Curls
11. Smith Squats (Deep)
12. Rope Pulley Hammer Curls
13. Deadlifts
14. 20 minutes cardio intervals

Full Body Programme "B"

1. 5 minutes cardio warm up
2. Cycle Crunches
3. Hack Calf Raises
4. Behind Neck Pulldowns
5. Leg Extensions
6. Incline Chest Press (any)
7. Seated Leg Curls
8. Smith Press Behind Neck
9. Decline Triceps Extensions
10. Preacher Curls

11.   Walk the Gym Lunges (holding plates)
12.   Behind Back Wrist Curls
13.   45 Degree Leg Press
14.   20 minutes cardio intervals

There may be exercises here that are not included in the gallery. If you do not know them. Contact us on the site and we will help. You can substitute any exercise for another as long as it is for the same bodypart and preferably of similar intensity. For example you could swap incline chest press for flat chest press.

PART 2 - Goal = Muscle Gain/Minimal Fat Storage - Duration 2 Months

Day 1 Upper Body - Carb-Boost Day

Day 2 Lower Body - Carb-Boost Day

Day 3 Carb-Boost Day

Day 4 Zero-Carb Day

Day 5 Upper Body - Carb-Boost Day

Day 6 Lower Body - Carb-Boost Day

Day 7 Carb-Boost Day

Day 8 Zero-Carb Day

And so on ....

Upper Body Programme "A"

Each upper body day we begin the day with hill sprints at the local park - this give a cardio workout and stresses the glutes and legs explosively. How often do you see a sprinter with poor hamstrings? The first day we warmup and do only one sprint adding one each time we visit the hill. We have both sustained injury in the doing these so we always build up gradually. They are tough but it feels great to get outside and push yourself. The hill is about 75 metres long.

1. 5 minutes Cardio Warmup
2. Wide Grip Pulldowns to Front
3. Hammer Chest Press Machine
4. Seated Low Pulley Rows
5. Inclined Dumbbell Flyes
6. Upright rows
7. Seated Dumbbell Shoulder Press
8. Seated Dumbbell Curls
9. Inclined Dumbbell Triceps Extensions
10.   Pulley Curls
11.   Triceps Kickbacks
12.   Rope Hammer Curls
13.   10 mins low intensity cardio cooldown

Lower Body Programme "A"

1. 5 mins Cardio Warmup
2. Hanging Leg Raises
3. Seated Calf Raise
4. Cycle Crunches
5. Standing Calf Raises
6. Lunges
7. Leg Press
8. Romanian Deadlifts
9. Leg Extensions
10.   Lying Leg Curls
11.   10 minutes low intensity cardio cool down

Upper Body Programme "B" - Pre- exhaust super sets - antagonistic for arms.

1. 5 minutes Cardio Warmup
2. Stiff Arm Pulldowns <u>no rest</u> Reverse Grip Pulldowns

3. Pectoral Flye Machine <u>no rest</u> Fit Elevated Press Ups
4. Dumbbell Lateral Raises <u>no rest</u> Machine Shoulder Press
5. Preacher curls <u>no rest</u> Triceps Extension Machine
6. 10 mins low intensity cardio cooldown

Lower Body Programme "B"

1. 5 mins Cardio Warmup
2. Leg Lowers
3. Hack Machine Calf Raise
4. Weighted Decline Sit Ups
5. Seated Toe Press
6. Leg extension <u>no rest</u> Recumberent Leg Press - Super Set
7. Hack Squats
8. Seated Leg Curls
9. 10 minutes low intensity cardio cool down

All exercise are done for 5 sets and the reps are kept between 8 and 12.

PART 3 - Goal = Fat Loss/Muscle retention(show prep) - Duration 2 Months

We really start to step up the training now. The diet takes a slightly different turn also. The aim now is to work each muscle more about 4 different exercises now and feed less(carbs) thus losing more bodyfat. Hopefully not much to lose by this stage. Depending on condition, as the target date draws closer (it can be for any reason, a holiday, a wedding or a show), the carb-boost day is eliminated until the carb load stage of preparation is reached. The initial plan is always to drop carb-boost for the second month, however if one reaches a lean condition earlier than anticipated then leave it in.

Day 1 Chest and Back - Targeted-Carb Day

Day 2 Abs and Calves - Targeted-Carb Day

Day 3 Shoulders - Targeted-Carb Day

Day 4 Biceps, Triceps and forearms - Targeted-Carb Day

Day 5 Legs - Carb-Boost Day

Day 6 Chest and Back - Targeted-Carb Day

Day 7 Abs and Calves - Targeted-Carb Day

Day 8 Shoulders - Targeted-Carb Day

Day 9 Biceps, Triceps and forearms - Targeted-Carb Day

Day 10 Legs - Carb-Boost Day

......And so on ....

I will now show you TWO sample workouts for each of the five sessions, "A" & "B" - remember though you can use almost any similar exercise to substitute as long as it is for the same bodypart and of comparable intensity. We love to use the push/pull system for upper body workouts. The beauty of push pull is that it keeps your exercise poundages high as you workout opposing muscle groups. This is great for motivation. We like to train chest and back together for the awesome pump in the torso, likewise for biceps and triceps. Lower Back gets trained indirectly with legs. In a 10 day cycle as above we try to change the session as much as possible. Maybe supersetting one session and straight sets the other. variety is the spice of life. To be honest we do what fancy on any day as long as it fits the framework of the routine for that day. This is supposed to be fun.

Chest & Back "A"

Always perform at least 5 minutes cardio to warmup overall body.

1. Pectoral Flye Machine
2. Wide Grip Pulldowns to Front
3. Smith Machine Inclined Press
4. Seated Low Pulley Rows
5. Cable Pulley Pec Flyes

6. Angled straight Arm Pulldowns
7. Vertical Chest Press Machine
8. Bent Over Low Pulley Rows

Chest & Back "B" - Superset.

1. Pectoral Flye Machine + Wide Grip Pulldowns to Front
2. Vertical Chest Press Machine + Seated Low Pulley Rows
3. Smith Machine Inclined Press + Angled straight Arm Pulldowns
4. Cable Pulley Pec Flyes + Bent Over Low Pulley Rows

As this session is normally done during a fat cutting cycle, the workout should deplete carb stores somewhat. Walking at 100/120 BPM (beats per minute) is done now to burn body fat.

Abs & Calves "A"

1. Hanging Leg Raises
2. Seated Calf Raises
3. Weighted Sit Ups
4. Standing Calf Raises
5. Cycle Crunches
6. Seated Toe Press

Abs & Calves "B" - Performed Superset Fashion

1. Cycle Crunches + Seated Toe Press
2. Weighted Sit Ups + Single Leg Calf Raises
3. Leg Lowers + Seated Calf Raises

As this session is normally done during a fat cutting cycle, the workout should deplete carb stores somewhat. Walking at 100/120 BPM (beats per minute) is done now to burn body fat.

Shoulders "A"

1. Press Behind Neck
2. Upright Rows
3. Single Arm Low pulley Lateral Raises

4. Seated Rear Deltoid Lateral
5. Barbell or Disc Forward Raises

Shoulders "B" - Performed Superset Fashion

1. Dumbbell Lateral Raises + Machine Shoulder Press
2. Bent over Lateral Raises + Upright Rows
3. Forward Raises + Seated Dumbbell Press

As this session is normally done during a fat cutting cycle, the workout should deplete carb stores somewhat. Walking at 100/120 BPM (beats per minute) is done now to burn body fat.

Biceps, Triceps and forearms "A"

1. Preacher Curls
2. Machine Triceps Extensions
3. Seated Dumbbell Curls
4. Decline Triceps Extensions
5. Rope Hammer Curls
6. Triceps Pushdowns
7. Behind Back Behind Back Wrist Curls.

Biceps, Triceps and forearms "B" - Performed Superset Fashion

1. Barbell Curls + Triceps Pushdowns
2. Preacher Curls + Machine Extensions

As this session is normally done during a fat cutting cycle, the workout should deplete carb stores somewhat. Walking at 100/120 BPM (beats per minute) is done now to burn body fat.

Legs "A"

Always perform some bodyweight squats and lunges just as a warm up on leg day.

1. Lunges

2. Squats
3. Romanian Deadlifts
4. Leg Extensions
5. Seated Leg Curls

Legs "B" -- Performed Superset Fashion

1. Leg Extensions + Recumberent Leg Press
2. Hack Squats + 45 degree Leg Press
3. Lying Leg Curls + Walking Lunges

As this session is normally done during a fat cutting cycle, the workout should deplete carb stores somewhat. Walking at 100/120 BPM (beats per minute) is done now to burn body fat.

Every Old Sock Needs an Old Shoe. Just as Every Good Workout Schedule Needs a Complimentary Diet, that delivers results with optimum health as a priority.

Here are the habits we have settled on, nothing wildly original just used in an effective original way.

The following is Gary's eating plan I(Julie) just quite simply eat less but follow a similar schedule.

Now I will explain our nutrition regime that works together with our workout plans to produce the desired results. It is important when looking at these plans that you realise that Julie is approximately 70kg(15%) and I am approximately 115kg(15%) at this time early in the maintenance section, part 1. Any amounts of food consumed should be tailored to meet your needs at that time. The way we each eat is generally the same, it's just the amounts that vary for our lean tissue requirements.

Zero Carb Day - 5/6/7 Feeds depending on appetite.

Upon Rising (5am) - 4 Universal Ripped Fast Capsules with Water and cup of tea. Walk dogs for about 1 hour.

Feed 1 - 6 omega eggs

Feed 2 - Whey protein with scoop of salt and sugar free peanut butter

Feed 3 - Chicken and handful of almonds

Feed 4 - Whey protein with scoop of salt and sugar free peanut butter

Feed 5 - Fish (salmon) & veg

Feed 6 - 6 omega eggs

Feed 7 - Whey protein with scoop of salt and sugar free peanut butter

Carb - Boost.

Upon Rising (5am) - 4 Universal Ripped Fast Capsules with Water and cup of tea. Walk dogs for about 1 hour.

8am - Feed 1......Breakfast Shake ..... Enough made for 2 Post workout shakes(minus the Banana). Julie Identical but in smaller shake containers available from "My Protein".

10am - Workout / Taken 30mins Before training - ECA/Multi Vits/Niacin/.

Noon - Feed 2 - Post Workout Shake 1

1pm - Feed 3 - Post Workout Shake 2

3pm - Feed 4 - Jacket Potato with protein source (fish/meat) and tinned tomatoes.

5pm - Feed 5 - Shake

7pm - Feed 6 - Cereals and skimmed milk or similar

9pm - Feed 7 - Calcium Caseinate - slow release protein before bed

Targeted Carb Day

The targeted carb day is one I (Gary) am using at the moment. I feel I am losing weight to fast and want to preserve muscle whilst still losing body fat. I tend to carb deplete very quickly. My day is as follows:

6am - ECA (2.58mile) walk every morning - I take ephedrine/caffeine and aspirin after having not eaten anything since 6/7pm the night before- the theory here is that I am burning fat as I walk (leisurely).

7am - Feed 1 - Protein Shake including fast and slow carbs

9am - Feed 2 - Protein Shake including fast and slow carbs

10am - Workout - Carbs provided by shakes.

Noon - Protein Shake including fast and slow carbs - This replenishment shake is sometimes repeated at 2pm.

The rest of the days feeds follow the zero carb diet.

Top Eight Habits of Successful Fat Loss

Many people who start a weight lose program start off enthused–ready to make some changes. They drop a few pounds in the first few weeks. Then it happens—week three roles by with no changes. Week four and they've gained back the few pounds lost in week one and two. Enthusiasm turns into frustration and all too often they give up. Does that scene sound familiar? Cheer up! There's good news. Many people have achieved success, and fortunately, they all share some common habits we can learn from to achieve success as well.

1) Motivation: They set a goal; write it down and resolve to achieve the goal. They break their goals into weekly, monthly, 3 month, 6 month and even annual goals. They make a declaration to lose X number pounds of fat and/or gain X number pounds of muscle. They know where they're headed and resolve to get there. They reinforce this plan daily and with declarations of success.

2) Plan: They follow a 'plan of attack' day-by-day, week-by-week and month-by-month and rarely allow themselves to miss workouts or skip meals. When life events interfere, and they must miss a workout or skip a meal, they get right back on the plan and do not allow the 'fall' to affect them.

3) Hydration: They drink liberal amounts of water. This is probably the most important thing you can do in almost any weight management plan. It's universal to all successful plans. Why? Water helps you to remain mentally sharp and focused. Water helps your brain and body function optimally. Water is the vehicle your body uses to rid itself of its toxins and metabolize stored fat. It gives you more energy and keeps you feeling positive and up-beat. The human body is composed of 50 to 65 percent water. Many programs recommend as much as 12 to 16, eight ounce glasses of water a day with no ill effects what-so-ever.

4) Cardio: They understand that walking is about as pure a fat loss exercise that you can get. Even five minutes a day is a great start. Those who have successfully lost weight often walk for 30 to 45 minutes 4 or more times a week. Beyond 60 minutes there seems to be a point of diminishing returns.

5) Resistance training: They know there is no greater fat-furnace than possessing muscle. Muscle tissue revs up metabolic activity. Muscle burns calories all day and all night, even when you're resting. Your metabolic rate is directly connected to how much lean muscle tissue you hold.

You must produce and retain lean muscle tissue within your body through weight training to lose fat effectively. In fact, your goal should be to stimulate muscle growth. You accomplish this with pushing or pulling a progressively heavier workload. Put in simple terms; lift more weight than your muscles currently can lift.

6) Stable Blood Sugar: They know the body needs protein several times a day. Every three hours or so is ideal. Lean protein causes the release of glucagon. Glucagon burns fat, builds lean mass and suppresses insulin. Insulin is the most powerful fat storing hormone in our body. A good strategy is to start your day with a protein shake to balance out your blood sugar and flood your system with dopamine. Dopamine is your "feel good, I can do anything" brain-body messenger. That's what happens when you eat protein. Eating carbs, on the other hand, puts you in a depressed, anxious state.

7) Slow Burning Carbs: They have found vegetables to be the best source as you get the highest amount of fibre and nutrients with the least effect on blood sugar with these, so this is always a first choice. Fruit is your next best choice and whole grains would be your third. Aim for about 15-25 grams per meal, but ideally keep your total carbohydrate intake to no more than 100 grams per day or about 400 calories from carbs. This would mean about 2-3 cups of vegetables (depending on the type of vegetable) or 1/2-1 cup of fruit or 1/2 cup of whole grains per meal.

8) Essential Fat: Essential Fats are very important, but they are also very calorie dense. Your best choices for healthy fats are: avocado, raw almonds, fish oil and olive oil .

These eight tips will soon have you on your way improving the way you look and feel.

A Simple Running programme.

⇒ Week 1 Run one min, walk 90 seconds. Repeat eight times. Do three times a week.

⇒ Week 2 Run two mins, walk one min. Repeat seven times. Do three times a week.

⇒ Week 3 Run three mins walk one mins. Repeat six times. Do three times a week.

⇒ Week 4 Run five mins, walk two mins. Repeat four times. Do three times a week.

⇒ Week 5 Run eight mins, walk two mins. Repeat three times. Do three times a week.

⇒ Week 6 Run 12 mins, walk one min. Repeat three times. Do three times a week.

⇒ Week 7 Run 15 mins, walk one min, Run fifteen mins. Do three times a week

⇒ Week 8 Run 30 mins continuously. Do three times a week

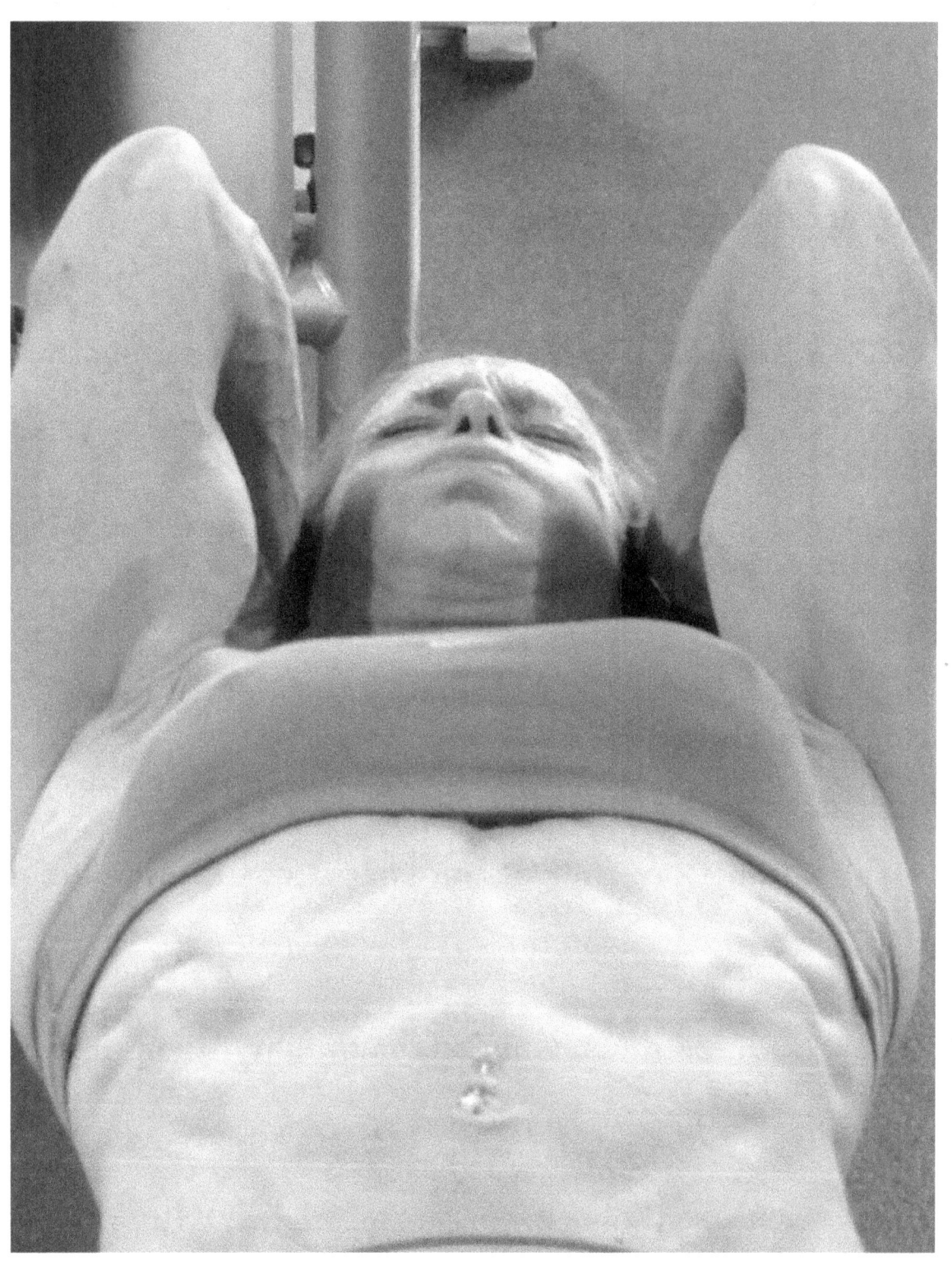

Exercise Descriptions.

It is very important that you develop your exercise form and habits correctly and to that end all gyms have qualified instructors to help you with the finer points. The pictures in our gallery are for most part quite self explanatory and I have decided that rather than go through the process of explaining again what you can clearly see and also have reinforced by an instructor, I will use the space to cover any points of particular interest and chit chat about anything that may be of help in your gym adventure. I hope my rambling will give those of you that are new to gyms an insight into gym culture and those of you that are existing gym members more of an appreciation as to what an amazingly interesting and diverse culture you have become part of. Any exercise that requires special explanation will be thoroughly explained. We will also be making demonstration video clips available of most if not all of the exercises covered here plus many that have not been included.

LEGS

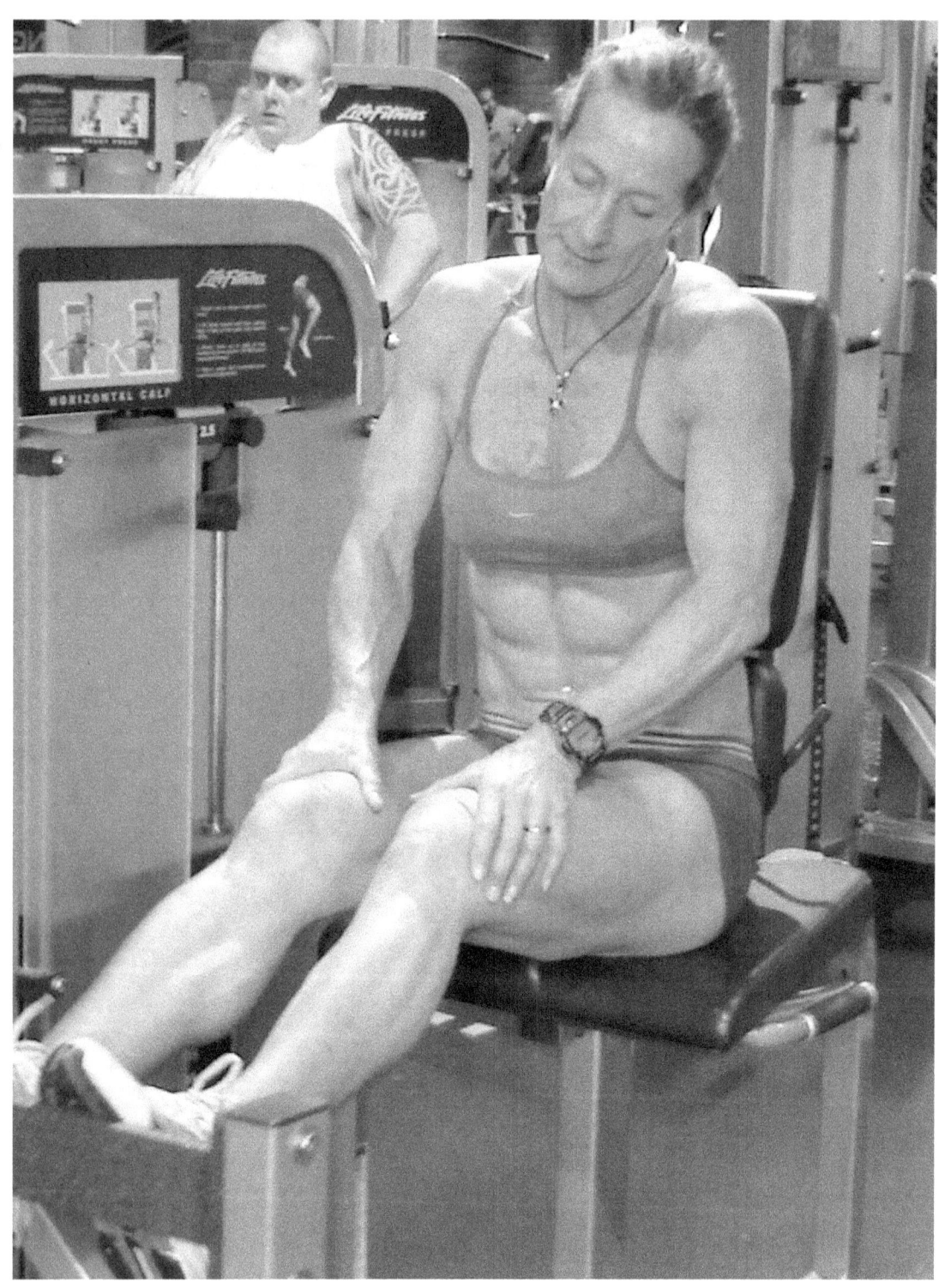

Weighted Barbell Step Ups

Important to remember here is to make sure the step or bench you are using is secure and safe. Initially don't use any weight as it will take a little while to get used to the exercise. When you are ready to use a barbell, place it across your shoulders or have a spotter place it there for you. You will complete all of your repetitions with one leg and then the other. As shown in the pictures, Julie is working her left leg. Her left foot is fully on the step and remains that way until 15 reps are completed, you may place your right foot on the step at the top of the rep initially to maintain balance but as you become more proficient your resting leg will go from the floor to the position Julie demonstrates thus keeping tension on the working leg. The working leg must have the heel on the

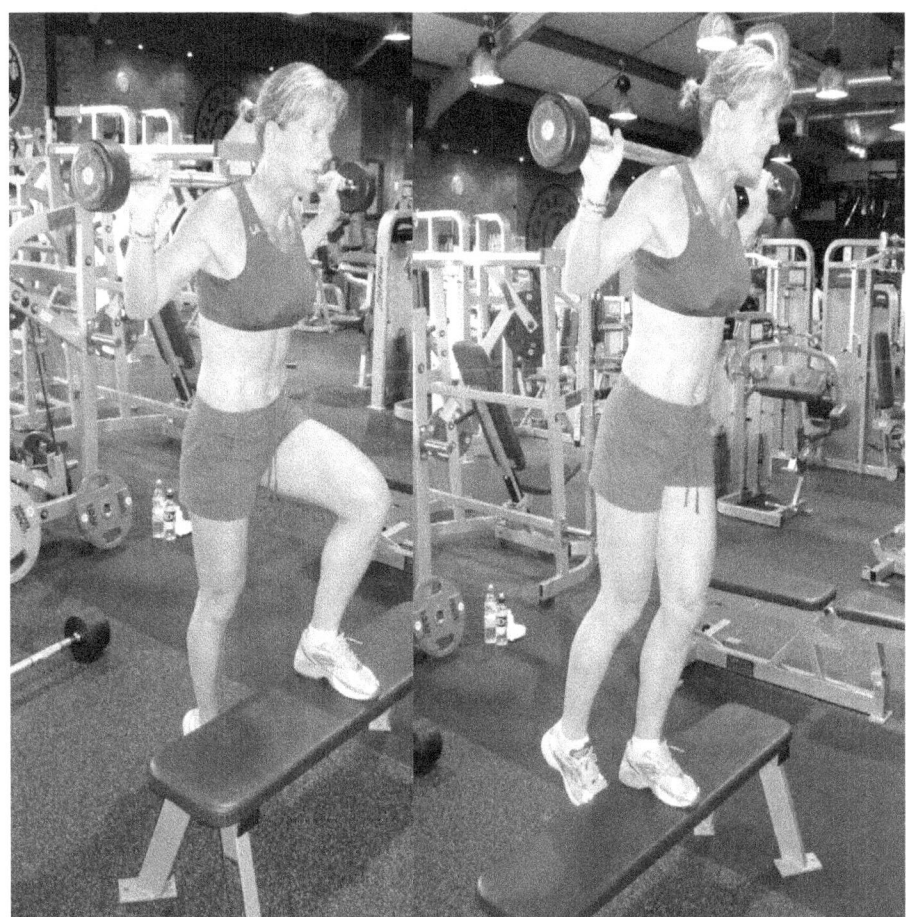 platform at all times and there should be no bounce from the bottom of the movement by the secondary leg. Work both legs.

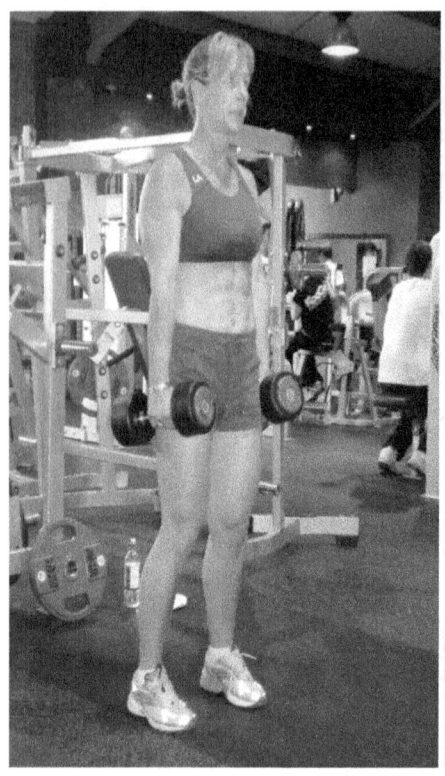
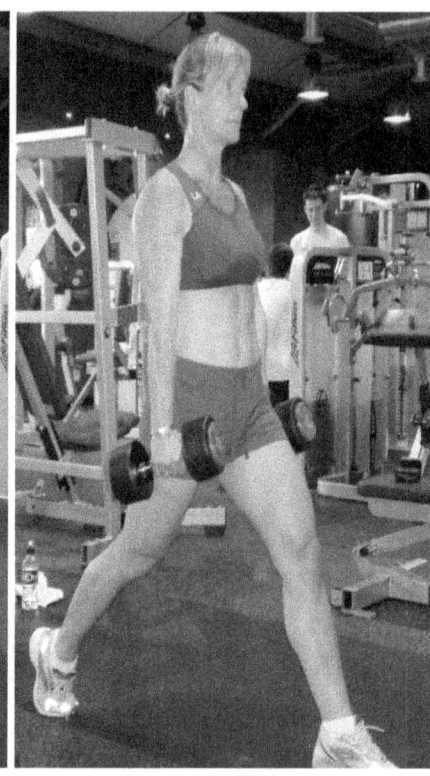

Weighted Dumbbell Lunges

When performing dumbbell Lunges we find it helpful to break the movement up into 3 parts, this helps to control the movement through each phase of the exercise. We again work each leg for the required number of repetitions before changing legs. However if you prefer you may alternate legs throughout the set. Again we tend to aim for 15 reps. Posture is important and you will notice Julie keeps her head in alignment throughout the set. Phase 1 - Begin with a large controlled step which will take you to position midpoint 1 – Phase 2 - next a controlled descent which should find you in the position of midpoint 2 - Phase 3 - and finally a powerful drive to take you back to the starting position.

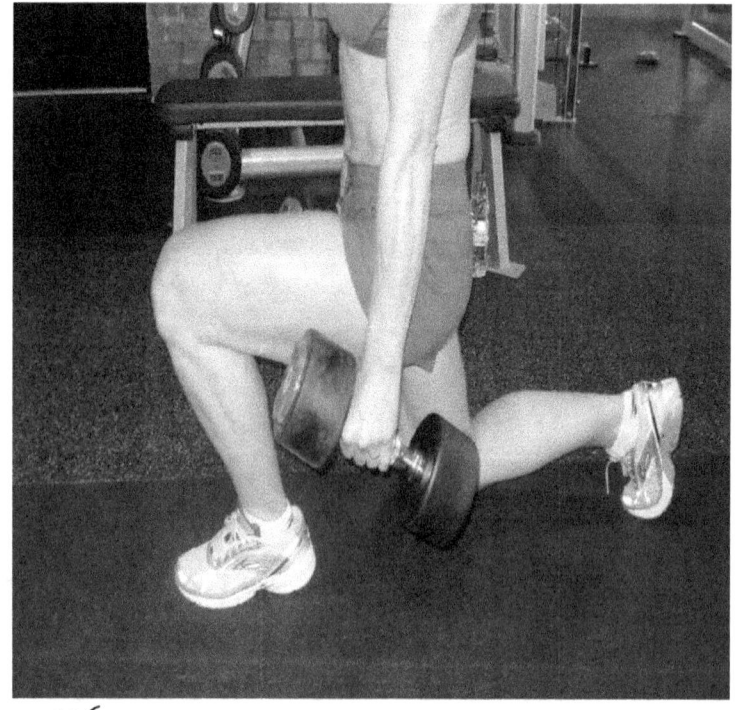

Barbell Bench Front Squats

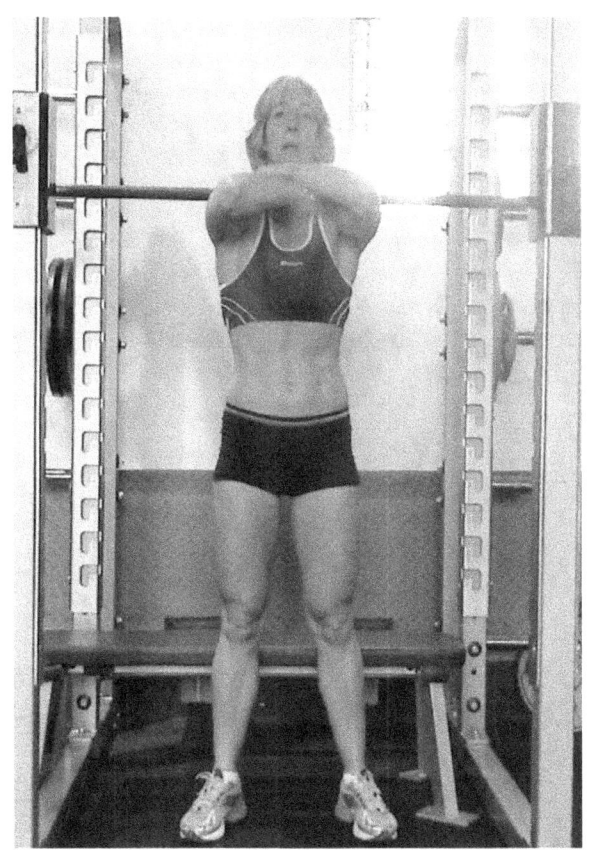

Front Squats are an advanced exercise and should only be attempted when you are confident in your ability. Ideally instructed by a gym professional. The position for the bar is quite uncomfortable as it is shoved into your wind pipe. The bar sits between your throat and shoulders whilst your hands cross over and keep it pushed into your wind pipe. The movement is the same as back squats however any forward motion of the torso and the bar wants to fall

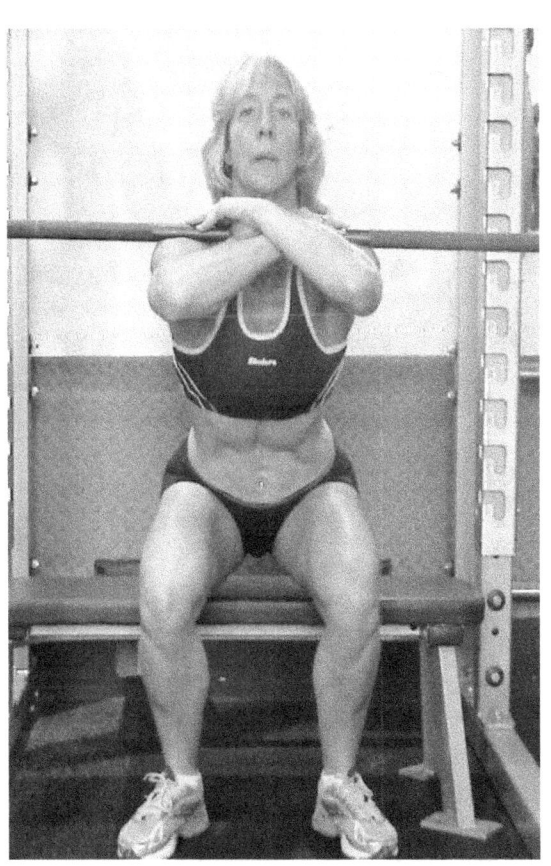

forward. Good posture and an upright position are vital to good front squatting. Front squats are a great exercise for your quadriceps which is why I have included them here but please be safety conscious and proceed with caution until you find your groove. Begin by warming up with no weight and always make sure you are in full control of your movements as any momentum <u>will</u> result in injury eventually.

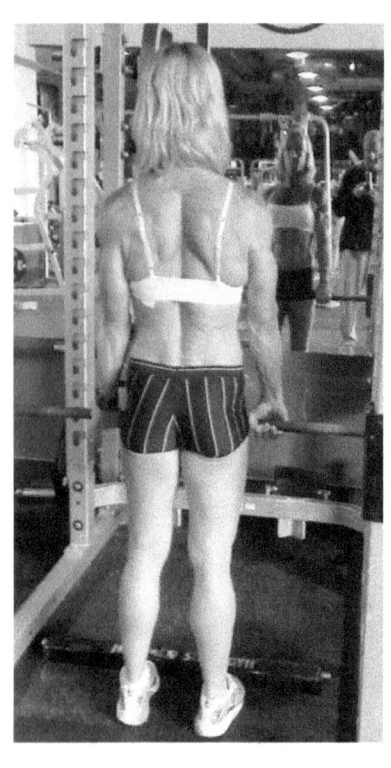

Romanian Deadlifts

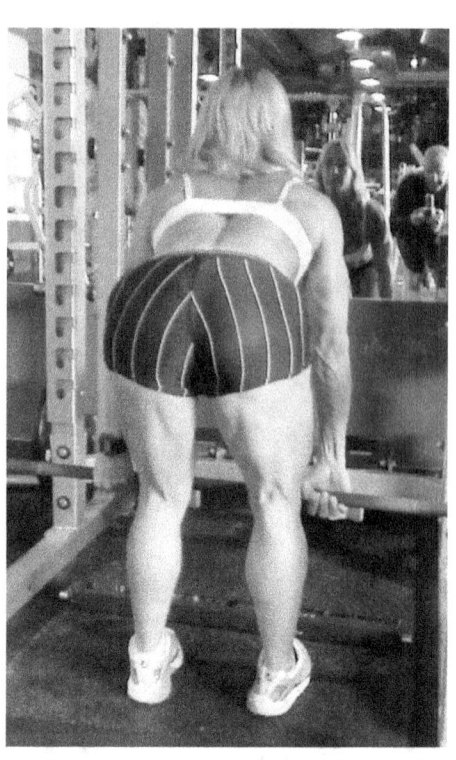

Romanian or Straight Leg Deadlifts are an advanced exercise and should only be attempted when you are confident in your ability. Ideally instructed for the first time by a gym professional. A flat bar or 2 weight discs are placed under the ball of each foot to obtain more of a stretch in your hamstrings and glutes. Although the name suggest straight legs there has to be a tiny amount of softness at the joint, not locked rigid. The bottom position for most people is about the level of your knees at which time you push back with your hips before returning to the upright position. Your back retains its natural curvature throughout the movement. You will notice that Julie has adopted a pronated grip with one hand and a supinated grip with the other, this grip is more effective when the weight increases.

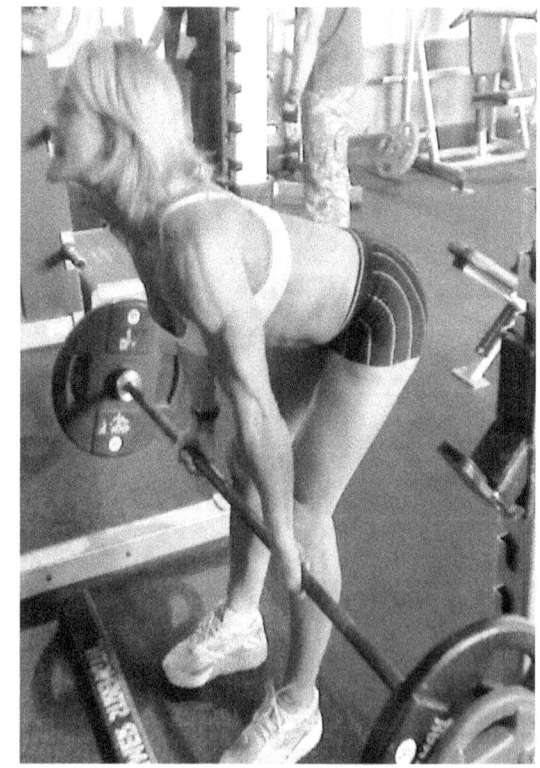

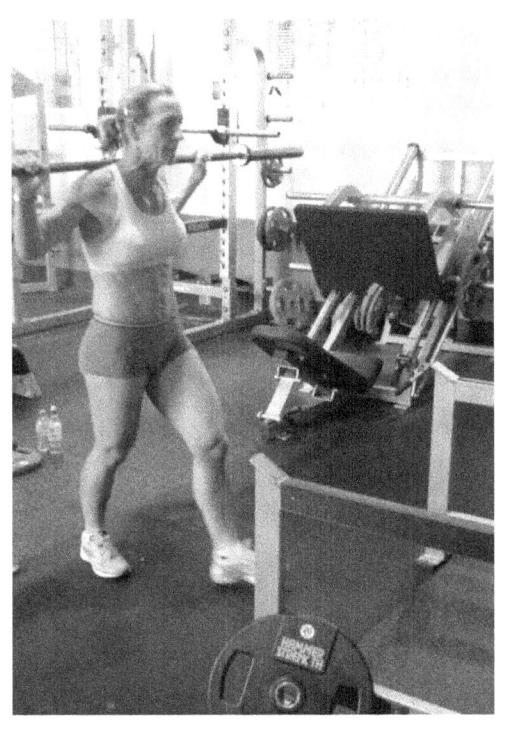

Barbell Lunges

When doing barbell Lunges we find it helpful to break the movement up into 3 parts, this helps to control the movement

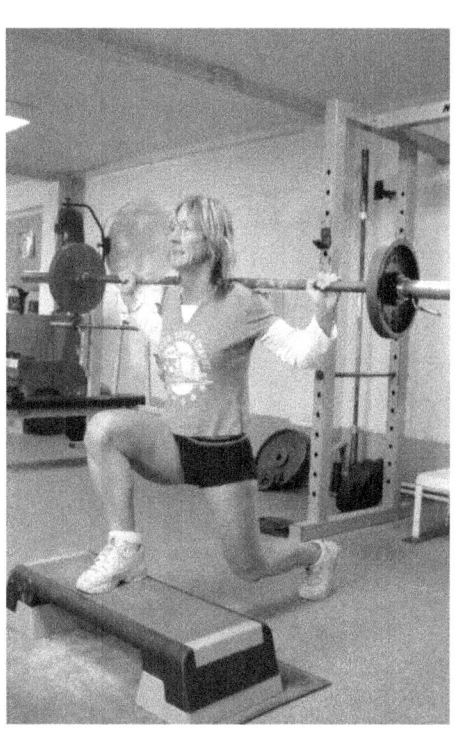

through each phase of the exercise. We again work each leg for the required number of repetitions before changing legs. However if you prefer you may alternate legs throughout the set. Again we tend to aim for 15 reps. Posture is important and you will notice Julie keeps her head in alignment throughout the set. Phase 1 - Begin with a large controlled step – Phase 2 - next a controlled descent which should find you in the position of midpoint - Phase 3 - and finally a powerful drive to take you back to the starting position. We have also shown a variation of lunging onto a step.

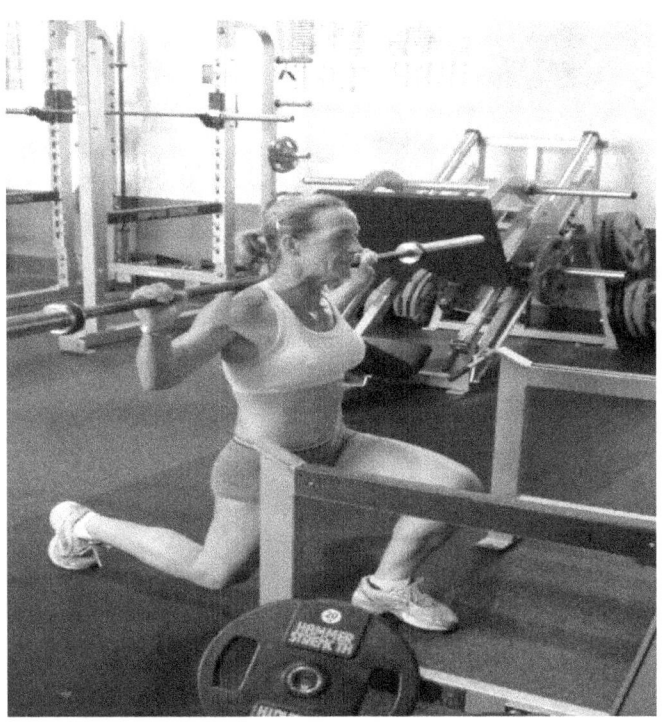

45 degree plate loaded leg press

Plate loaded leg press – start light and work heavier but make sure you keep a full range of motion and a smooth movement. This is one of the exercises that commonly does

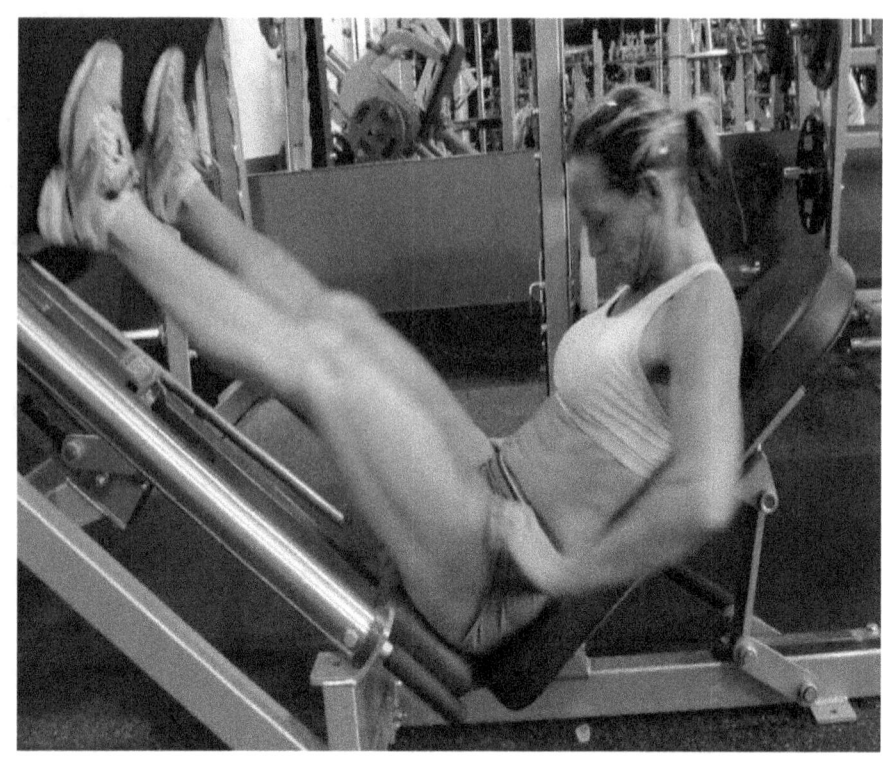

tempt gym users to load too much weight on and cheat with partial movements. Keep your feet flat on the plate and breathe deeply on each rep. Higher reps 15/25 work well and keeps the weights you will be using down to a sensible level.

Make sure you fully acquaint yourself with the machine before using any weight. In fact this advice rings true for all exercises. Leg press is not really a good substitute for squats or lunges but is worth using periodically for a welcome change and to add some variety.

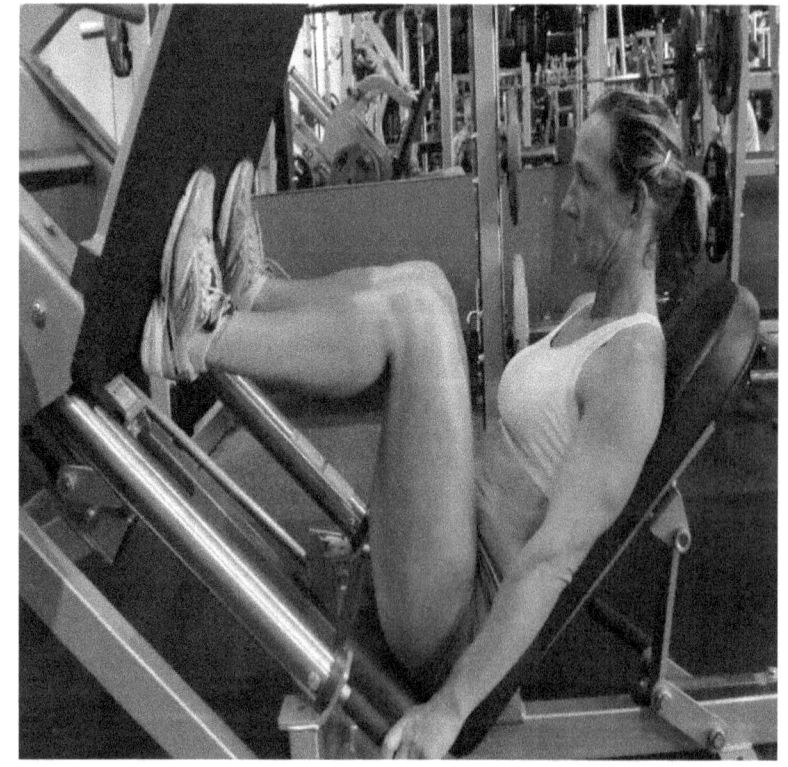

Leg Sled

This is one of the exercises that commonly does tempt gym users to load too much weight on and cheat with partial movements. Keep your feet flat on the plate and breathe

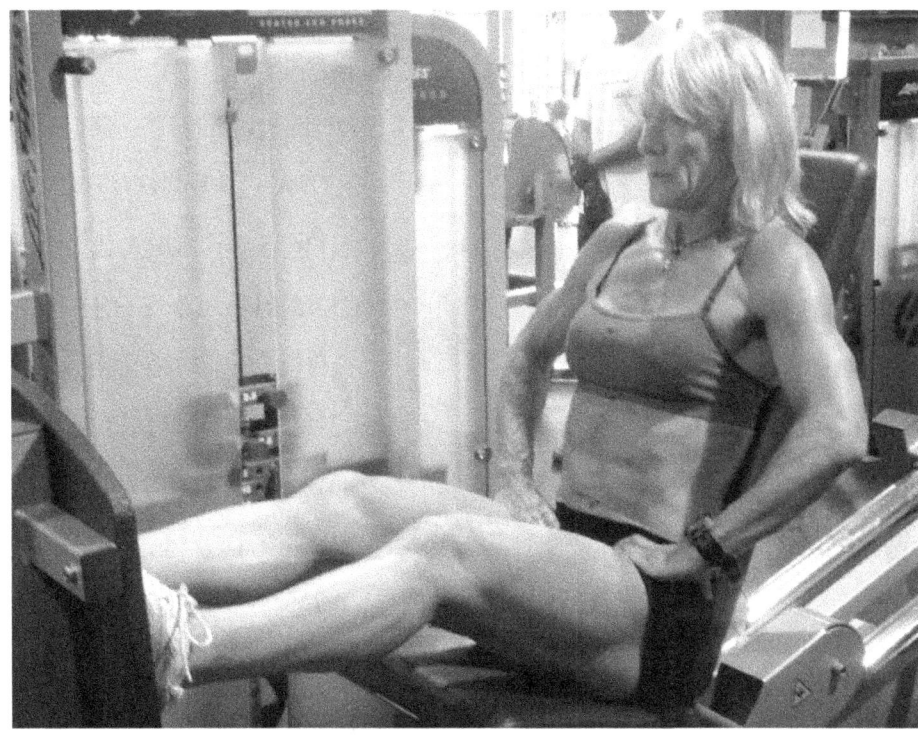

deeply on each rep. Higher reps 15/25 work well and keeps the weights you will be using down to a sensible level. Acquaint yourself with the machine before using any weight. In fact this advice rings true for all exercises. Leg sleds and presses are not really a good substitute for squats or lunges but are worth using periodically for a welcome change and to add some variety.

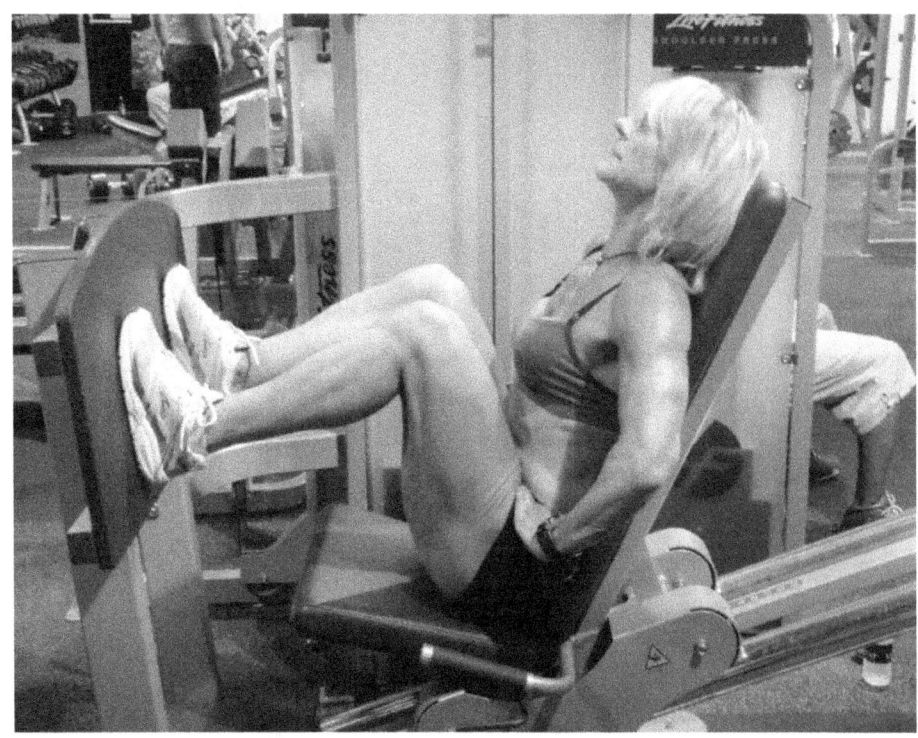

Barbell Back Squats

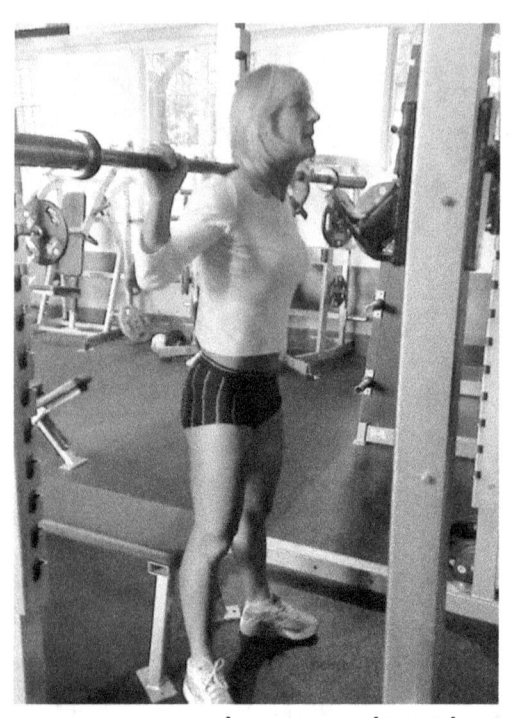

Back Squats are performed with the bar held high on your back, a little uncomfortable at first but after a couple of sessions you don't even notice the feel of the bar on your back. Foam may be wrapped around the bar if you really feel the need. Eyes are held on a fixed point quite high on the wall and you may squat down to a bench as Julie is doing if you need your depth consistent, eventually dispensing with the bench and going very deep. At first while you are using light weights you may be able to lift the weight to your shoulders, however you will very soon progress to a point where you will be squatting more than you can lift this way. Most if not all gyms have at least one squat rack that will enable you to do this safely. Begin by warming up with no

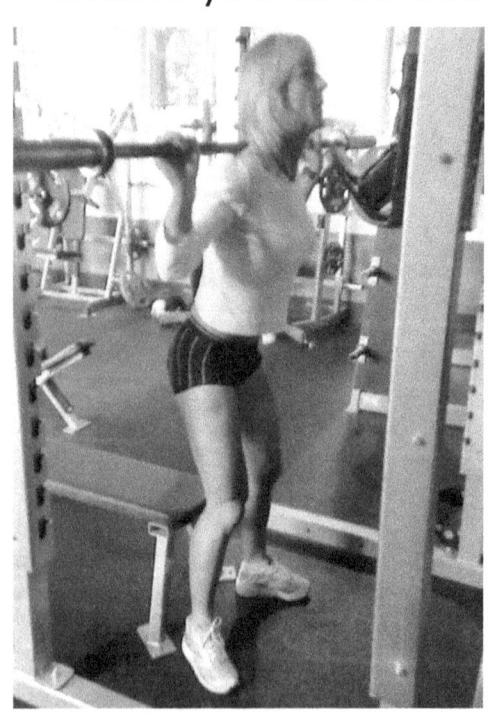

weight and then an empty bar and always make sure you are in full control of your movement as any momentum <u>will</u> result in injury eventually.

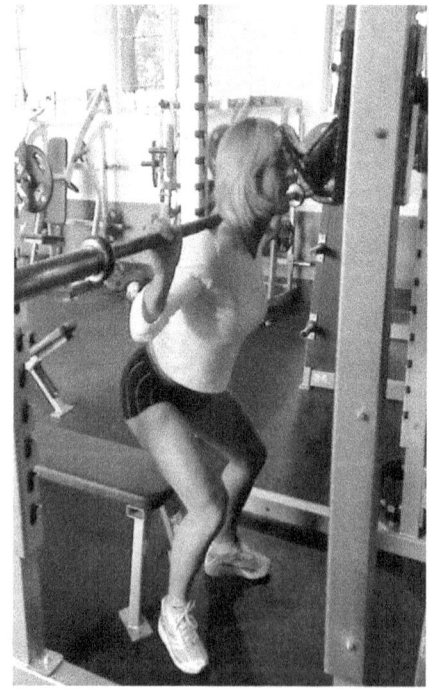

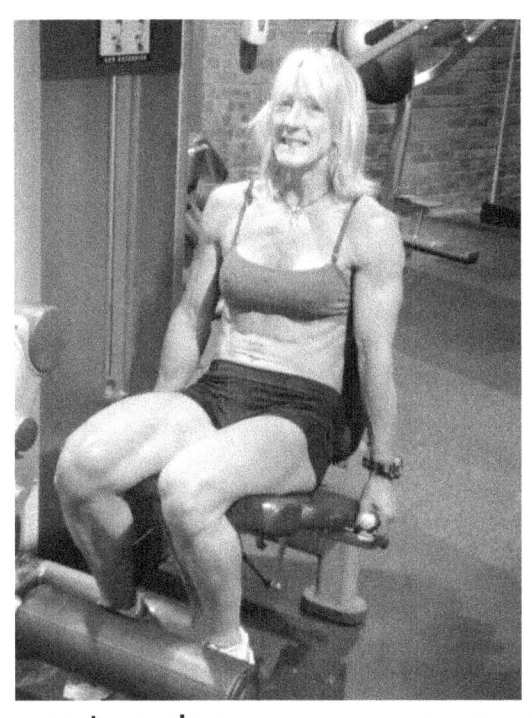

Leg Extensions

Leg Extensions work the quadriceps, frontal thighs in isolation. As part of a well balanced leg workout

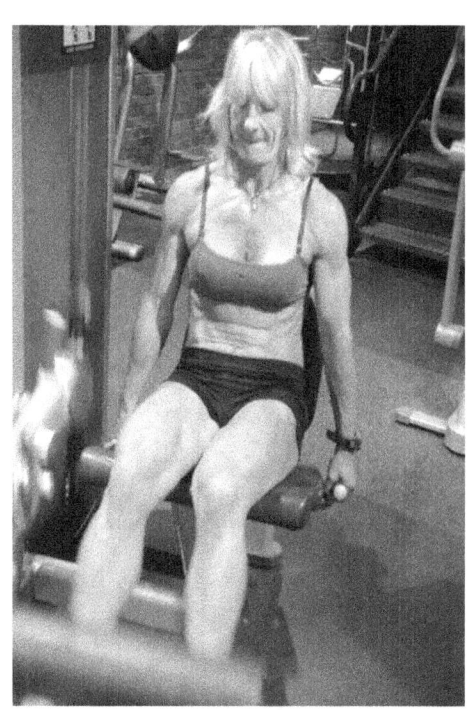

extensions are very good, however they should not be used as the staple exercise of any programme. Always do multi joint moves such as squats and lunges which require balance and an element of synchronicity first. Used to finish off your

thighs, leg extensions are very good. A nice controlled movement without any kicking is optimum in this move and again reps in the 12/20 range work well. The weight you use is of little importance, the form must be controlled with a nice squeeze in the muscle at the point of contraction (top).

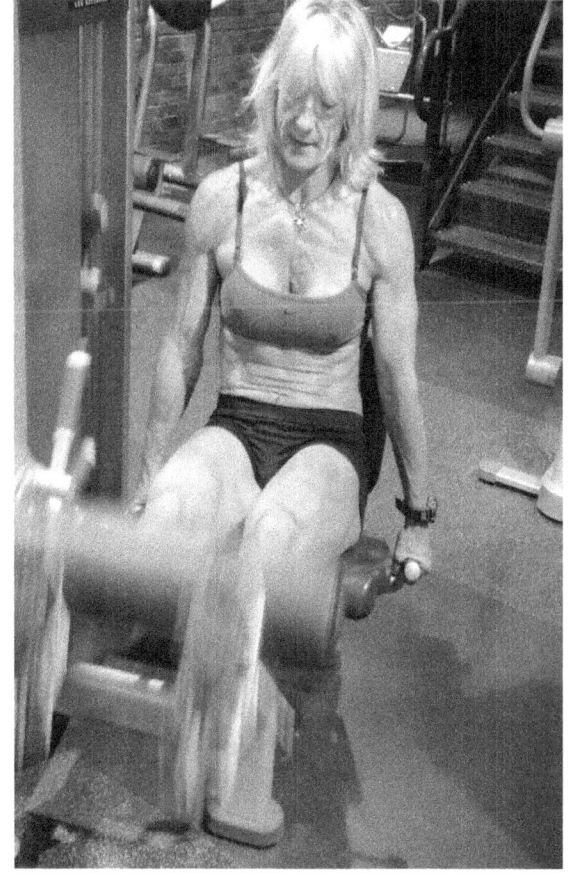

Dumbbell Jump Squats

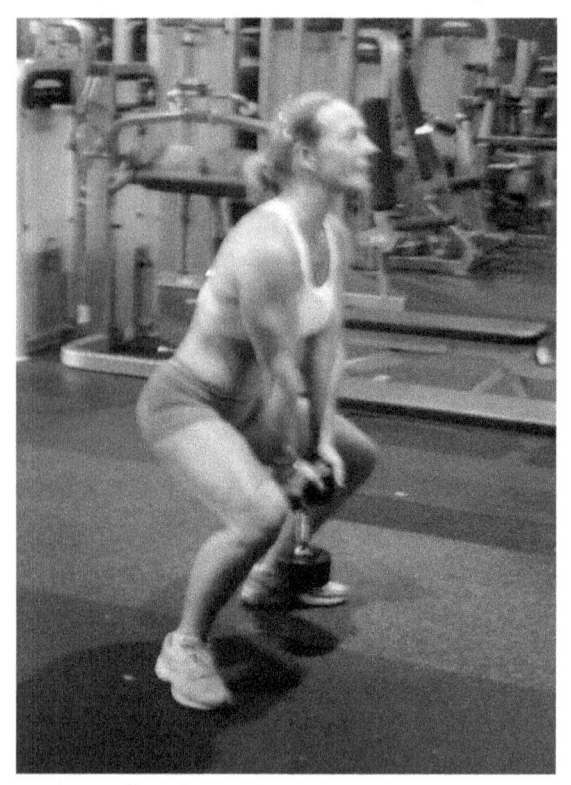

Julie is just a blur here because she is jumping so high or at least that what she says. Many track and field athletes do this exercise or the barbell equivalent. The key here is to remember when you first learned to jump as a child how you were taught to soak up any impact by bending your legs at the right moment. If you cannot jump lightly or do not know what that means then you probably shouldn't add this to your workouts. Holding the dumbbell as Julie is, you go from a controlled deep squat to an explosive leap as if you have sat on a wasp and he has

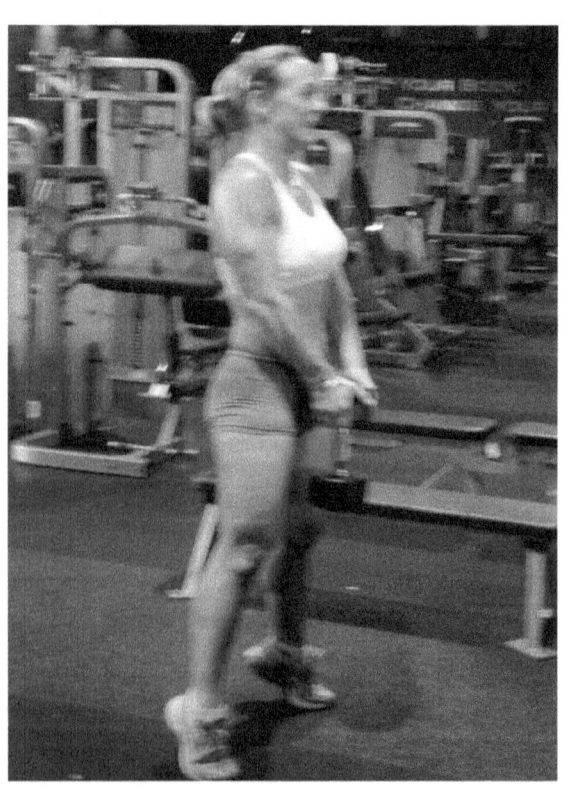

stung your backside. Control and power combined for this one. Land as softly as you can if you can hear yourself landing that is probably an indicator that the impact may be too great. Land quietly or pick another exercise. Begin by warming up with no dumbbell and always make sure you are in full control of your movements as any surplus, messy momentum will result in injury eventually.

Hack Squats

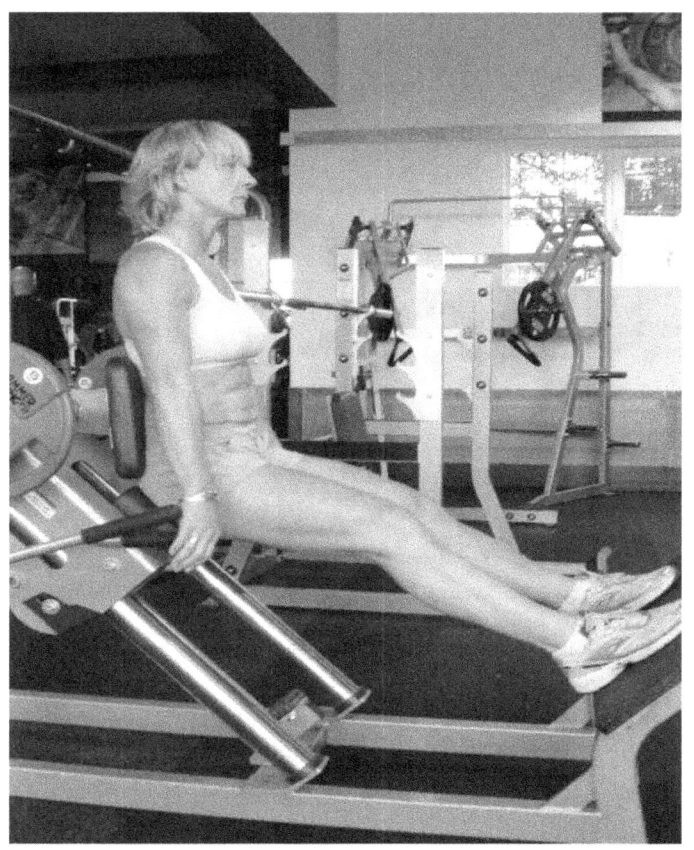

The Hack Squat named after George Hackenscmidt who first introduced the exercise by holding a barbell at arm's length behind his back and performing deep squats, very awkward. Nowadays there are many hack squat machines although the similarity to the original exercise is virtually non – existent. Our gym has a machine where the weight is resting on your hips and I have to say compared to most of the shoulder support machines it is very comfortable. The pictures paint the words for me on this one. Full range and in control please. Begin by warming up with no weight and always make sure you are in full control of your movements as any momentum <u>will</u> result in injury eventually.

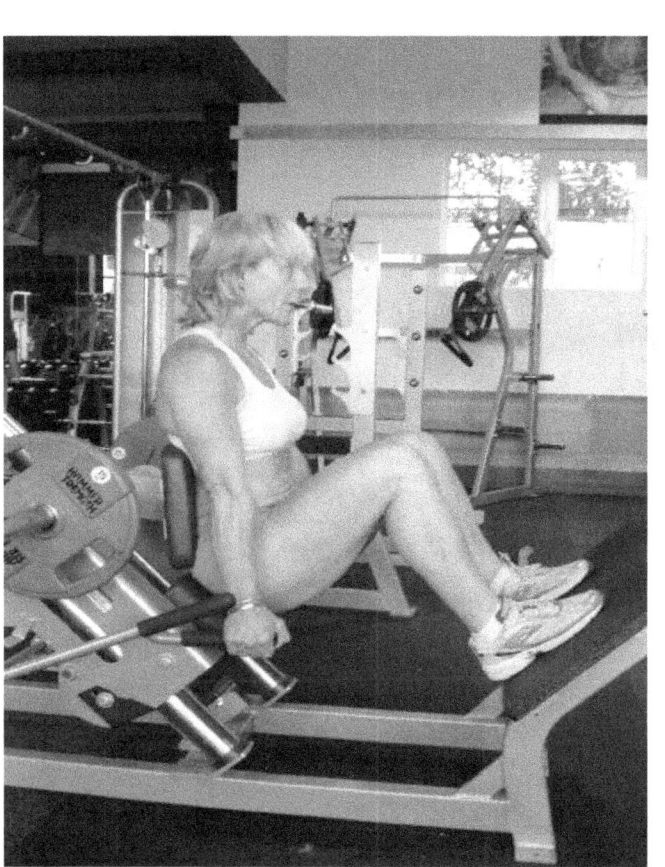

Good form - Stay Safe!!

Lying Leg Curls

Leg Curls, work the hamstrings (rear thighs) in isolation. As part of a well balanced leg workout curls are very good, however they should not be used as the staple exercise of any

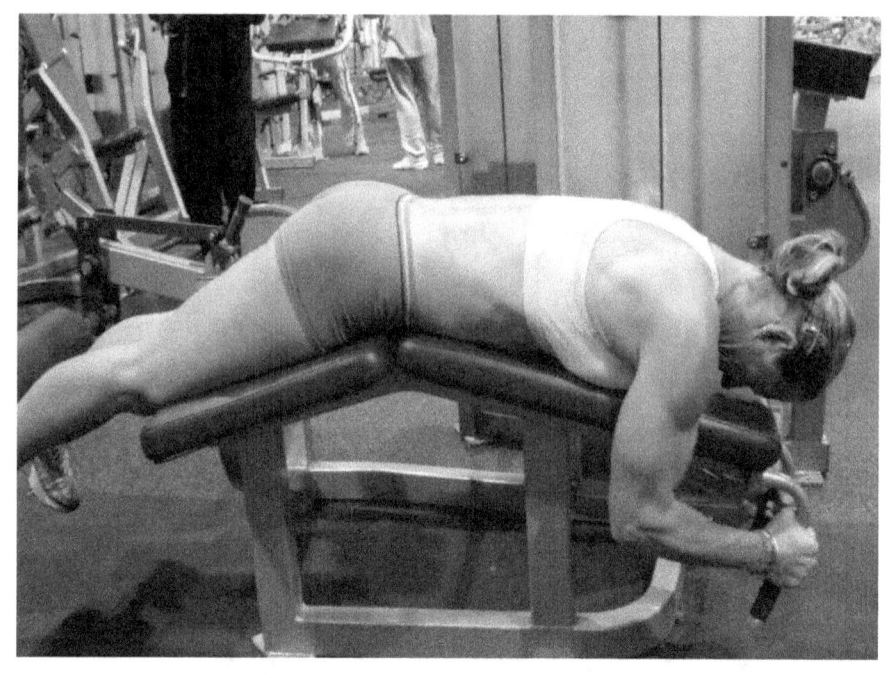

programme. Always do multi joint moves such as squats and lunges which require balance and an element of synchronicity first. Used to finish off your thighs, leg curls are very good. A nice controlled movement without any kicking is optimum in this move and again reps in the 12/20 range work well. The weight you use is of little importance, the form must be controlled with a nice squeeze in the muscle at the point of contraction (top).

Begin by warming up with no or light weights and always make sure you are in full control of your movements as any momentum <u>will</u> result in injury eventually.

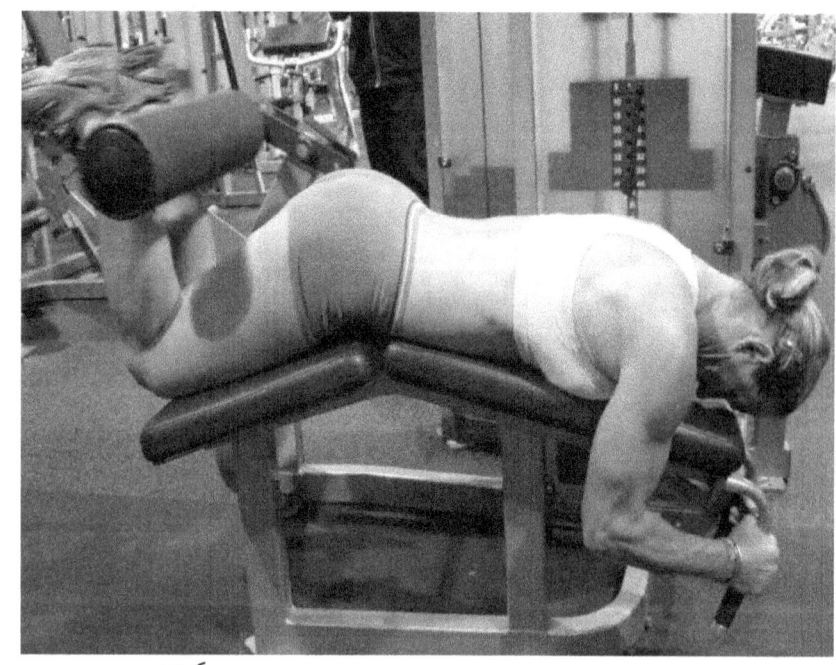

Seated Toe Press

At Gold's where we took these workout pics there is a purpose built machine for this exercise, however the exercise may 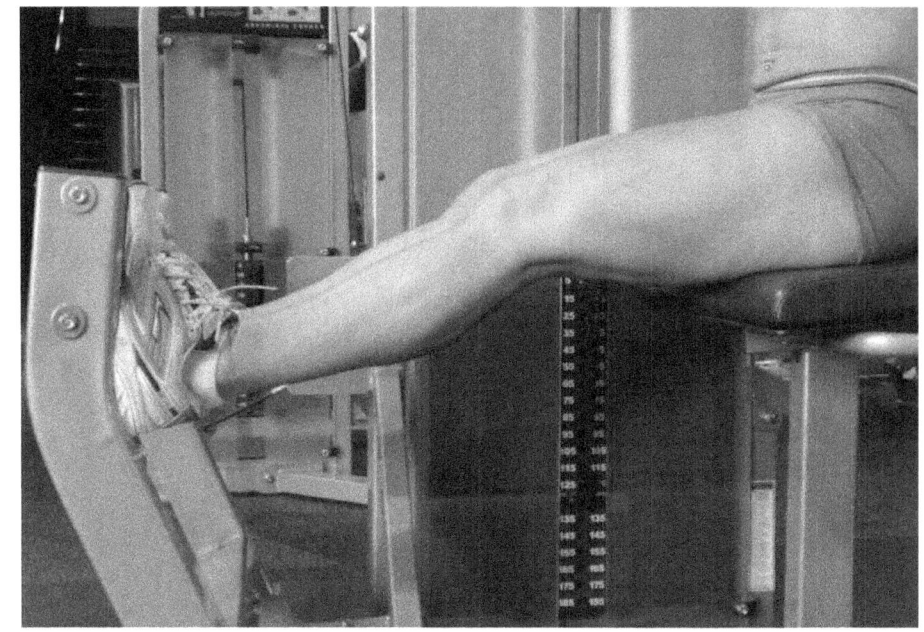 be done on any leg press machine if the design allows. The movement as with all calf work is a simple pointing of the toes and then a return to stretch your calf by letting your toes stretch up towards your knees. Legs held straight or just slightly soft at the knees is the desired leg position. Reps for calves tend to be traditionally higher as we use them constantly to walk and run and the muscle fibres are constructed in such a way to need higher reps 15/25 and generally a substantial weight. Begin by warming up with no

or light weights and always make sure you are in full control of your movements as any momentum <u>will</u> result in injury eventually.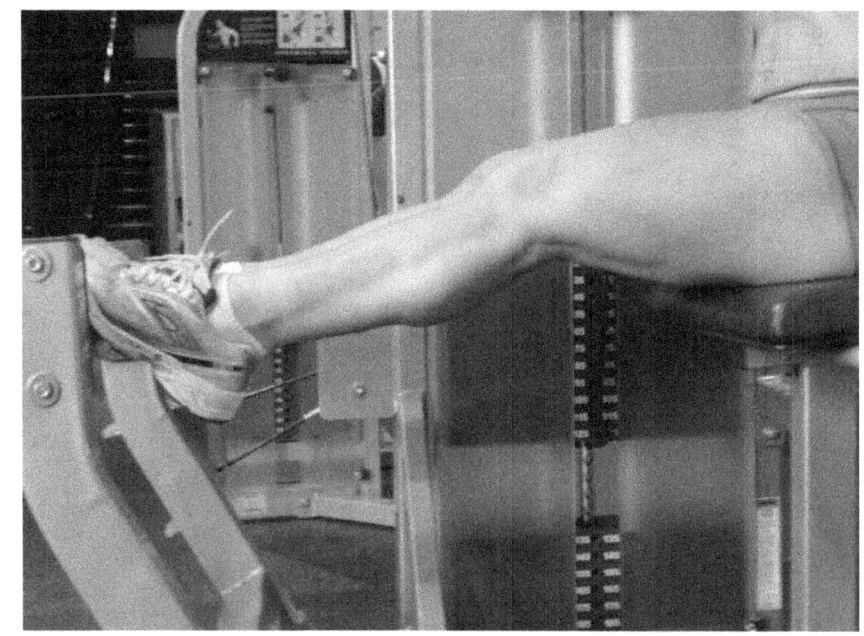

Seated Leg Curl

As part of a well balanced leg workout curls are very good, however they should not be used as the staple exercise of any programme.

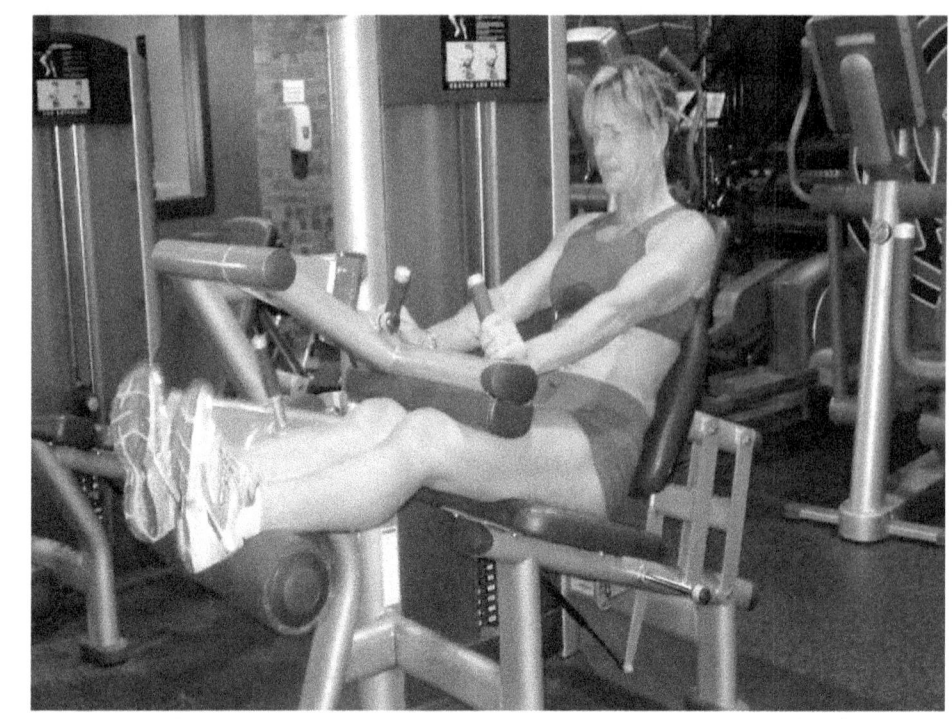

Always do multi joint moves such as squats and lunges which require balance and an element of synchronicity first. Used to finish off your thighs, leg curls are very good. A nice controlled movement without any kicking is optimum in this move and again reps in the 12/20 range work well. Begin by warming up with no or light weights and always make sure you are in full control of your movements as any momentum <u>will</u> result in injury eventually.

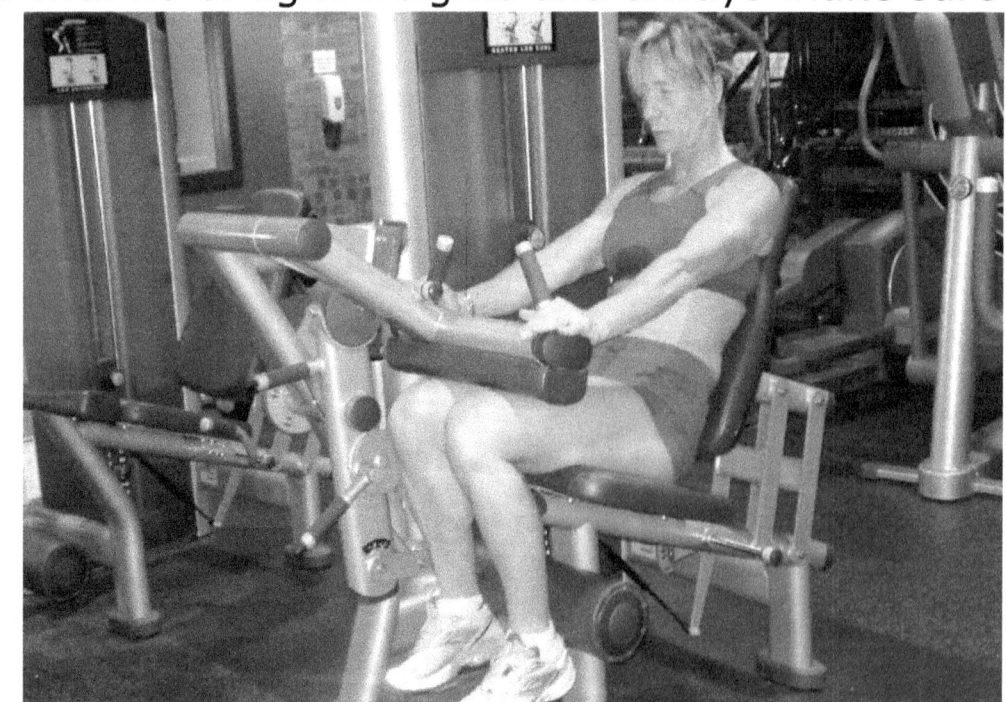

Hip Adduction

This exercise is very popular with women as it can be felt directly in a place where they perceive they need work. Granted this exercise works the inner thigh but it DOES NOT burn fat from that area directly. As you may tell from Julie's face we seldom use the adductor machine, whilst it is good at isolating the adductors we feel we get enough adductor work from the rest of

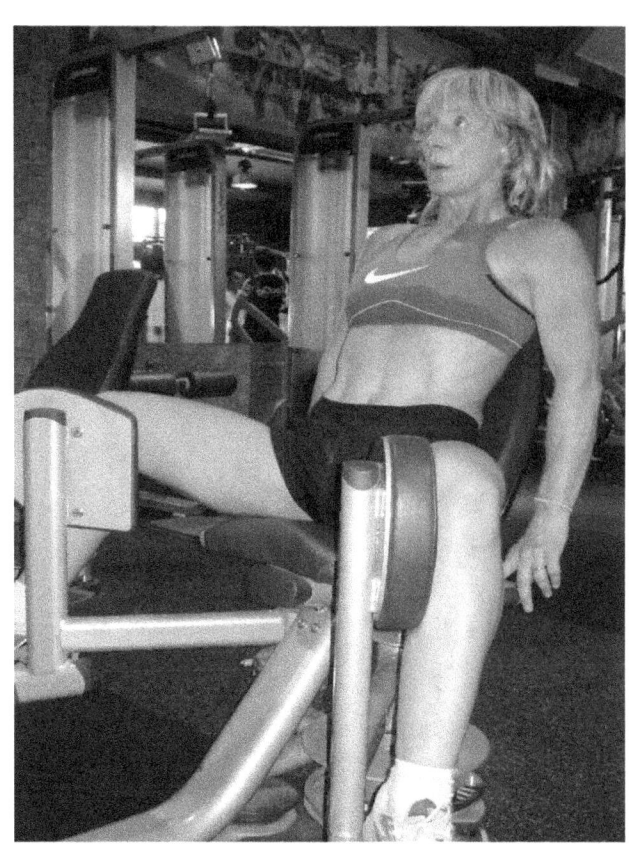

our workout, from lunges squats etc. However it is a good way to finish and every now and again we spice up our workouts by doing the stuff we don't normally do. We found that having not done it for a while it certainly hit the spot and once we stopped walking like John Wayne we included it in our routine for a few weeks. One thing I would say though if it feels good you should add it to your workout, as belief is half the battle, if you believe in your exercise plan it will work.

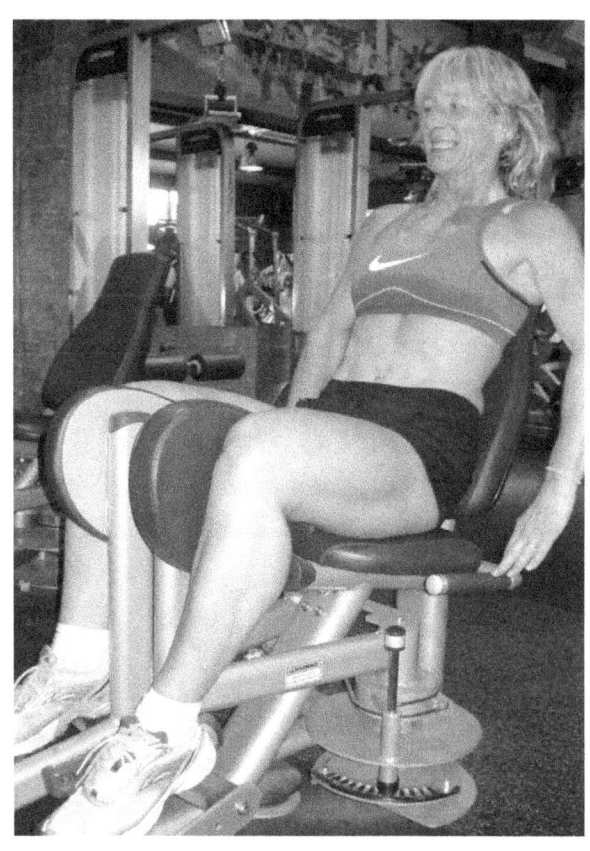

Hip Abduction

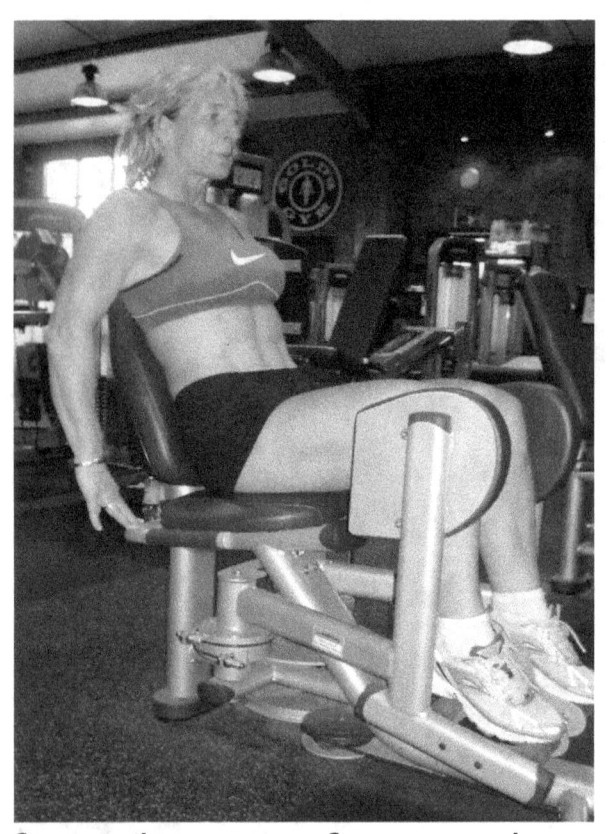

This exercise is very popular with women as it can be felt directly in a place where they perceive they need work. Granted this exercise works the hips but it DOES NOT burn fat from that area directly. As you may tell from Julie's face we seldom use the adductor machine, whilst it is good at isolating the abductors we feel we get enough abductor work from the rest of our workout, from lunges, squats etc. However it is a good way to finish and every now and again we spice up our workouts by doing the stuff we don't normally

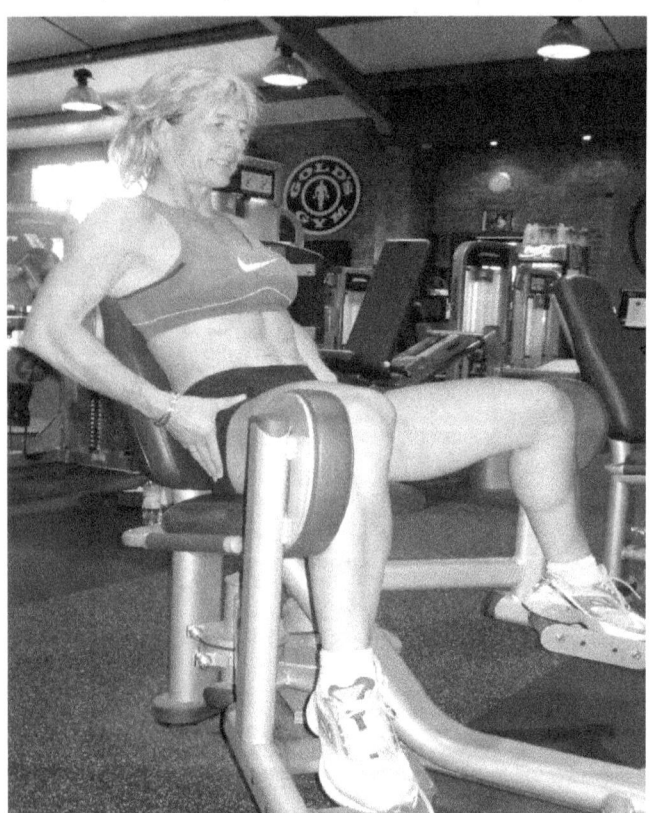

do. We found that having not done it for a while it certainly hit the spot and once we stopped walking funny we included it in our routine for a few weeks. One thing I would say though if it feels good you should add it to your workout, as belief is half the battle, if you believe in your exercise plan it will work.

Seated Calf Raise

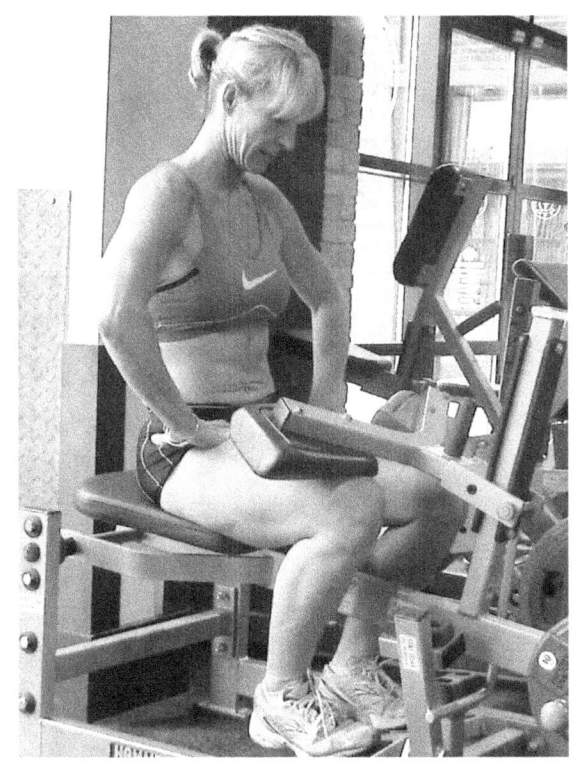

Seated calf raises hit your calf in a different area than when your legs are straight and both seated and standing calf raises inclusion in any leg workout would work very well. The machines can be quite awkward but hit the spot pretty well. We use much variety in our calf work to fight off any boredom. With calves it seems that hereditary factors are crucial, Julie would have great calves even if she didn't work them directly just from her running and the indirect work they receive in her other exercises. Other people are not so lucky and whilst it is always possible to improve, if you calf muscles sit high on your calf naturally you will never produce muscle in a place

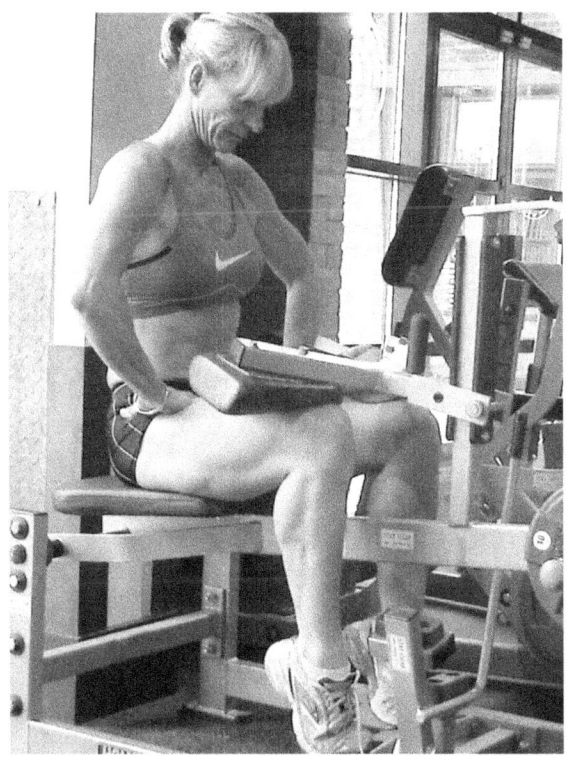

where it does not exist. You can only develop what you have. Many bodybuilders resort to implants when nature has left them found wanting in the calf department. It is rare for any person to have it all so to speak and to strive for that perfection will give little peace of mind. Love yourself and your unique potential.

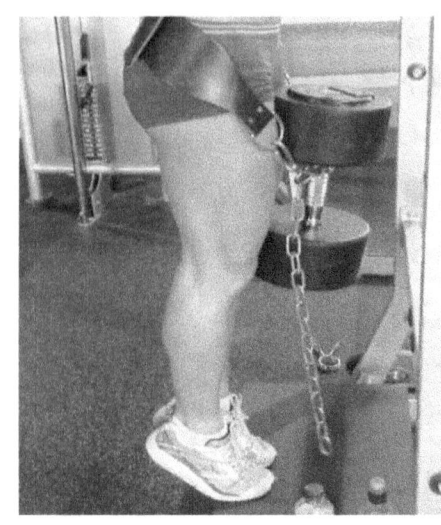

Standing Calf Raise

Our gym has no standing calf raise so we use a dipping belt with weight attached to do our standing

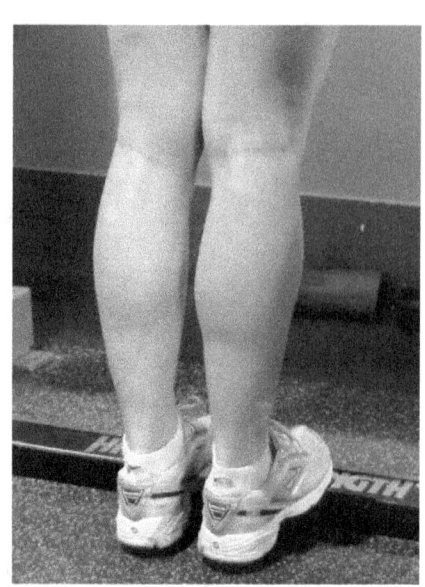

calf raises. The belt is positioned as shown around the waist and finding a step, we use the back of another bench we are able to obtain a good stretch (bottom) and contraction (top). The pictures here are self explanatory. Keeping control and A rep range of 15 is about right. I normally go for between 15 and 30 while Julie aims for about 15 on average. Once again as we increase the weight with each set our reps drop, we ensure never to drop below 8/10 on leg work. We are not weight lifters and

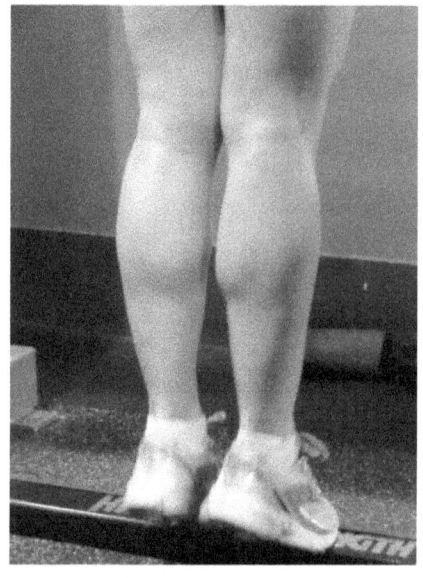

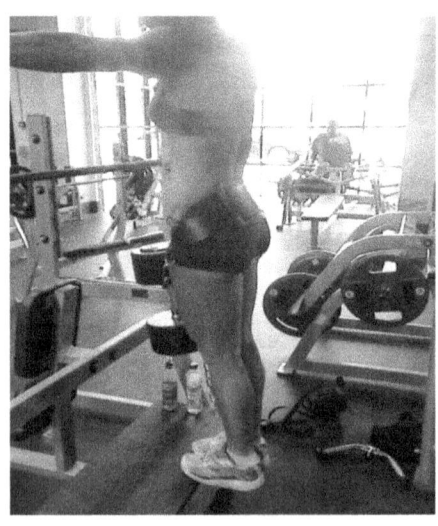

this suits our purpose perfectly. Legs are hard work and that is why so many people tend to miss them out -

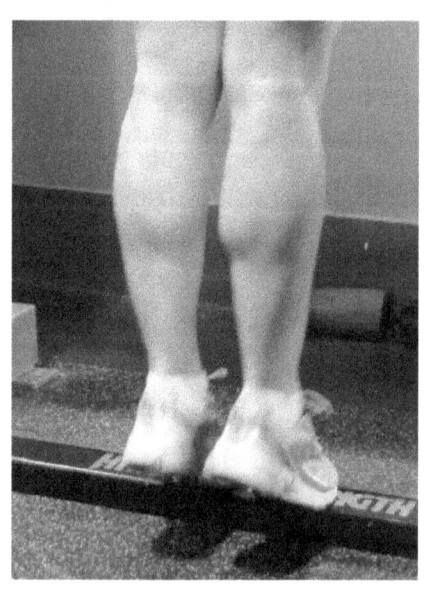

Hack Machine Calf Raise

The hack squat machine we have at our gym can be used to add some variety to our calf work. It is safe as we don't need to release the carriage lever and should we slip off the plate the carriage would stop a short way down. Safety is of paramount importance particularly when you are using equipment for a purpose other than that for which it was designed. On this machine the weight is supported primarily by your hips. Again as with all calf work sink your heels deep down and then up on to your toes as high as possible, this will be different for each individual. We keep our knees soft which is just short of full locking out of the joint, we feel this gives us a more powerful contraction (top).

Good Form – Stay Safe!!

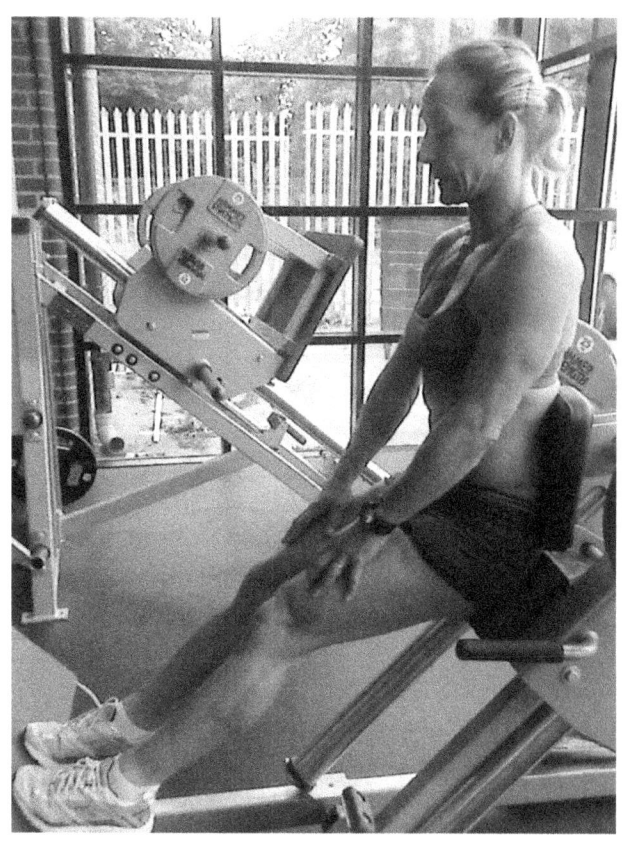

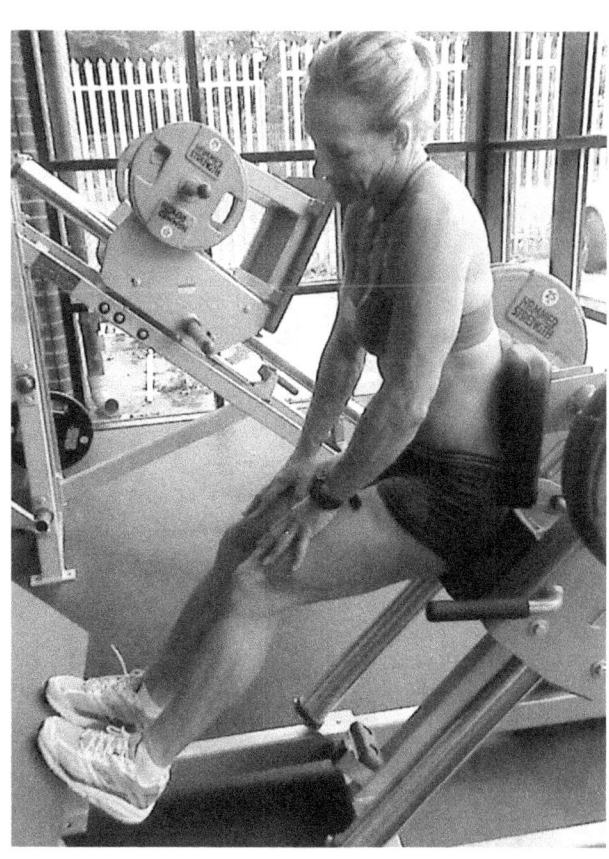

Dumbbell Squats

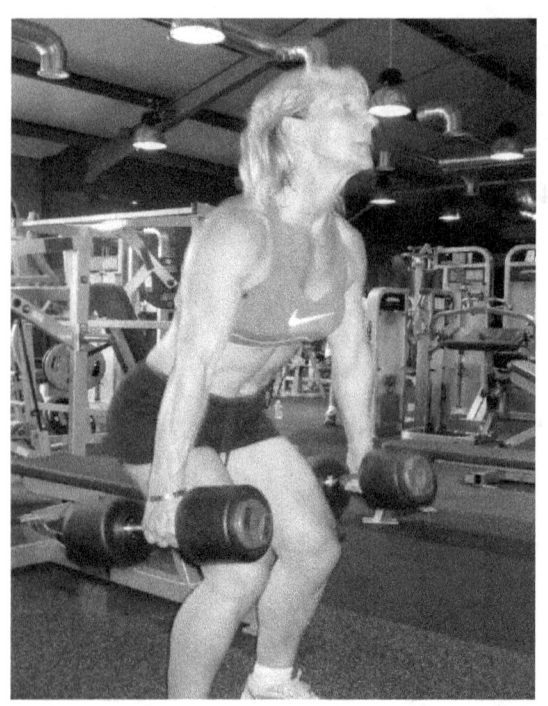

These could just as easily be called dumbbell sit downs. Any squatting movement can be thought of as just sitting down if it helps to give you that mental link to something familiar. Again good posture is of paramount importance. Your stance will need to be reasonably narrow to facilitate the path of the dumbbells. Feet flat on the floor at all times, initially just squat as far as you can comfortably, your range of motion will improve with practice. Ultimately you are aiming to go nice and deep as I demonstrate in the midpoint picture above. However you are working primarily your legs, so do not lean forward from the waist in order to go deeper. If you keep your eyes fixed on a point high on the wall or mirror in front of you, you will maintain the alignment

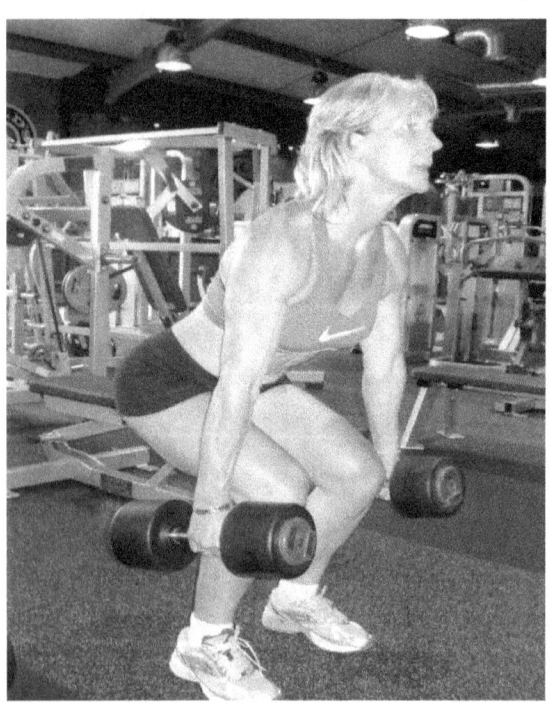

of your head thus keeping your chest high and back in the correct position. Just sit down and stand up. As with most leg work we are again aiming to achieve 15 reps per set. You will be very breathless as with most leg work, large muscle groups require much oxygen. Legs are hard work and that is why so many people tend to miss them out -

BACK

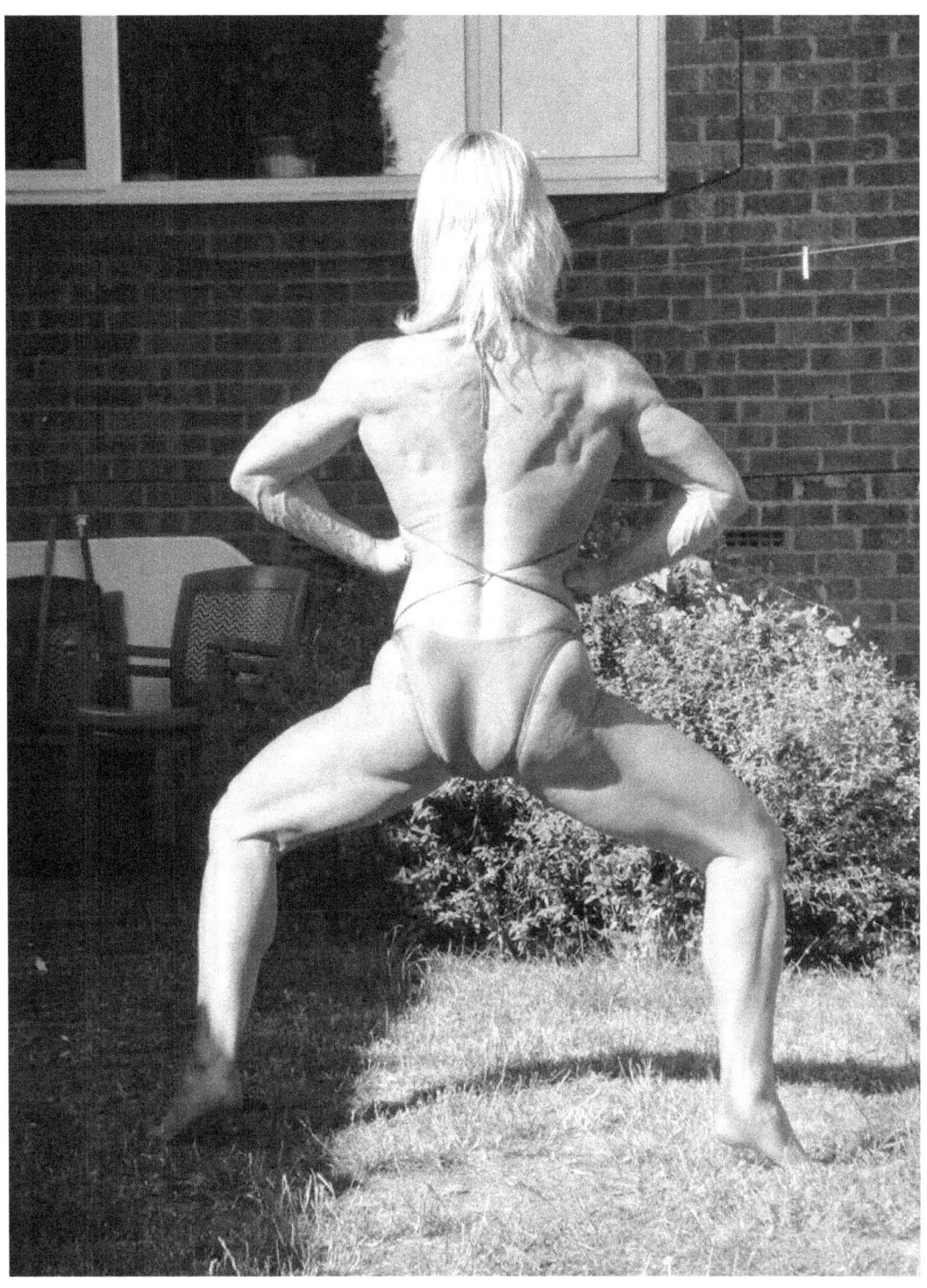

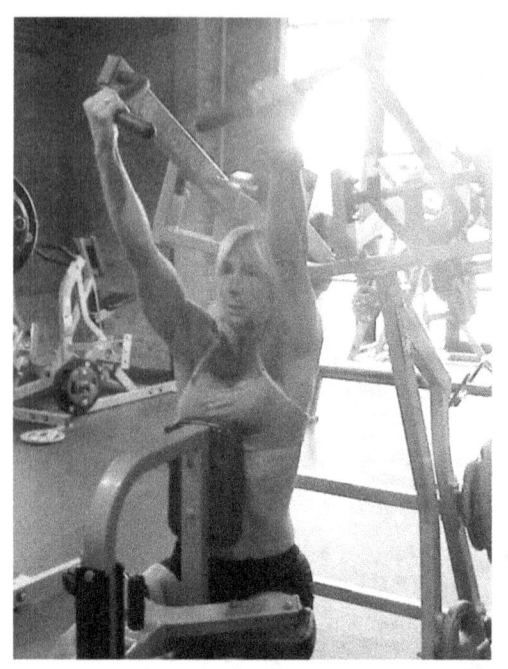

Hammer Pulldowns

Good posture here is your chest held high and your head in a neutral position, maintaining the natural curvature of your spine. The only motion should come from pulling your arms into your torso as you squeeze your shoulder blades together. Please remember absolutely no motion from your waist, no leaning backwards. You will notice your posture improving both in the gym and in everyday life, not the ridiculously exaggerated "I have a role of carpet under each arm" posture, but more the impressive slouch free, proud, graceful movement of a trained toned body. As usual start light and work up to a weight that really tests you without losing your form. If you cannot attain the Midpoint position that I have without leaning backwards the weight is too heavy.

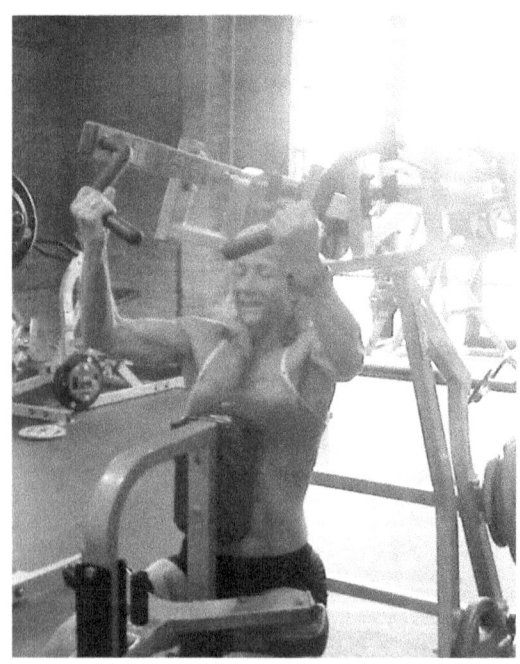

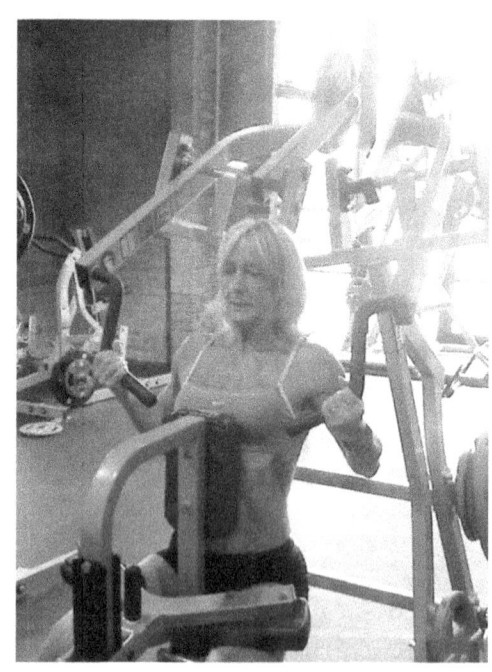

Wide grip Pulldowns to Front

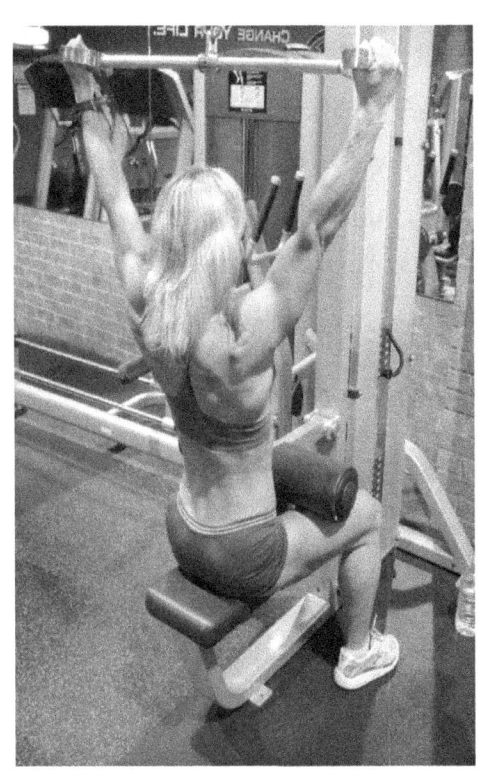

Do you remember when you were told to sit up straight as a child? Well that is exactly how you need to be when you are training your back in all seated exercises. Your chest held high and your head in a neutral position, maintaining the natural curvature of your spine. The only motion should come from pulling your arms into your torso as you squeeze your shoulder blades together. Please remember absolutely no motion from your waist, no leaning backwards. You will see many gym users swaying about whilst training back in order to facilitate using more weight, ignore their example and stick to what you know is correct form. You will notice your posture improving both in

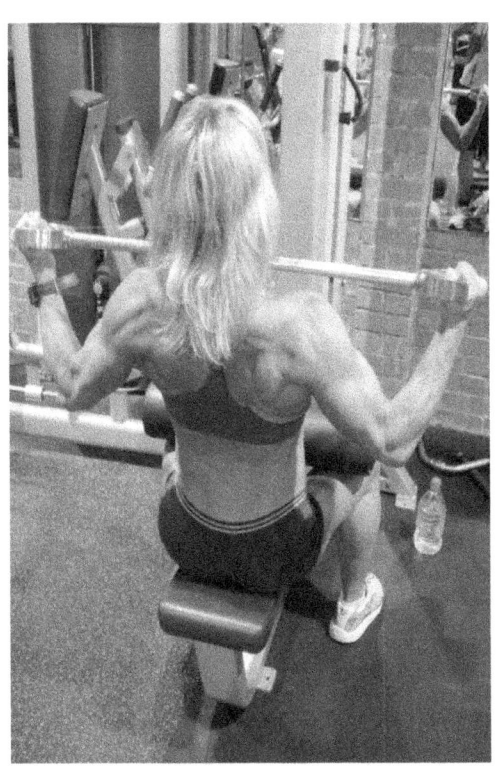

the gym and in everyday life, not the ridiculously exaggerated "I have a role of carpet under each arm" posture, but more the impressive slouch free, proud, graceful movement of a trained toned body. As usual start light and work up to a weight that really tests you without losing your form. If you cannot attain the Midpoint position that Julie has without leaning backwards the weight is quite simply too heavy.

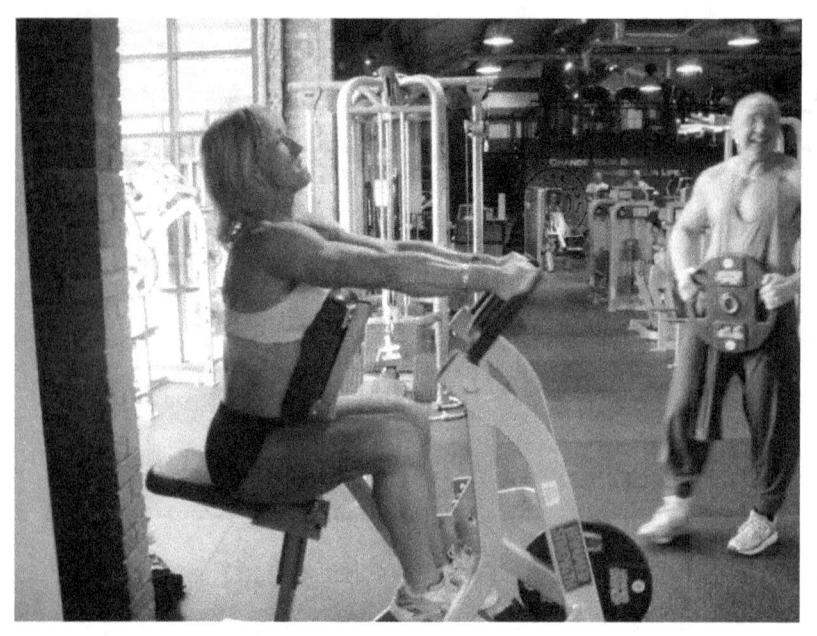

Seated Close grip Machine rows.

You will notice with back work that even though the angle of pull changes between rows and Pulldowns the position you need to maintain is identical. Do you remember when you were told to sit up straight as a child? Well that is exactly how you need to be when you are training your back in all seated exercises. Your chest held high and your head in a neutral position, maintaining the natural curvature of your spine. The only motion should come from pulling your arms into your torso as you squeeze your shoulder blades together. Please remember absolutely no motion from your waist, no leaning backwards.   You will notice your posture improving both in the gym and in everyday life. As usual start light and work up to a weight that really tests you without losing your form. If you cannot attain the Midpoint position pictured below without leaning backwards the weight is quite simply too heavy.

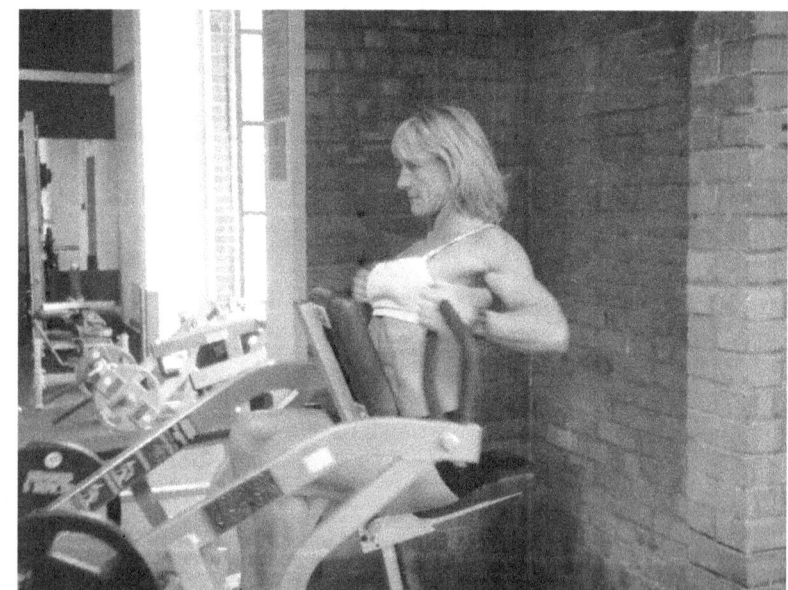

Palms up, close grip Pulldowns

Do you remember when you were told to sit up straight as a child? Well that is exactly how you need to be when you are training your back in all seated exercises. Your chest held high and your head in a neutral position, maintaining the natural curvature of your spine. The only motion should come from pulling your arms into your torso as you squeeze your shoulder blades together. Please remember absolutely no motion from your waist, no leaning backwards. You will notice your posture improving both in the gym and in everyday life. As usual start light and work up to a weight that really tests you without losing your form. If you cannot attain the Midpoint position that Julie has in the bottom picture without leaning backwards the weight is quite simply too heavy.

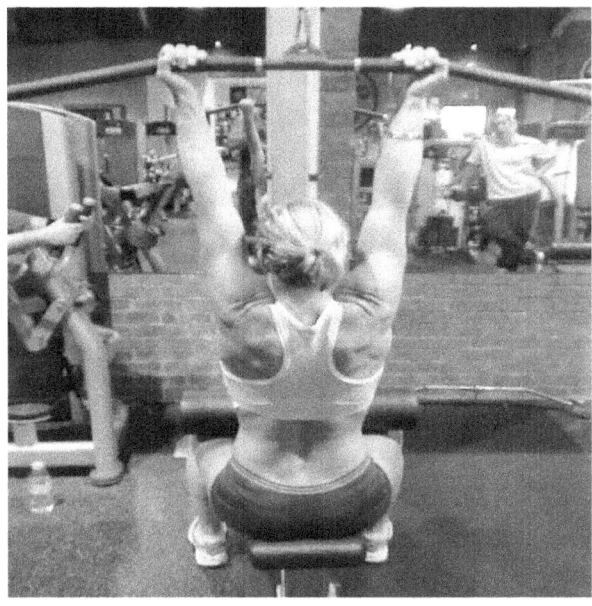

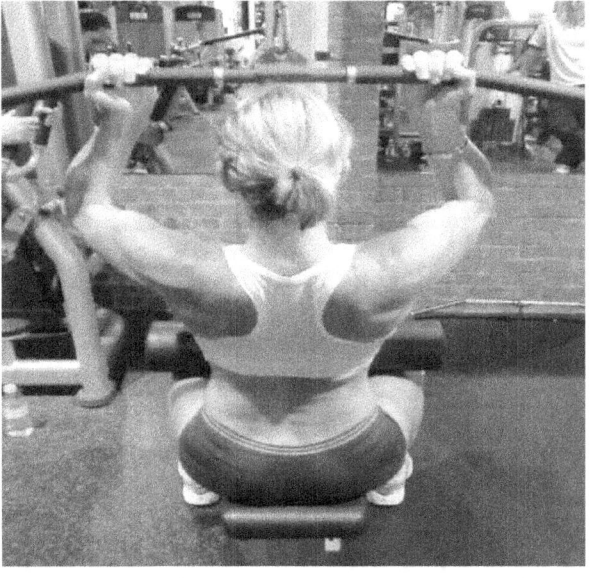

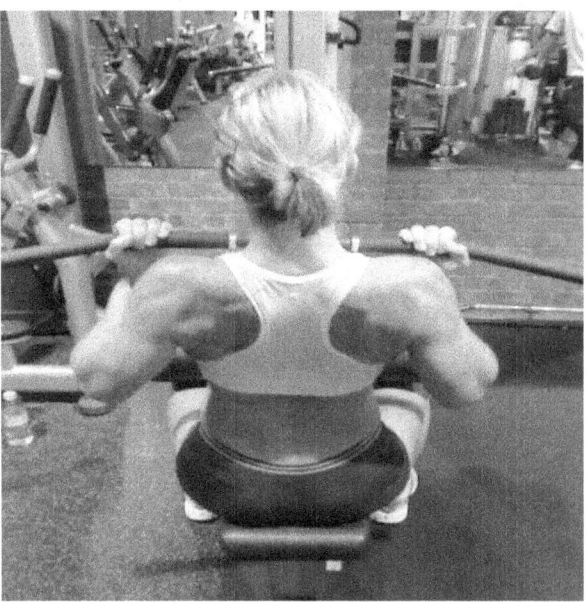

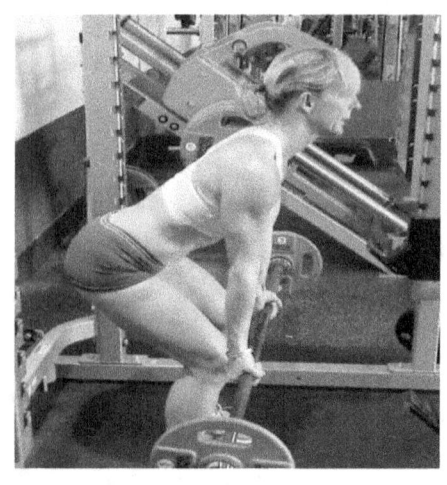

Palms up-Bent over - Barbell Rows.

As with Deadlifts I can't stress enough the importance of a good strong

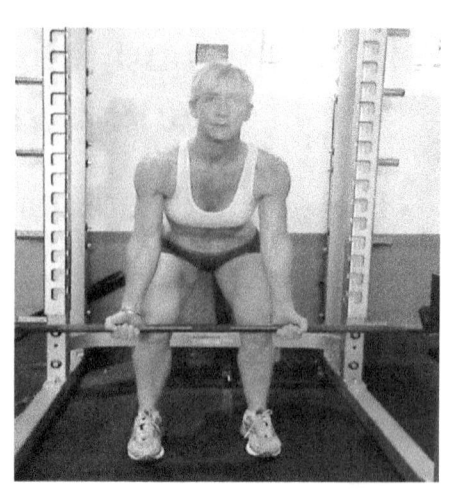

exercise starting position, with rows you will need to hold your position throughout the set. Julie holds this position she does not let the weight pull her down or swing backwards to assist the lift. One moment of carelessness or mis-placed bravado and you are hurt. Certain exercise are unforgiving if you abuse them, this is one such exercise. A nice smooth rhythm, fully extending the arms at the bottom and squeezing your shoulder blades together at the top will yield optimum results. This is one of the exercises that will build you a great core strength base if worked correctly. Basic Squats, deadlifts, Rows, Presses, curls, dips and pull-ups will create a great foundation for any fitness or physique goal. Remember in the early days of strength training there were none of the "fancy" machines available today and yet the physiques were

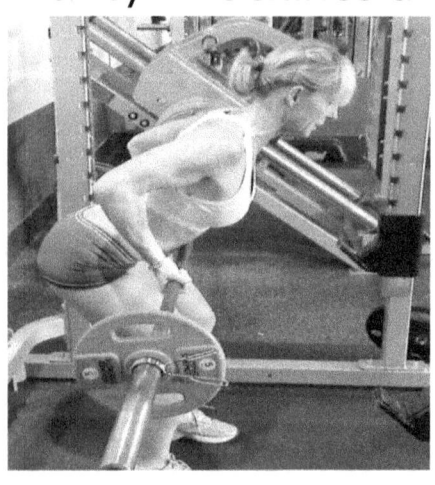

outstanding. Work the basics hard with strict form and you will succeed.

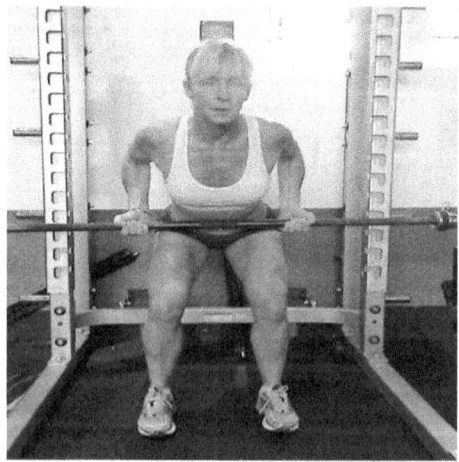

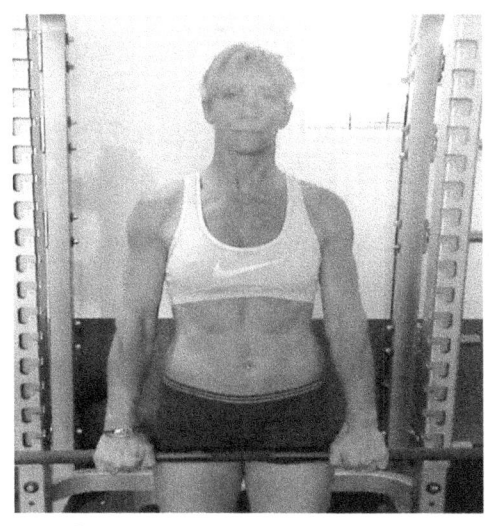

Barbell Shrugs

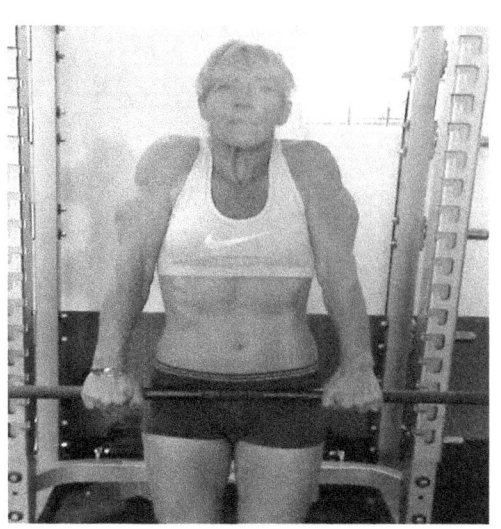

Shrugs are a trapezius exercise and not an exercise that we do very often at all in fact we do no direct trap work, relying on our back and shoulder work to give us enough trap stimulation. However many trainers do incorporate them into workouts and they do seem to be a favourite of many. Julie is demonstrating them admirably just stand straight and shrug your shoulders keeping your arms and body still, you can shrug up rotate your shoulders back and then down but it is not essential. One word of caution here if developed to much your traps can give the illusion that you have no neck, you may have seen powerlifters and Olympic lifters with massive traps giving the illusion of having lost their neck. Also big traps an make you look round shouldered and detract from your shoulder width. I think the answer is work them in moderation and you will be fine.

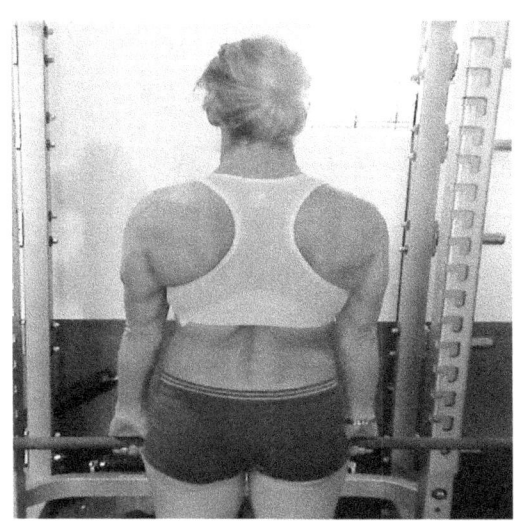

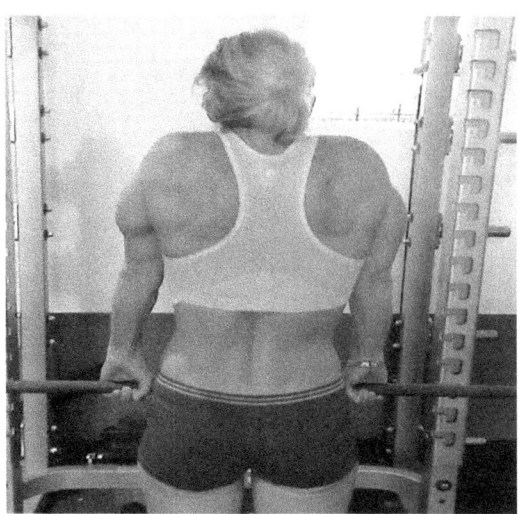

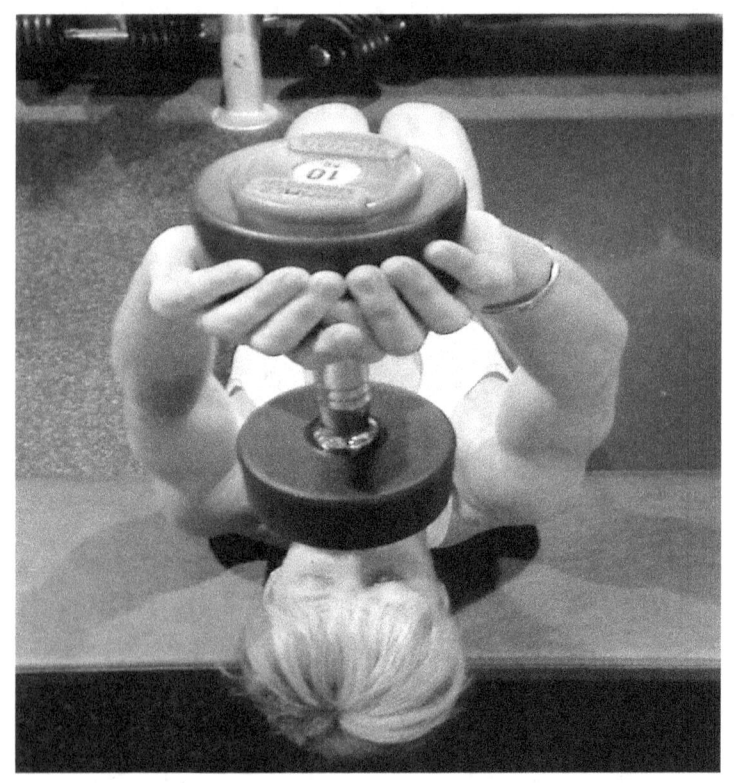

Across Bench Pullovers

Dumbbell pullovers are an exercise that doesn't really fall under any body part, we use them in back workouts but I know some trainers use them in Chest and some don't do them because they are not really specific enough for them. Many trainers want to know exactly what they are getting for their efforts. I have always liked them, I first did them 35 years ago. They partially work the chest and for me mostly back but again only partially, add to this an incredible stretch right

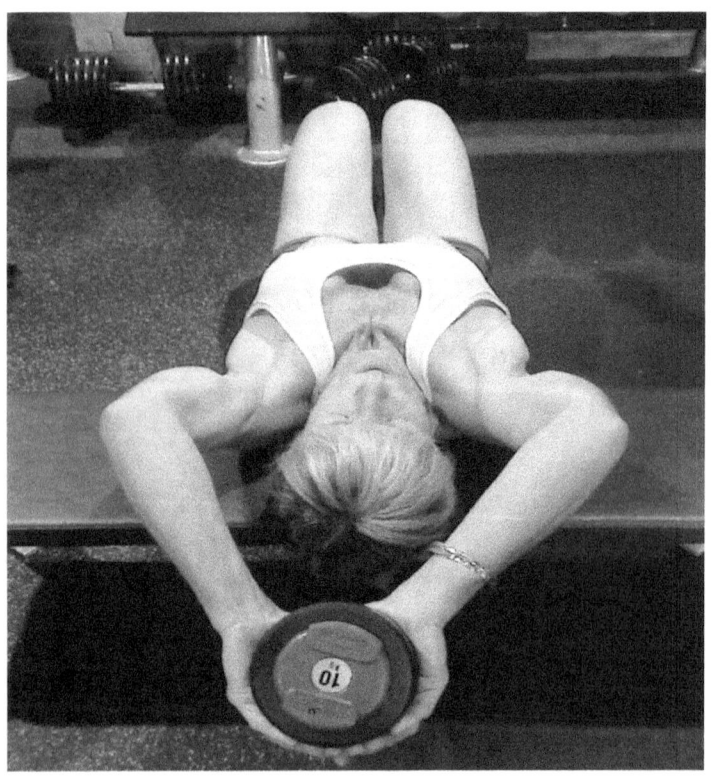

through your torso and for me they are worth doing. Pullovers finish for back where straight arm Pulldowns begin. Always get somebody to hand you the weight, keep your hips down low almost on your heels all the time and mind your head.

Good Form – Stay Safe!!

Deadlifts

We have included Deadlifts in the back section but could just as well have included it in with the leg exercises. Deadlifts are a great compound exercise, working many body parts and when performed well they are a great addition to any workout. You will feel them mostly down quite low on your back and as such ultimate respect has to be played to your form and function. Sloppy form will eventually result in injury and an injured lower back is not top of anybodies Xmas list. However, good form and a progressive approach to adding weight will strengthen your lower back and make any problems with low back far less likely in your life. Adopting the starting position Julie has above allows you to ease, not jerk the weight from the floor using legs and back in synchronicity. The lowering is also done in controlled fashion. We recommend you don't use deadlifts

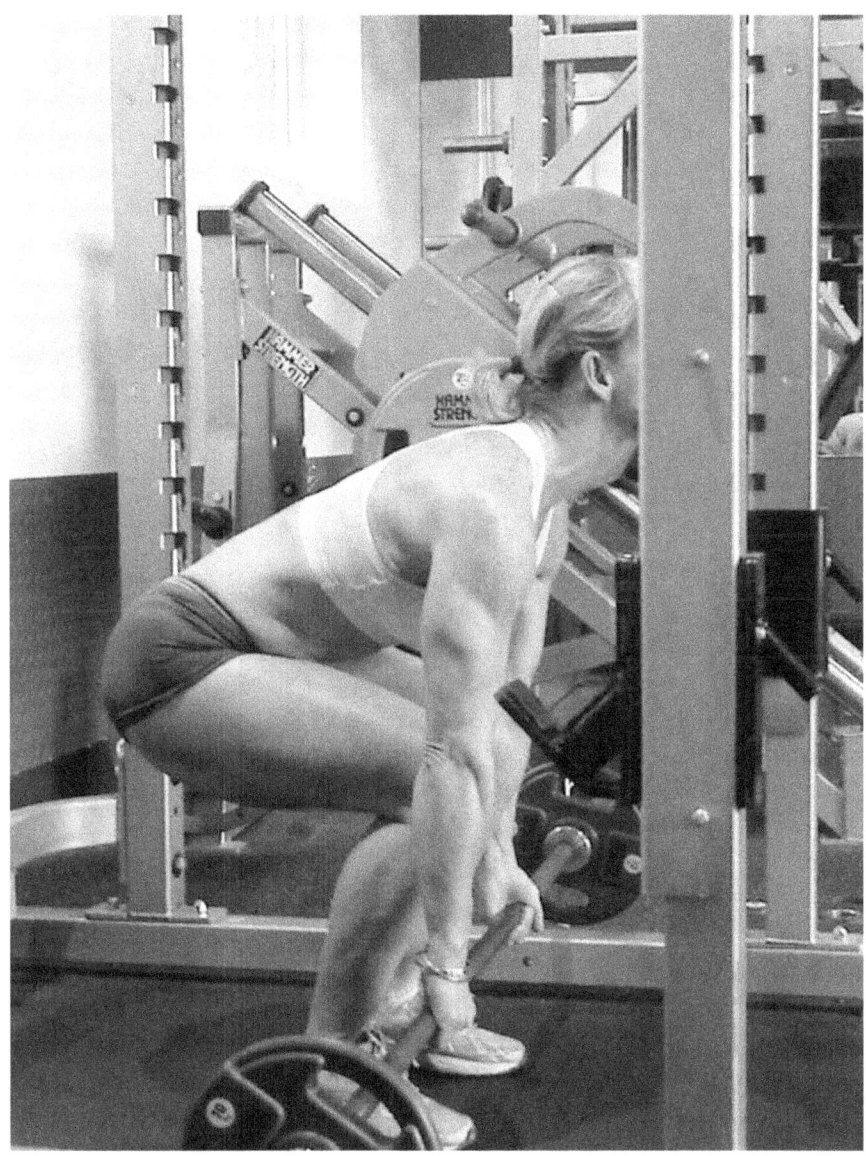

to show how strong you are and stick to about 8/12 reps per set any lower reps and you begin to get into the realms of powerlifting and hardcore bodybuilding, if this is your chosen path then your training will become more high risk as a matter of course. For the rest of us mere mortals 3/5 sets of 8/12 reps with a challenging weight will fit the bill perfectly. Many casual trainers avoid deadlifts as they are very hard work and "only for the big guys" but with care they are well worth the effort for all of us.

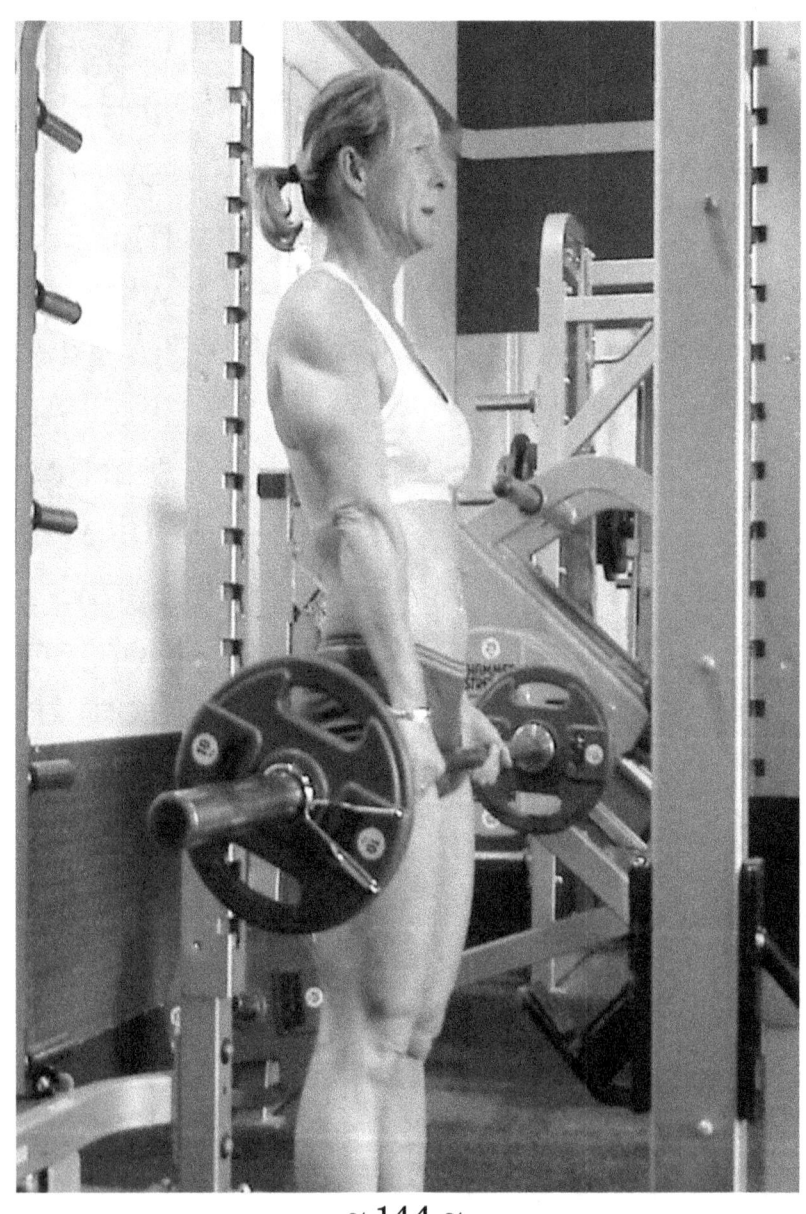

Pull Ups

With Pull-ups you can use many different grips and you may do them with bodyweight, bodyweight added,(by way of a belt around your waist with weight attached) or assisted. They may also be performed, assisted by kneeling on a pad of the machine which supports 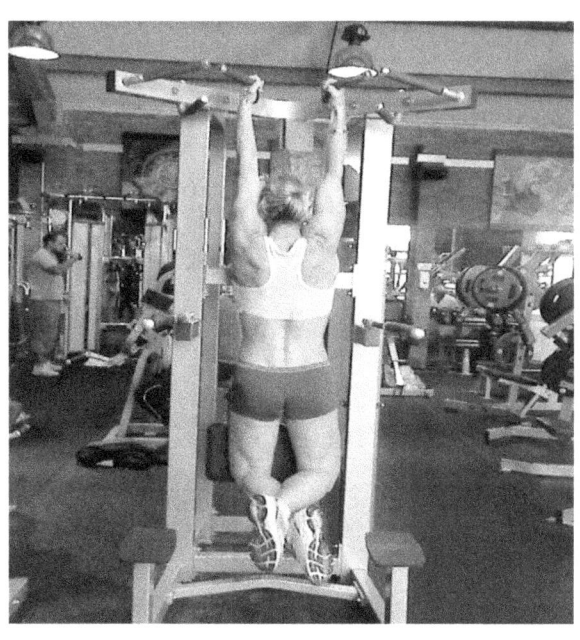 some bodyweight. Julie is using bodyweight. Pull-ups are a great exercise for your Lats (wings) and also work your biceps to quite a large degree. Pull-ups are a challenge and many people start at 1 or 2 and add reps on each visit or weekly. They are suited as most weight training is to people with short levers, you will see short people firing out many reps and tall folk squirming around just to get half a dozen. Pulldown machines evolved from pull-ups and make it possible for all shapes and sizes to get the benefit of this productive movement. At 18 and a half stone and 6'4" I hate them, but still do them occasionally just for a change. Pull-ups are responsible for many a guys V shape. A very good exercise.

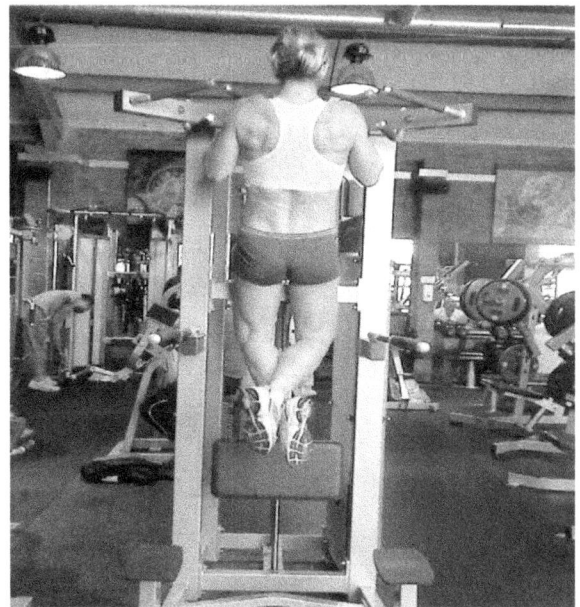

Good Form – Stay Safe!!

Angled Straight Arm Pulldowns

Once again in straight arm Pulldowns our back will work in pulling our arms into our torso, this time straight and around the shoulder joint. An angled position of as much as 45% is fine, hold the body position throughout the set. We work this set with either dumbbell or machine pullovers very often as this exercise starts where pullovers finish off. A great side effect is that holding this position 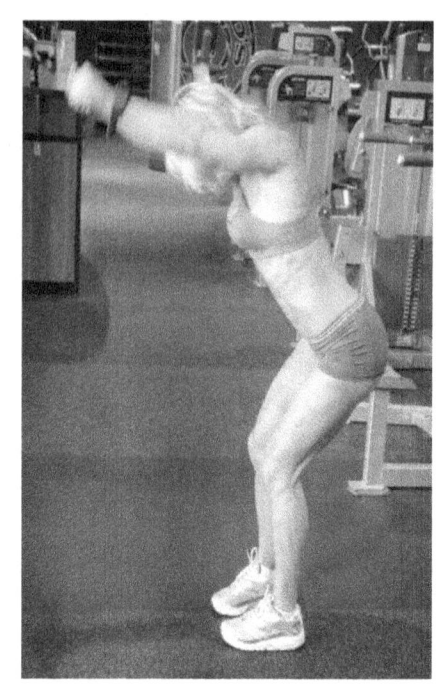 also works your abdominals very well in stabilising your body. Start light and really work to get your form spot on before adding much weight. You will have to work to maintain form as you move through the exercise and much of your body is involved in maintaining your posture. This is not an exercise where you will be able to use heavy weights, slightly higher reps 15/20 with immaculate form is the way to go with this one, really concentrate on your Lats as you work and you will feel the benefit. The start position Julie adopts has the weight taken up from the stack by about an inch, taking the strain and ready to go. This may take a while to master but a great exercise so worth the perseverance. Under no circumstances let too heavy a weight affect your being anchored in perfect form.

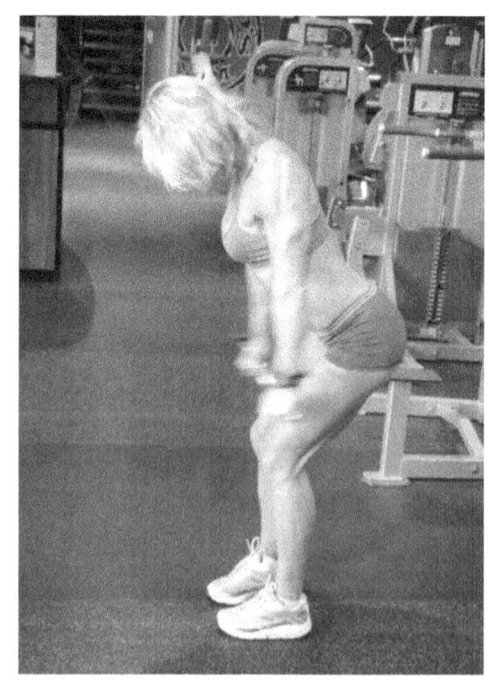

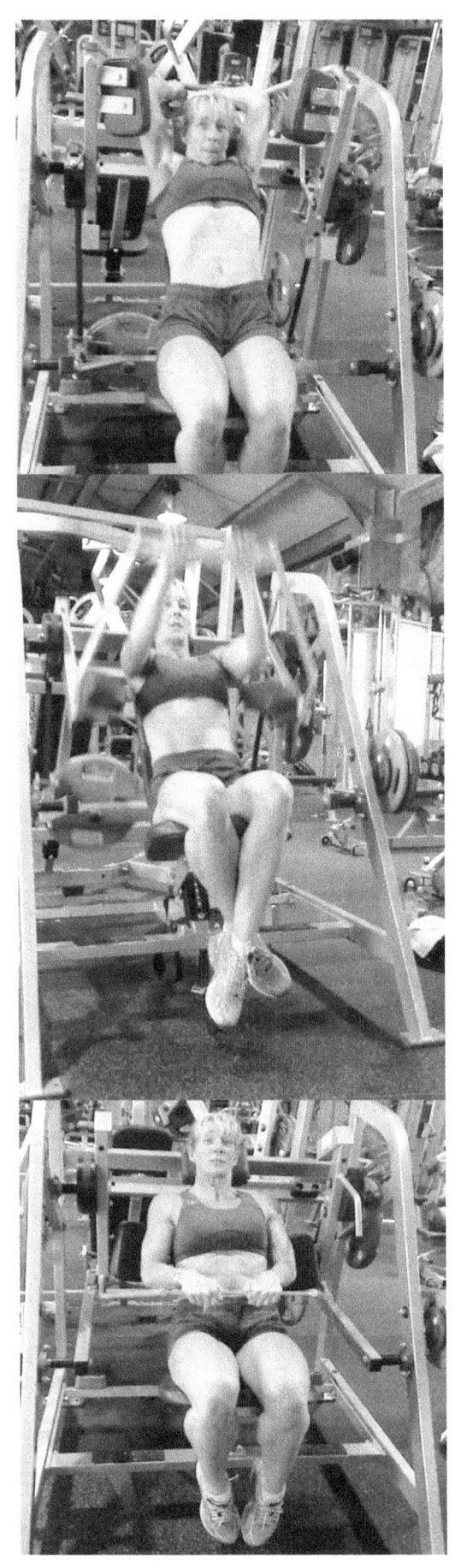

Hammer Machine Pullovers

Unlike Dumbbell Pullovers, Machine Pullovers are more of a complete exercise for your Lats (back) as from this seated position the tension remains with you until you hands are into your waist. On the machine we use and there are differing designs we load the weight at the back and there are pads to rest your elbows against, we tend not to use the pads as keeping the arms free just feels right for us. There is an adjustment at the seat and I suggest you take some time the first time you use any machine in order that you get the best position for your build. With pullovers taking a deep breath as you stretch up enables good expansion and stretch of the rib cage. At a young age this may result in a permanently larger chest cavity, however as you get older it is just a damn good torso stretch.

Good Form – Stay Safe!!

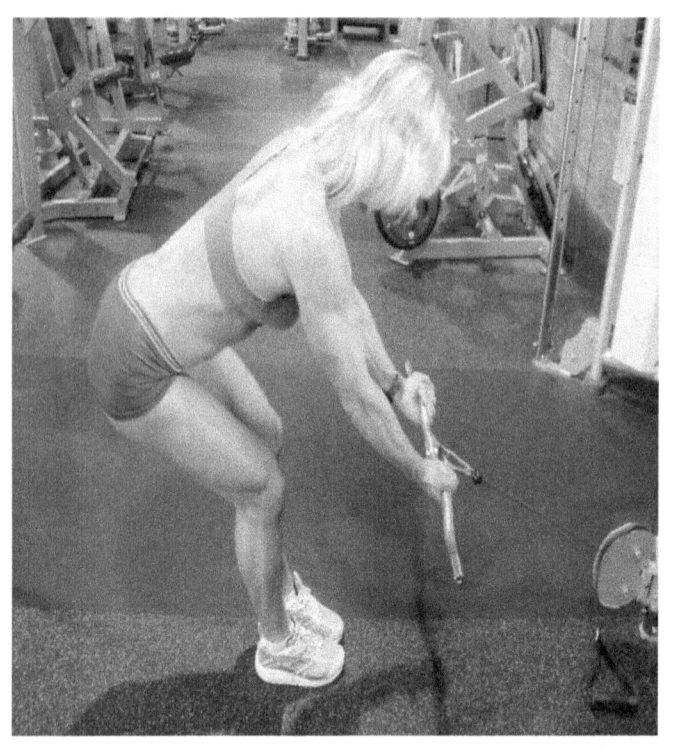

Bent over Low Pulley Row

As with Deadlifts I can't stress enough the importance of a good strong exercise starting position, with rows you will need to hold your position throughout the set. One moment of carelessness or mis-placed bravado and you are hurt. Certain exercise are unforgiving if you abuse them, this is one such exercise. A nice smooth rhythm, fully extending the arms at the bottom and squeezing your shoulder blades together at the top will yield optimum results. We suggest slightly higher reps 12/15 on bent-over low pulley rows than other basic rows and also make the most of the stretch the pulley allows

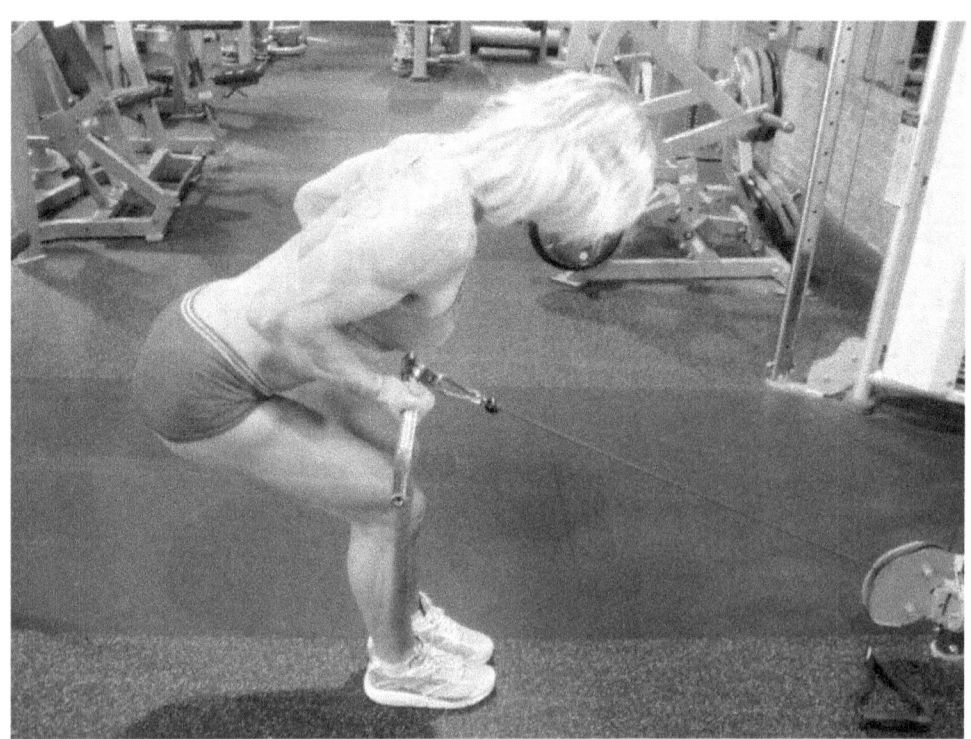

at the bottom. We work until we feel that we are losing form and then end that set. Work the basics hard with strict form and you will succeed.

Seated Pulley Row

Seated low pulley rowing enables you to use more weight than the bent over version as your body is anchored by your feet being against the plates. We need absolute minimal

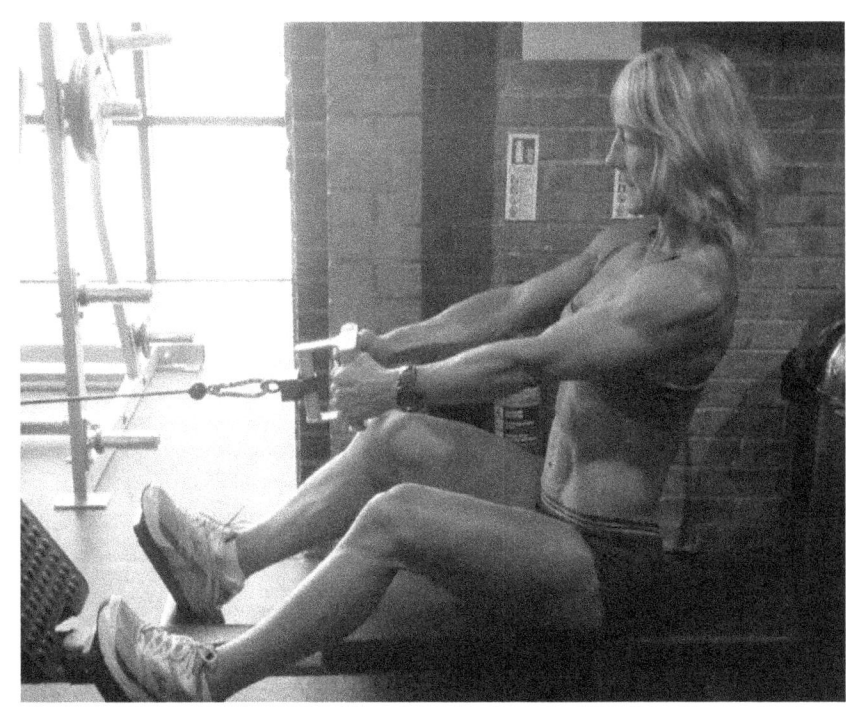

movement from the waist please as we are looking for a stretch from the Lats and upper back and not a bend forward from the waist. Sit up straight keeping your chest high and again aim to squeeze your shoulder blades together at the top or midpoint of the movement. There are many bars and different grips you will see used, maybe you can experiment a little to find what suits you best or even better change your grip every once in a while. Taking the strain for the first rep can be a little awkward but start light and you will get used to the equipment.

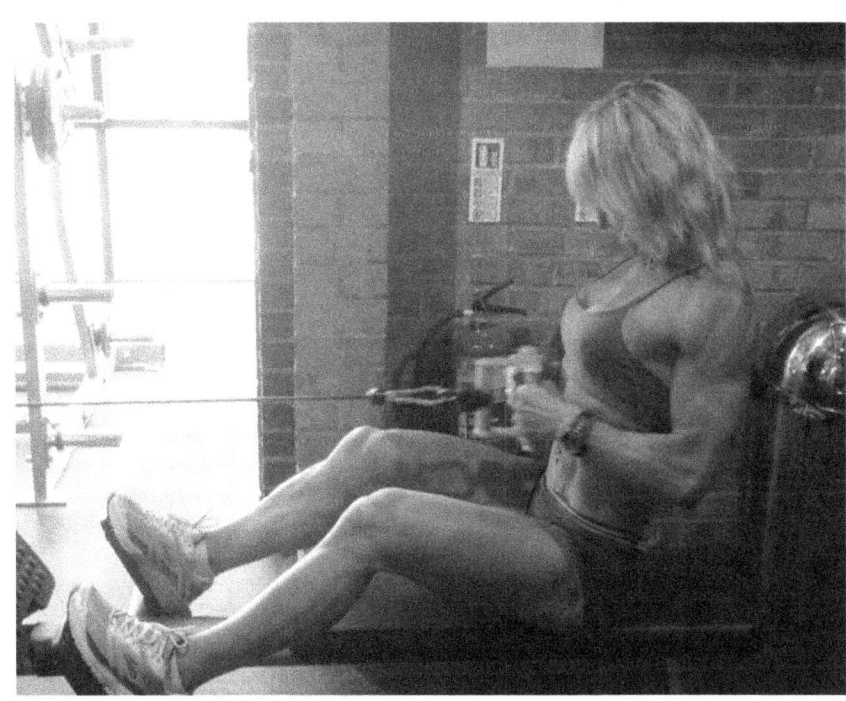

Single Arm Dumbbell Row

The use of a bench here enables you to keep very good form. Once again you can see Julie has a great back position and posture. As much as possible attempt

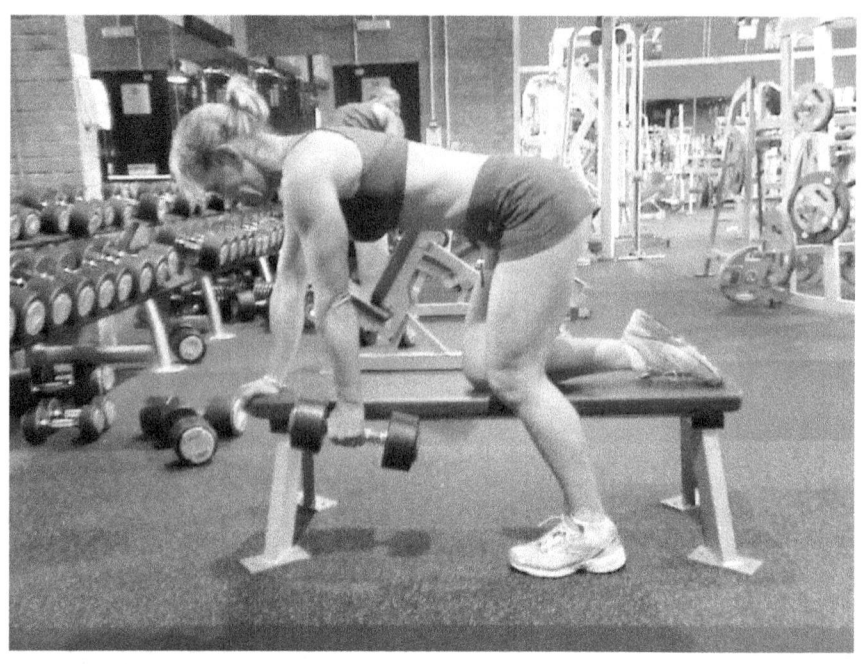

to keep your shoulders square to the floor when you row, the temptation is to twist at the waist as you pull up, resist this. Keep your Shoulders square, stretch at the bottom and squeeze at the top, almost as though you are sawing a piece of wood. A nice rhythmic set. To change arms either face the same way and step over the bench swapping arms and legs or turn around and face the other way. You probably think that is obvious but I have seen many novices turning

around all over the place and just working the same arm in a different position. You should alternate between left and right arms using the 8/12 rep range for each set.

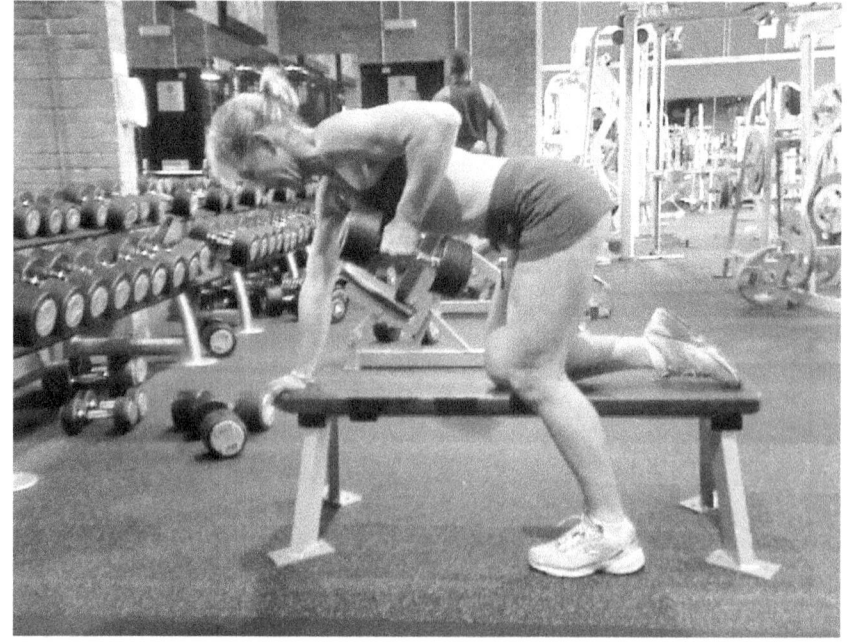

CHEST

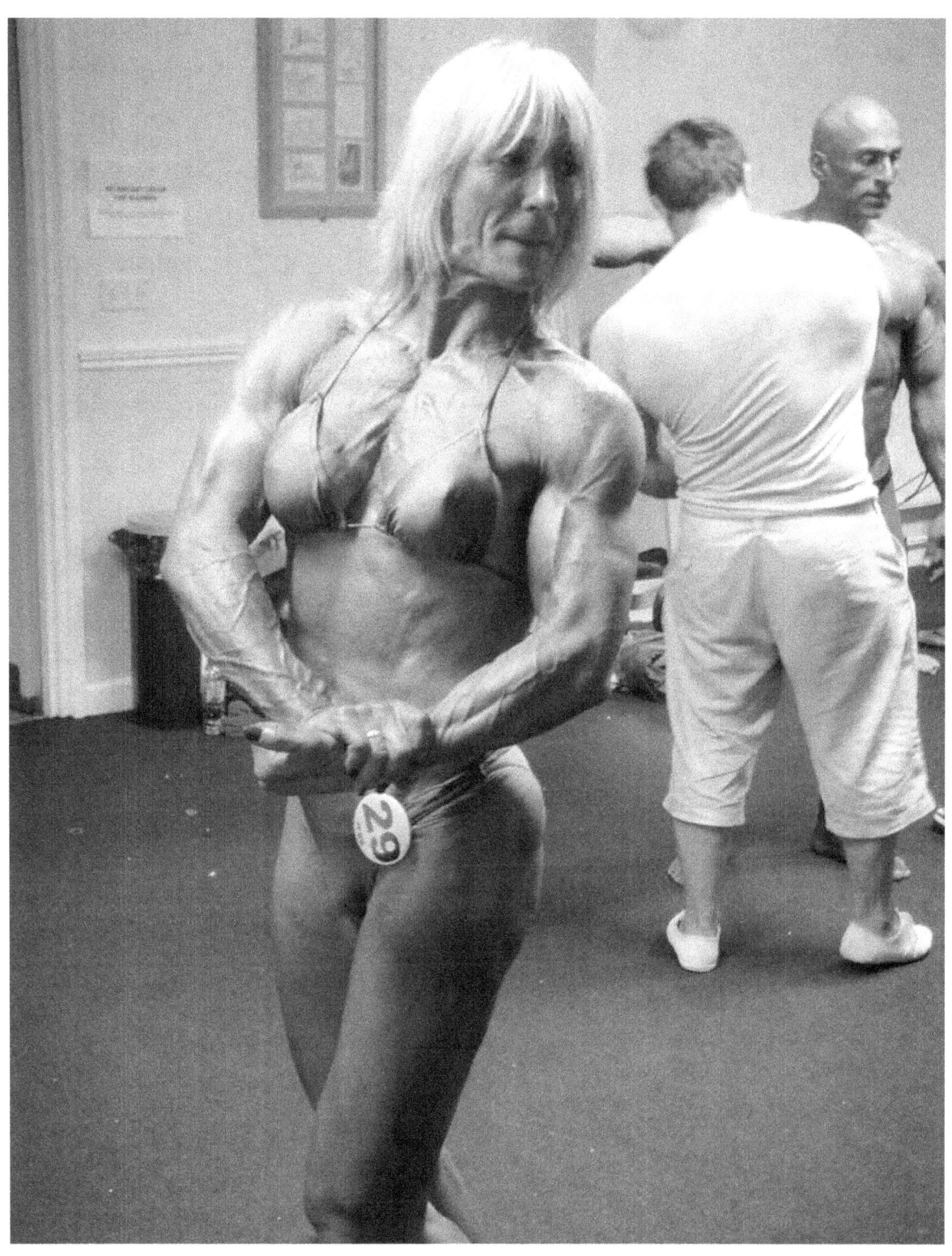

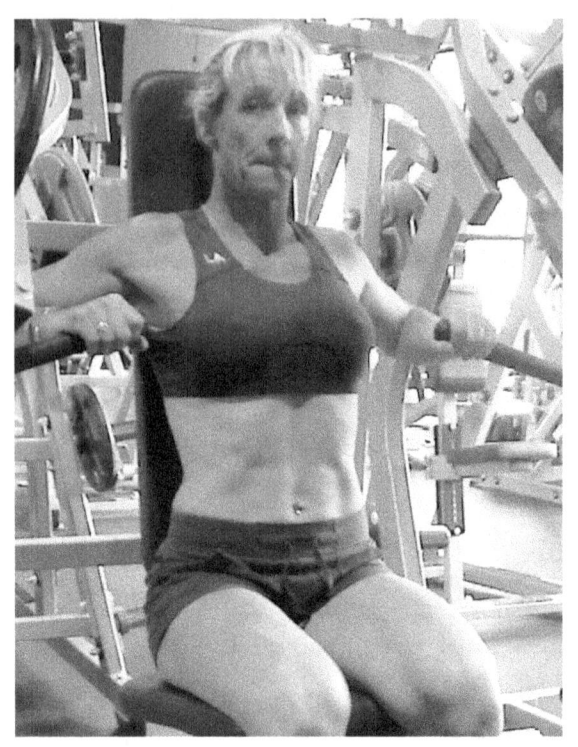

Hammer Chest Press

You will see from this gallery there are a great number of exercises and much variety for all body parts. Without entering into a debate about which are the best and worst, accepting that synchronising free weights works slightly more muscle groups in a single exercise I think it is fair to say that any exercise is better than none and each has its individual merits. At Gold's we have a lot of hammer equipment and whilst it is large and intimidating it is good to use and over time we are glad of the variety. The choices allow for change and that stimulates our workouts to keep them fresh. Most chest work as you will see is variations of either hugging towards or pushing away from

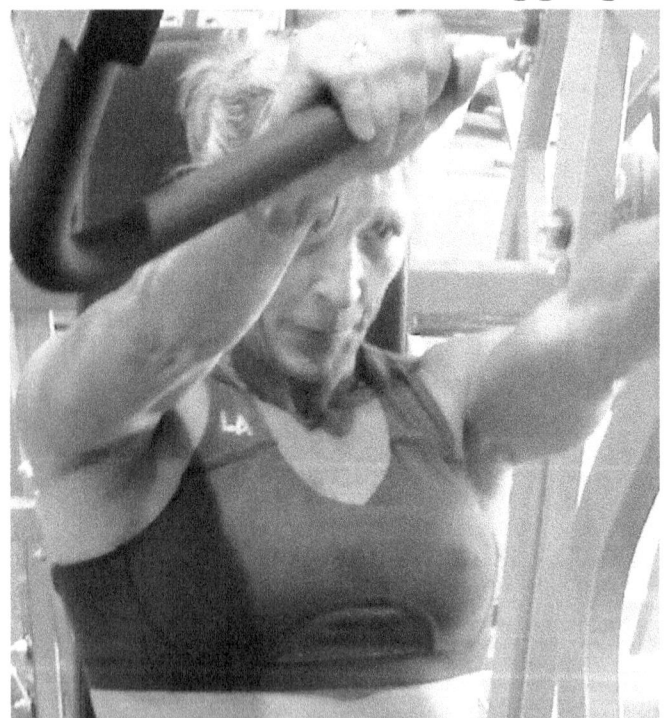

your torso, the angles change but that is just about the gist of it. You may have noticed I like to over simplify but I have discovered very few people are really bothered about the biomechanical details of how, as long as exercises work "the bit" they want to work.

Vertical Chest Press

I worked chest today and I combined it with my cardio for a quick paced change. I began with 5 minutes on the cross trainer, which is my favourite cardio machine of the moment although experience tells me that will change. I followed that with 4 intense sets on the pectoral Flye machine increasing the weight each set. I moved next to another 5 minutes on the crosstrainer. My next chest exercise was Hammer chest

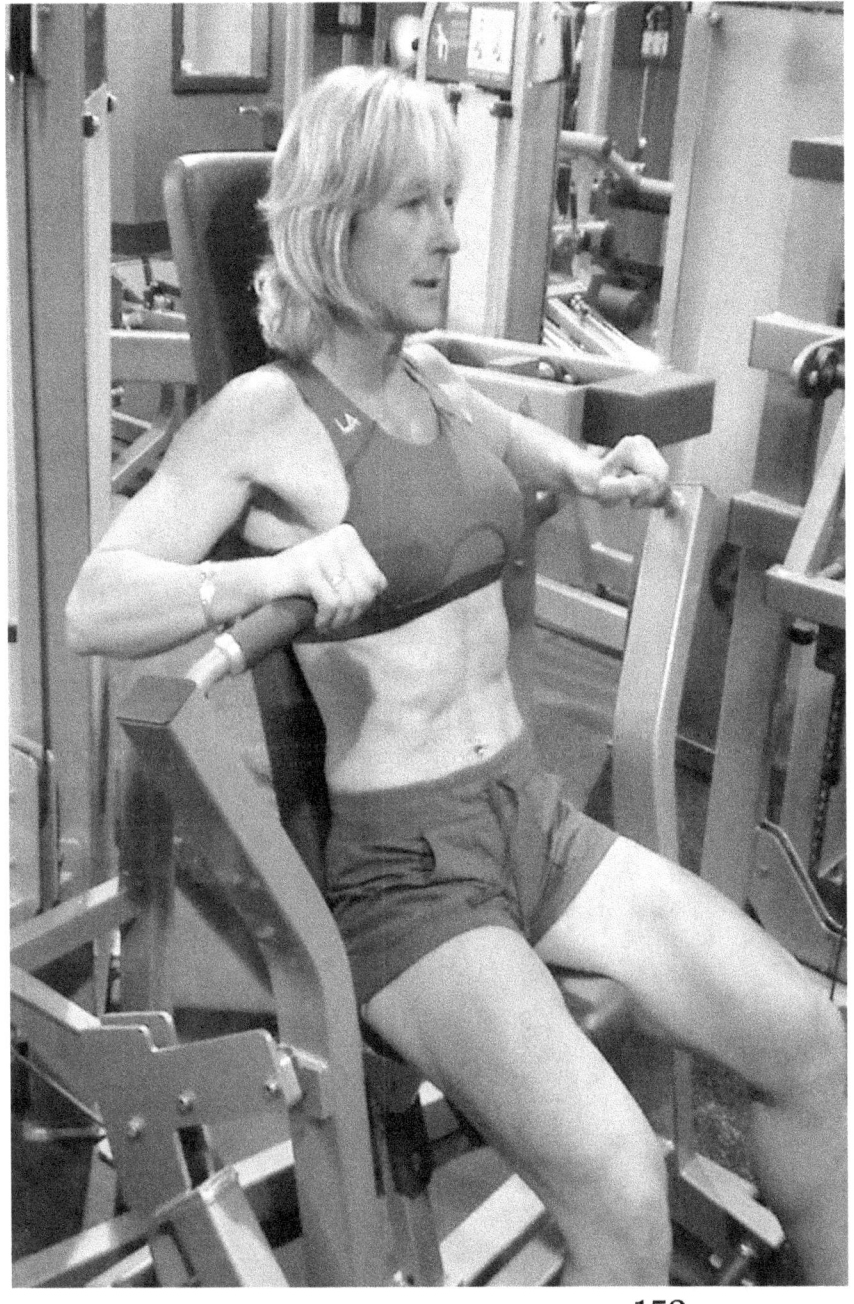

press, again performing 4 sets increasing the weight each set and resting only 60 seconds between sets. You guessed it another 5 minutes cardio followed. My third chest exercise was inclined dumbbell Flyes, just 3 sets of these with the same format increasing weight each set and resting no more than 60 seconds. Dum Dee Dum! Yep back to the cardio for another 5 minutes.

My fourth exercise for chest was seated selectorised chest press for a further 3 sets in the same manner. Back for my last 5 minutes on the cross trainer before finishing with 3 sets of press ups with my feet elevated on a flat bench. Ok I hear you say, sell that one to me. For us this workout ensures an elevated heart rate all the way through the workout, an important point for cardio fitness. The workout also breaks up the cardio into nice manageable pieces. As for the chest

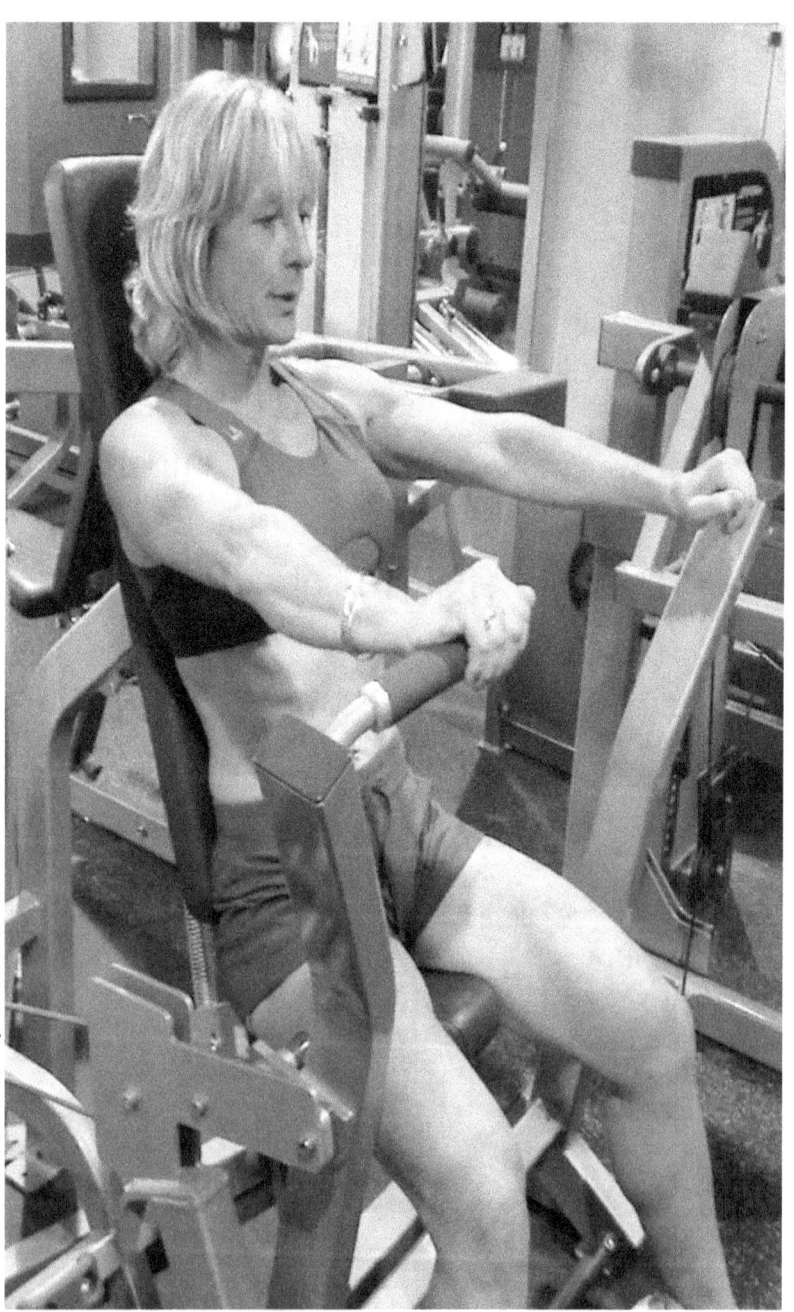

work the cardio breaks allow for enough recovery time to keep your weights up and work your chest thoroughly. The exercises you choose do have to lend themselves to quick and convenient completion of you sets. The entire workout takes about 45 minutes plus stretching time. I finished my entire workout in the time one group of guys spent on just one exercise - bench pressing.

Machine Assisted Dips

Dips are not an exercise that everyone can do without a little help, particularly if you are heavy, have long limbs or both. Luckily most gyms these days have a chin/dip assist machine such as the one pictured. This allows you to kneel on a pad and perform the exercise assisted by a selectorised weight stack. It is a great goal to target being able to dip unassisted. I remember when Julie couldn't do any dips without assistance. Now she adds weight by way of a dipping belt to increase her intensity. Fit happens! with perseverance and good consistent habits. When performing dips it is important to control your decent at all times, there is nothing to be

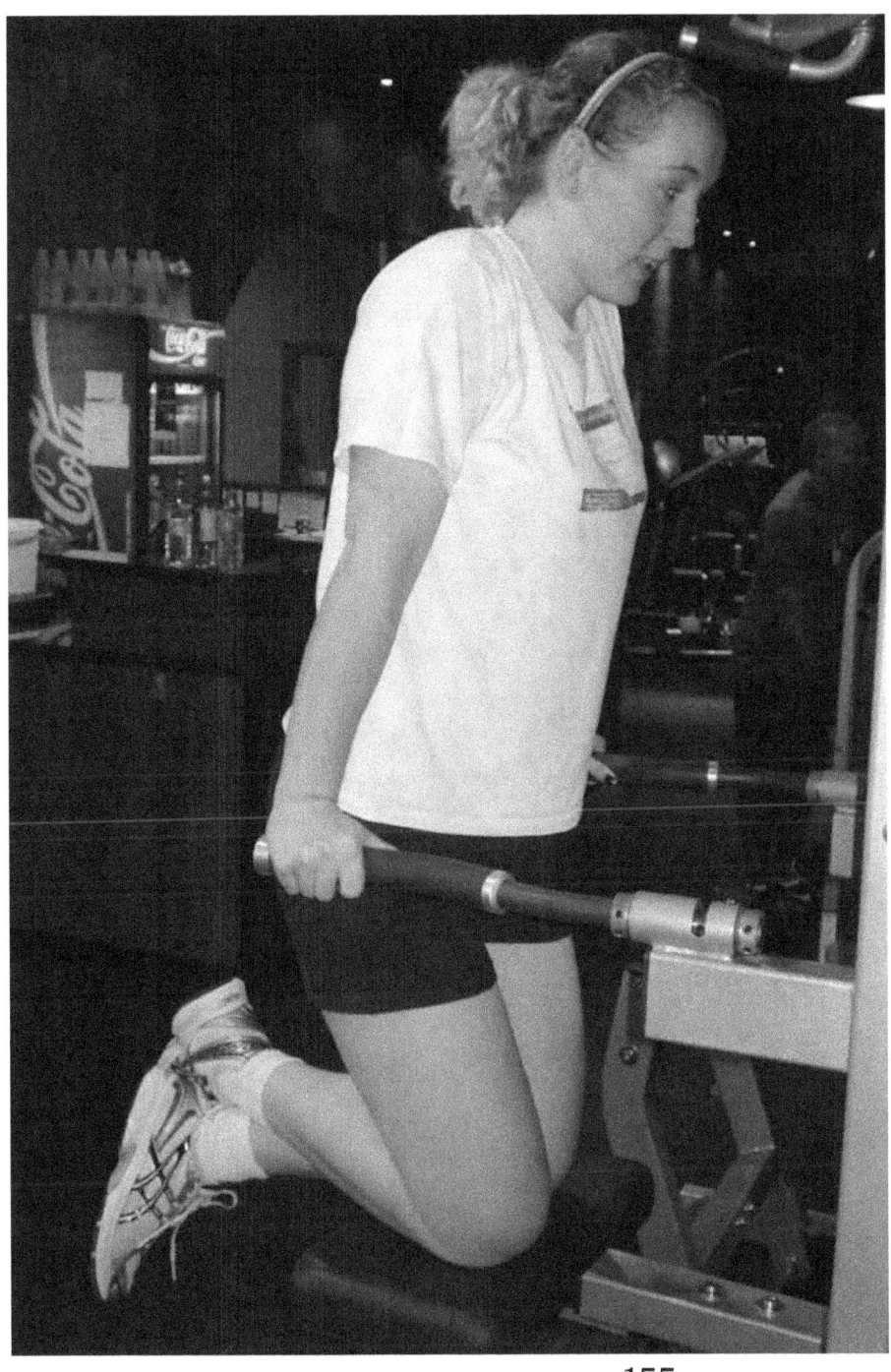

gained except injury by allowing yourself to plummet and then attempting to bounce back up. Dips heavily involve the triceps and shoulders and when combined with pull ups would be considered as a great upper body workout in true push /pull fashion. Initially at least it is wise to include dips early in your chest workout whilst you are fresh and your strength is at optimal levels. Lowering slowly and then driving back to full extension, keeping your body from swaying and rocking too much. Dips will take a little while to master but they are well worth the effort. A great upper body exercise, but with a high injury risk factor, please proceed with caution. The young lady in this picture is our youngest daughter, Shaunie.

Bodyweight Dips

A quick word on breathing may be in order here. It is important to breathe freely but not to get hung up on the technique. Worrying too much can cause a problem where there are none. My tip here would be to count your reps as that generally helps the novice to breathe correctly. In the picture above you can clearly see that Julie breathes out as she extends to midpoint lockout. Julie will count each rep at

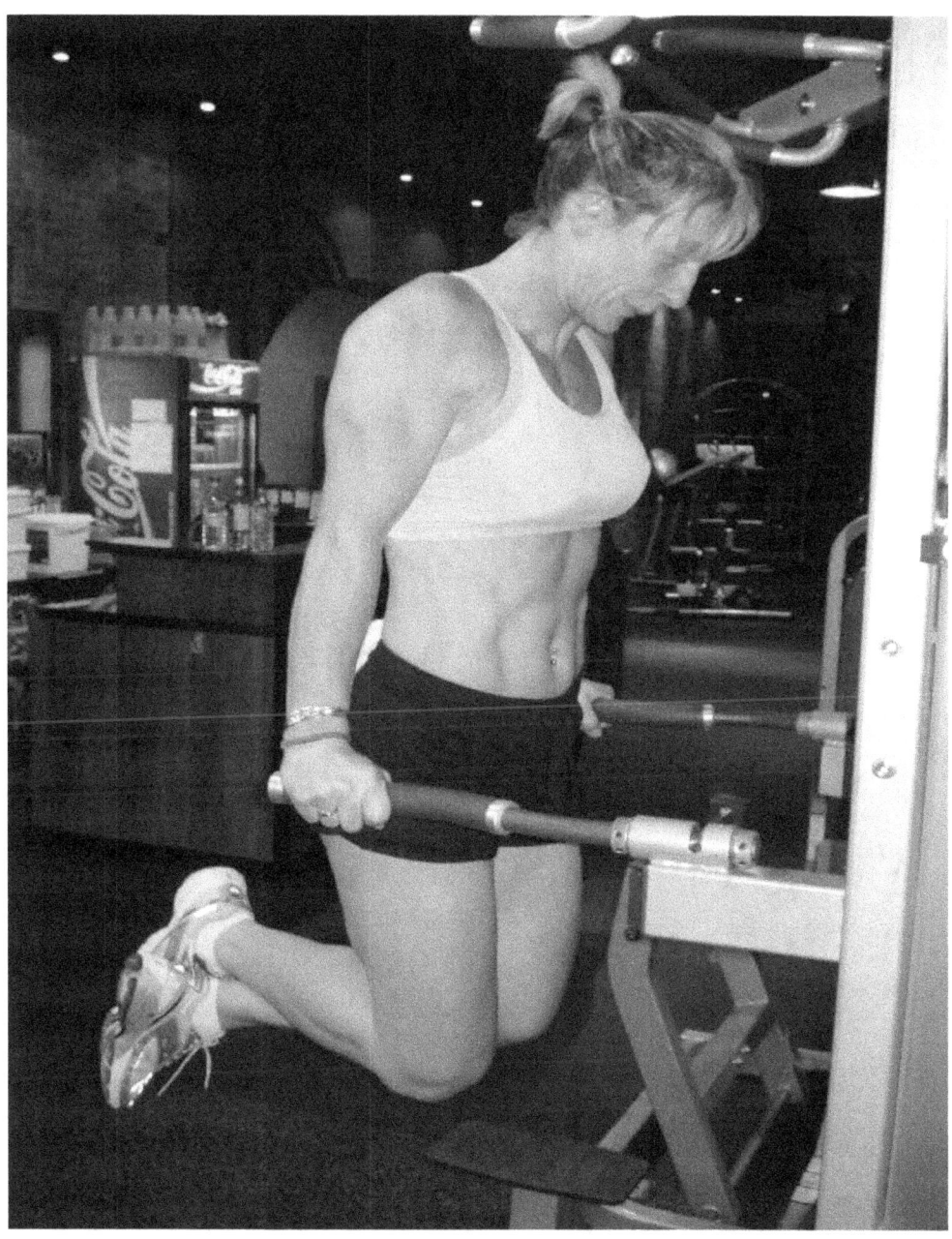

the conclusion of this position. The exercise tempo is controlled without being artificially slow. Most trainers and that includes you, will have a tempo and breathing rate they are naturally comfortable with, that is the tempo you should embrace.

Your tempo will slow toward the end of the set as you tire and the reps become harder to complete but there should still be a natural feel to the breathing and reps. At no time should you be gasping and trying to remember whether you need to breathe in or out. Just relax count those reps and go with your natural flow. Never hold your breath. Very soon your breathing and tempo will be imprinted on your subconscious and you will not have to think about it at all. Remember when you first learned to drive how awkward it felt and you had to think about everything, then one day it all came naturally and your subconscious did it all for you. Weight training is the same, it all feels awkward for a while and then one day it doesn't and it all happens much quicker than it did for driving.

Press Ups

When performing press ups there are a wide range of positions that will suit all strength levels. Elevating your upper body makes the exercise easier whilst going flat or even elevating your fit on a bench is more advanced. It is important to find the

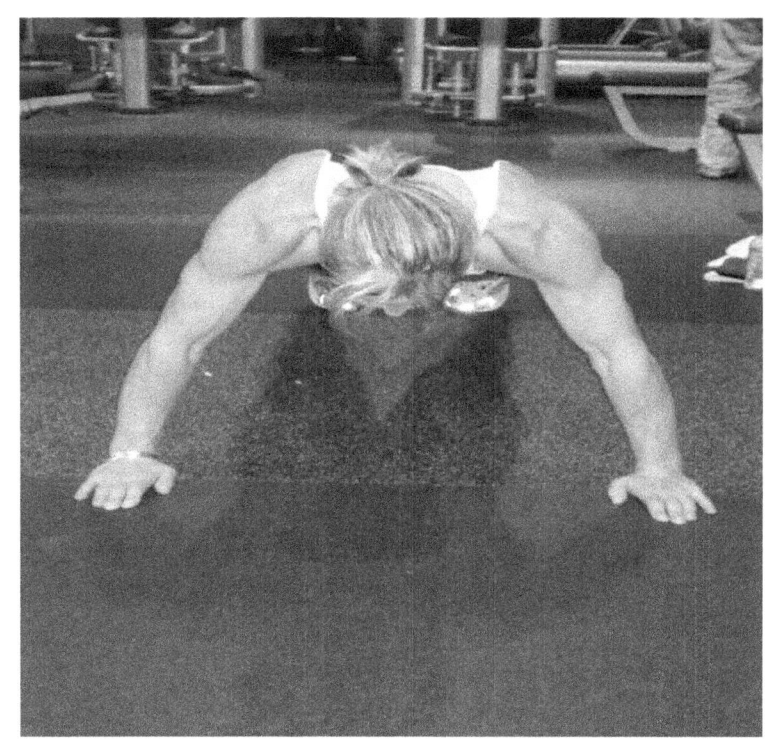

position that offers you optimum intensity. We often use press ups as a finisher for chest at the end of our workout. Another good use of press ups is the compound exercise in a pre exhaust super set for chest. In a chest pre exhaust you would perform flyes, chest hugs or cable flyes immediately

followed by press ups with minimal rest. Press ups are, after all is said and done just a bodyweight bench press and the angle can be varied just as with bench presses.

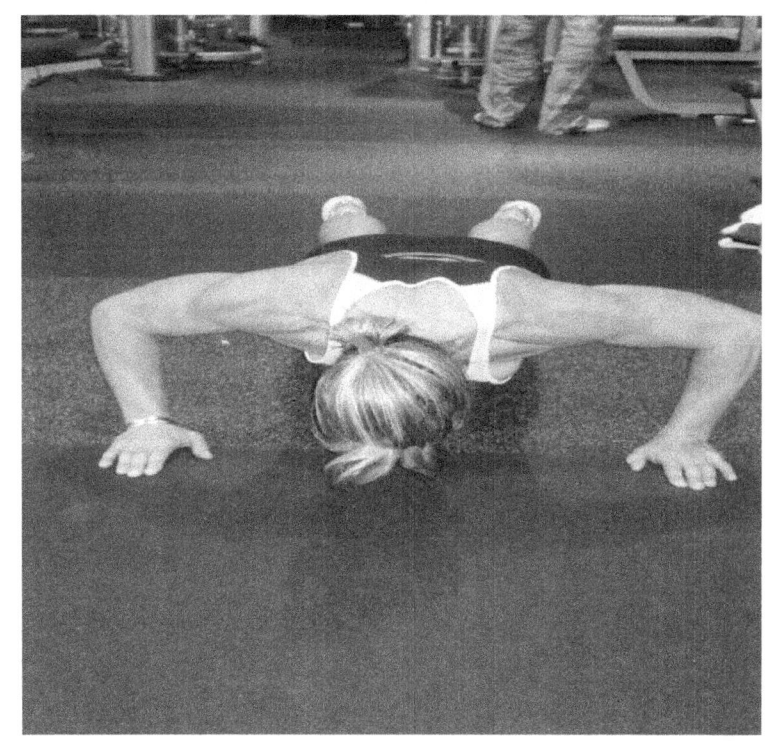

Panatta Inclined Press

Different makes of Incline press machines offer subtle differences in the movement. The Panatta version pictured here with Julie using it does feel very good and works the top of the chest very well. Golds gym have a Hammer strength version of the machine and both are good in our opinion. Although at first independent handles can feel strange that feeling quickly goes as one develops the balance needed to complete the movement. Heavy weights can be achieved as the balance and coordination needed is minimal. The

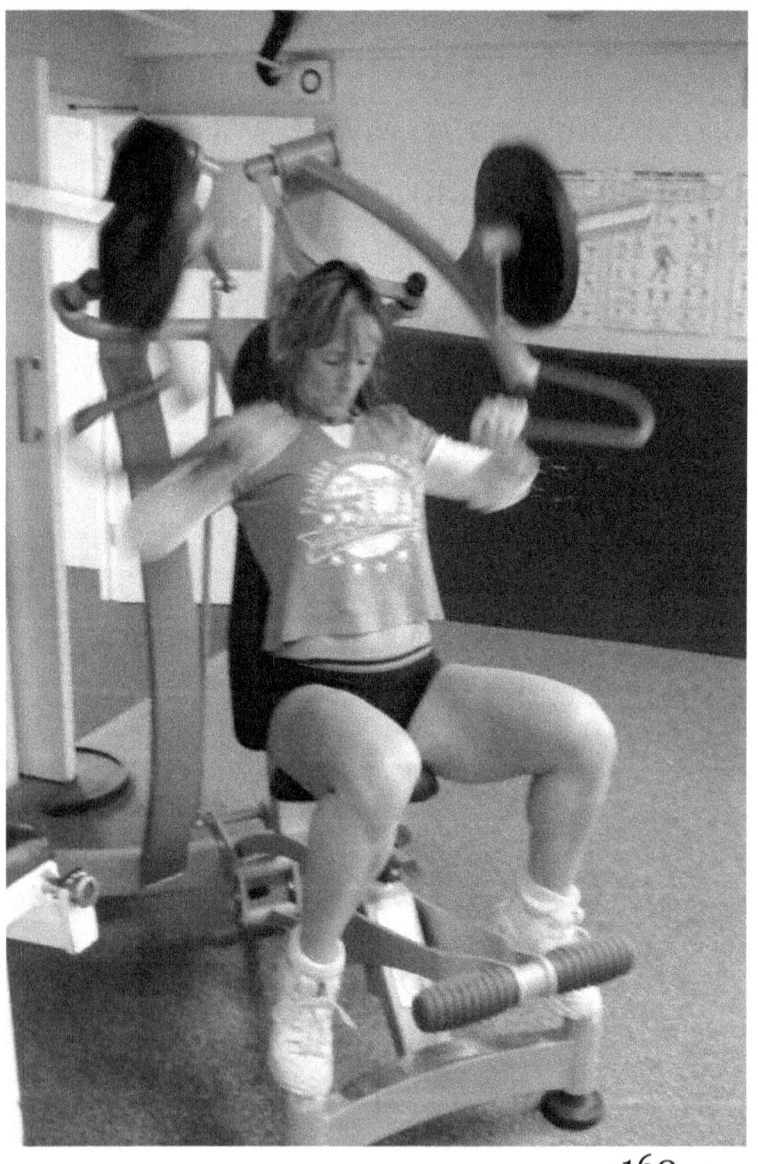

movement also activates the front of the shoulders (Anterior delts) and the back of the upper arm (Triceps). The free weights are loaded by hand on to the spindles as can be seen. Normal practice is to start with a moderate or light weight and work up with each set until the number of reps targeted requires supreme effort. The breathing pattern is to breath out as you straighten your arms. We find breathing is helped by counting your reps to yourself each time you press your arms out. When we began to train 35 years ago there were no, or very few machines and still it was possible to achieve great results. The machines available today offer amazing variety to workouts and at times we have seen them lead to confusion with trainers unable to settle on a good results producing workout, much like kids in a sweet shop or candy store. Variety and change is great but any routine must be given the chance to produce the required results before being changed. I have recently heard a young man who had began training legs with another trainer bemoan how the workout was boring and didn't work after just three sessions. I suspect the workout was not the problem at all.

Pectoral Flye Machine

This machine is absolutely my favourite for chest. The movement is smooth and the chest is targeted to perfection. The designer of this little beauty deserves a pat on the back. They have designed a chest machine that manages to isolate the chest like no other I have experienced in over 35 years of working out. I believe the seat needs to be set in a low position and the arms kept as straight as possible on the earlier light sets. The arms will naturally bend a little as you train heavier, and this gives you the best of both worlds a strict light chest burn early on and a heavy flye in the later sets. We aim for 5 sets usually starting light and very strict and then heavier and loosening form just a little. When I mention isolation, the term means to isolate just the muscle you are

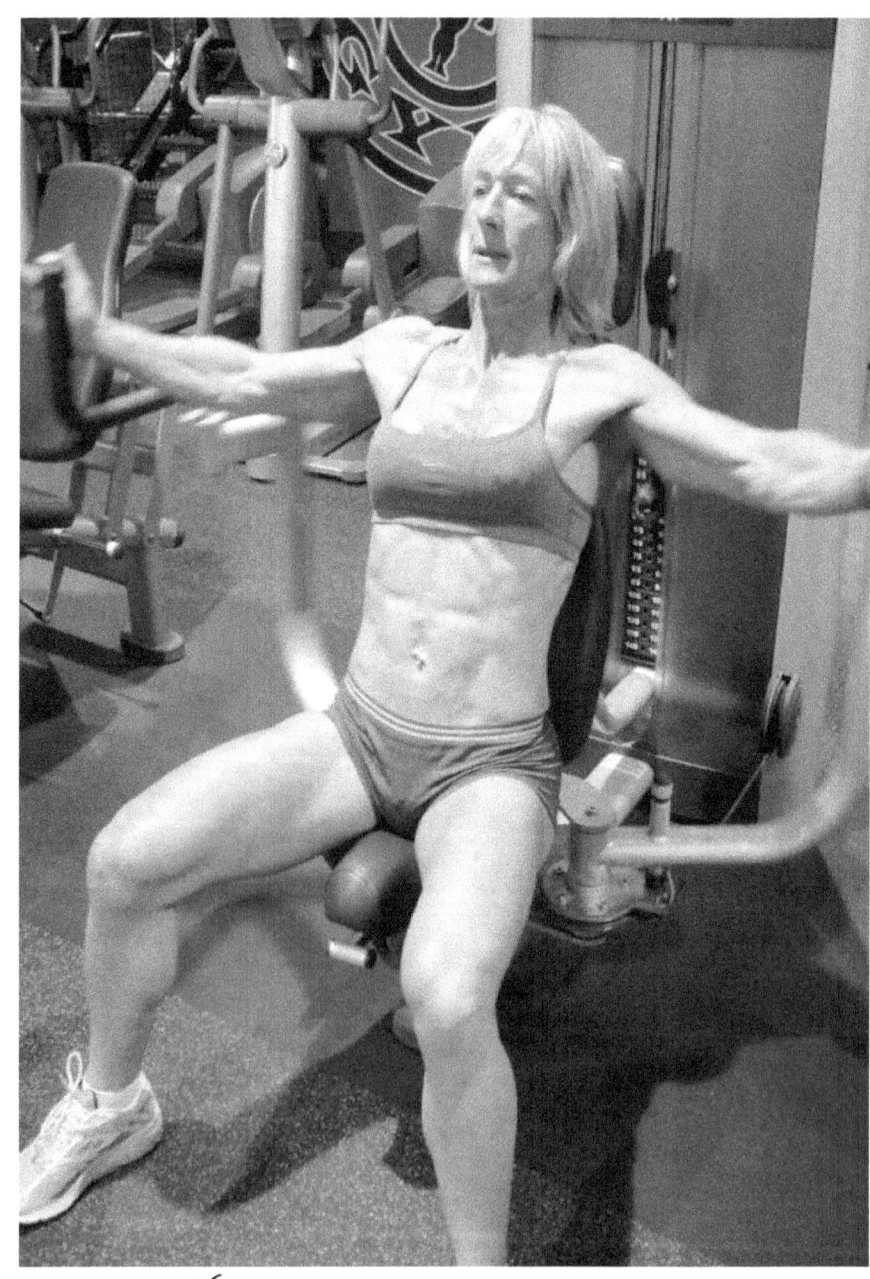

working. This isn't really possible entirely but compared to say dips or bench presses which along with chest heavily involve both shoulders and triceps. Flyes and cables activate a higher percentage of chest muscle compared to shoulders and triceps. Keep your chest high and sit up straight. Breath out as you bring your arms together and try to avoid throwing your head back as Julie is doing in the picture. That is a bad habit she has and despite endless nagging, once habits are developed they are very hard to change. Maybe she is praying the nagging will stop. Seriously here though, we all have little quirks that develop, but do try to stick with good form.

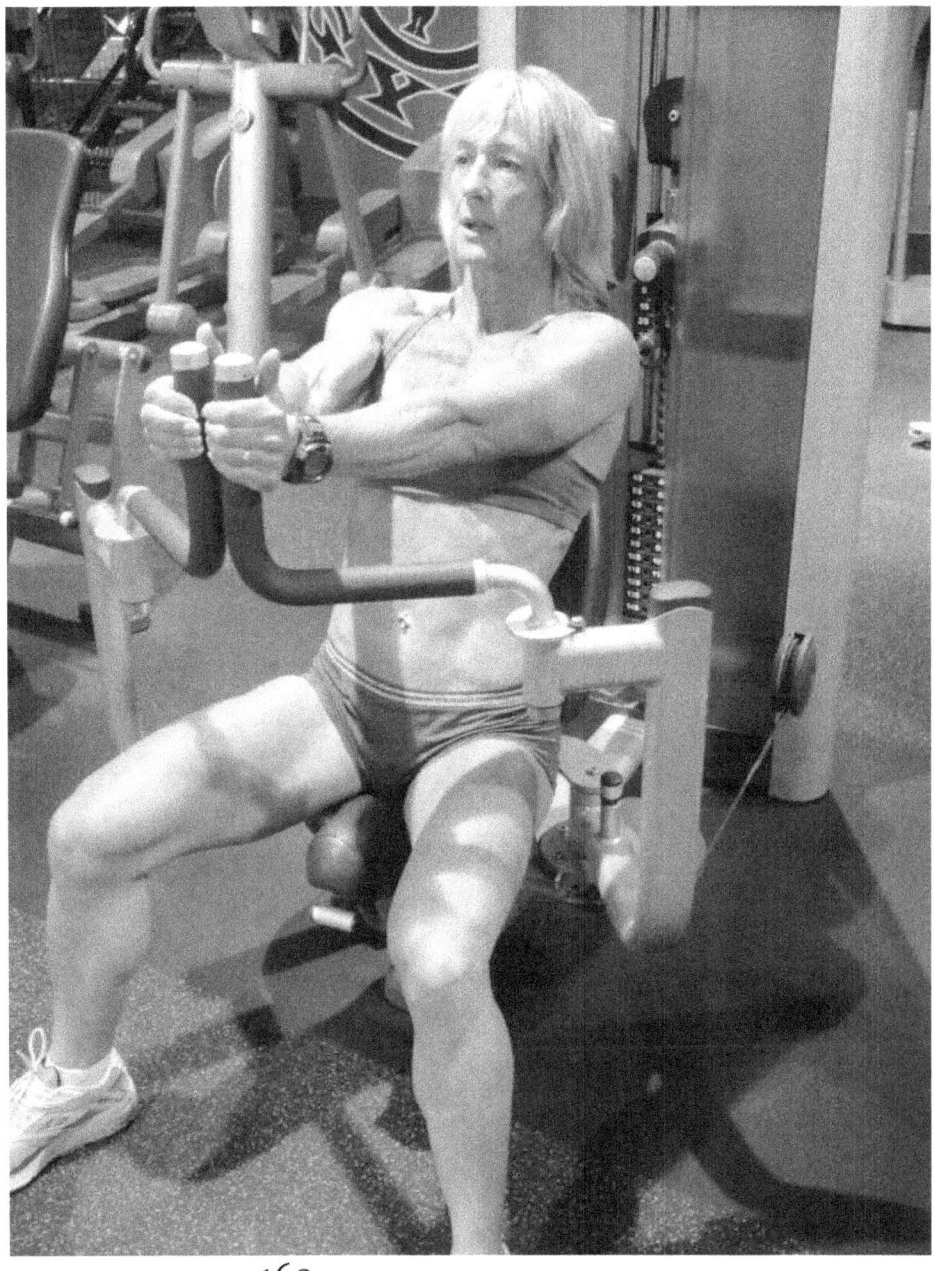

Inclined Dumbbell Press.

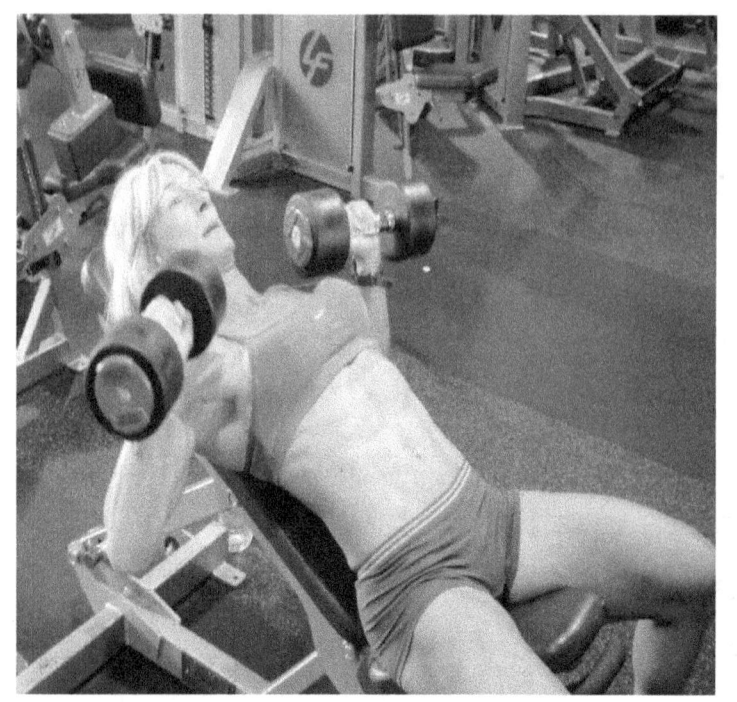

Dumb-bells are used to allow a greater range of motion and also a greater flexibility within the range of motion. For chest we normally set the bench at 30/45 degrees. As the bench becomes more upright then shoulders become the prime mover in this exercise so for chest 45 degrees maximum works best. We see so many trainers using dumb-bells and then only doing a partial movement, this sort of defeats the object of using them. You will make faster progress by performing a full range of motion with the correct weight than you will by lifting a weight that is too heavy and only doing half an exercise. This is a very common

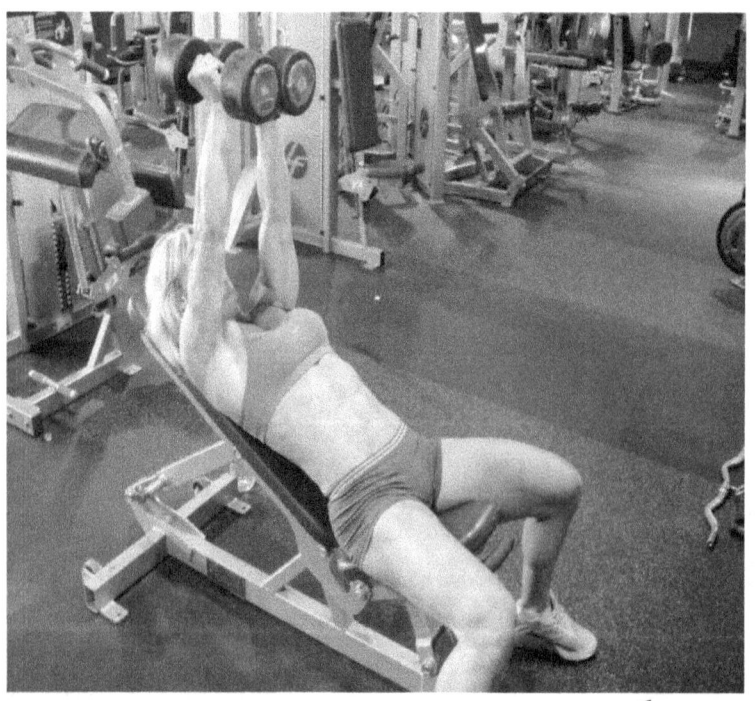

problem within gyms, with members competing to use the heaviest weights and exercise form going out of the window. To build a physique you MUST train your muscles perfectly, NOT YOUR EGO!

Pec Deck Flyes

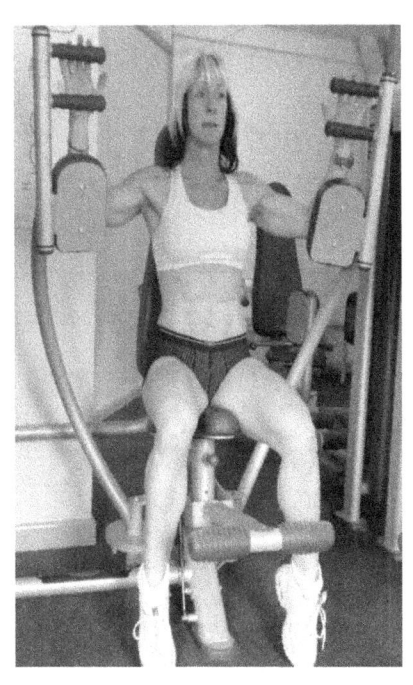

An isolation chest exercise. As with most isolation exercise it is important not o get too carried away with the weights being used but rather make sure you are able to feel the muscle working. Weightlifters are concerned with moving a weight from A to B. We are not weightlifters and are more concerned with activating as many muscle fibres as possible in a movement and this can be achieved often by using a more moderate weight. This is true with isolation exercises in particular. This is not to say that we don't have to work hard and to failure on at least the last set of each exercise because that is exactly what we need to do. The point is, that the more control we have of the movement the more fibres we will activate and this means progress. When performed correctly many isolation exercises will produce a deep burn in the muscle, if you have to cheat or use momentum to get the job done then you are missing out on the benefits that good form and tempo can produce and drastically increasing your chances of injury occurring. Your call really, ego or physique? In this picture, Julie may have the seat a touch too high, ideally your upper arm should be parallel to the floor.

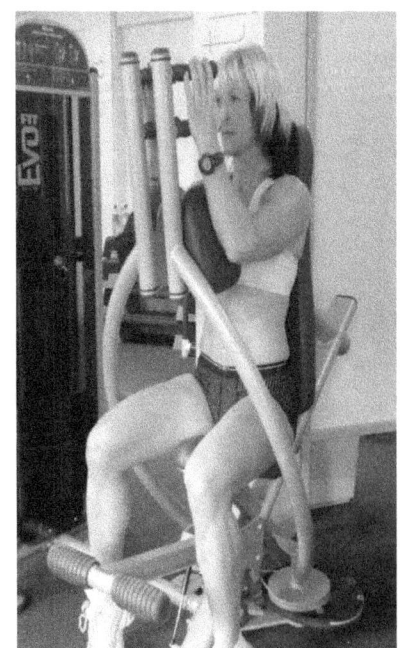

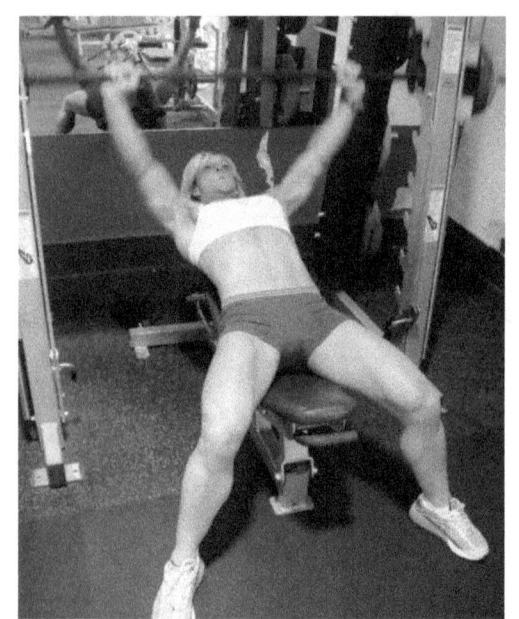

Smith Machine Inclned Press

The Smith Machine is useful for most exercises and is good to use from a safety aspect if you train alone. It is important to realise however that the exercises when performed on smith machine or any other machine for that matter lose many of the benefits that having to balance and coordinate free weights will provide. Often the bar is counterbalanced so that the starting weight of just the bar is very light, enabling beginners to use it safely. If it isn't counterbalanced, the weight of the bar plus running gear can be in excess of 30kilos so beware when using for the first time. Before using a smith machine you will need to familiarise yourself with just how it works and set the bench angle and position before you load any weight on to the bar. We like to spin the bar forward when we finish to hook it back on. To do this we have to turn the bench to face

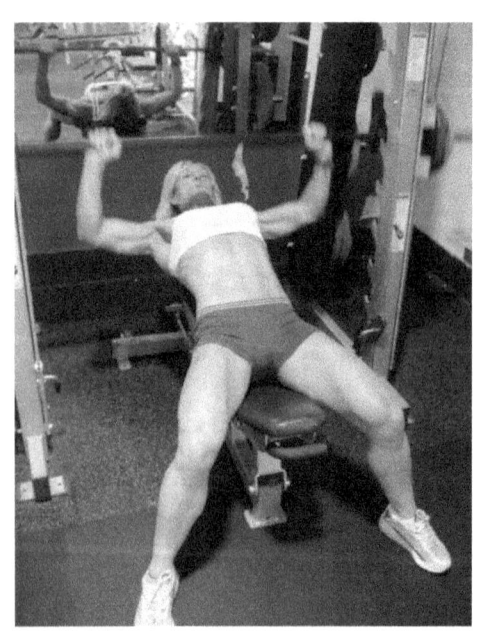

away from the mirror. These minor adjustments are important and you should always take the time to set yourself up correctly.

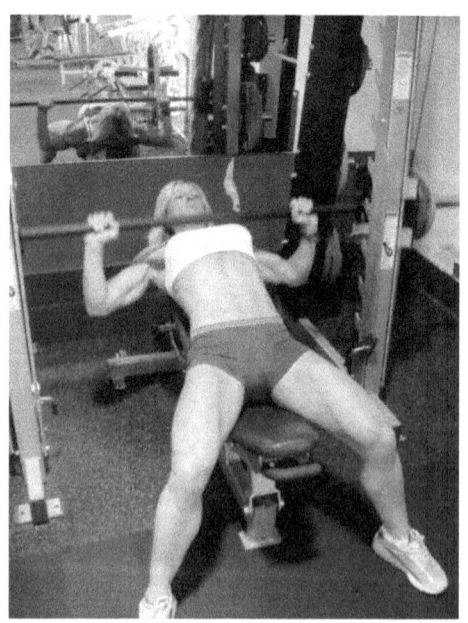

Cable Pulley Pec Flyes

Almost always positioned in front of a mirror, cable flyes are great for pulling your best faces, although please refrain from screaming on each rep as this is unnecessary and very annoying to other trainers, if you really want to get noticed, don't scream just wear skin tight pink lycra. As with the other isolation chest exercise don't get carried away with the weight and concentrate more on the feeling in your chest.

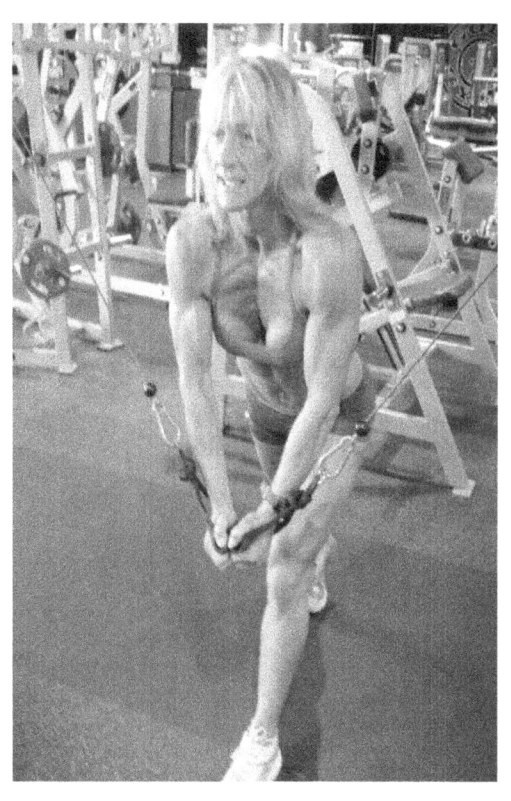

Keep the exercise under control, even exaggerated control. Stretching and squeezing your pecs on each rep. The more you emphasise the stretch and contraction the more you will benefit from cable flyes. Julie stands with her fit staggered, this is her preference. Many trainers keep both feet together. Whichever you choose make sure you are central in the pulley with a solid stance. The rep range on these and other isolation exercises is often a little more than compound exercises. We would advise an average of around 12 reps per set, concentrating hard.

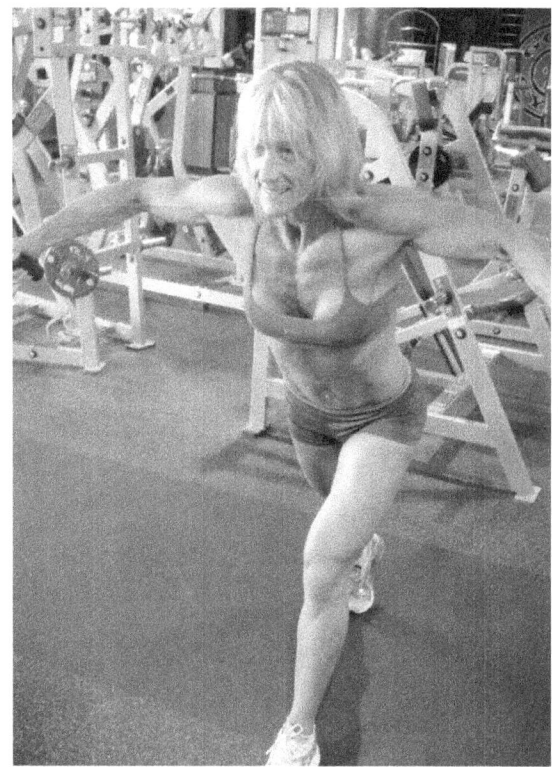

Barbell Bench Press

The favourite exercise of many trainers. Most asked question: How much can you bench press? To be totally honest it is not an

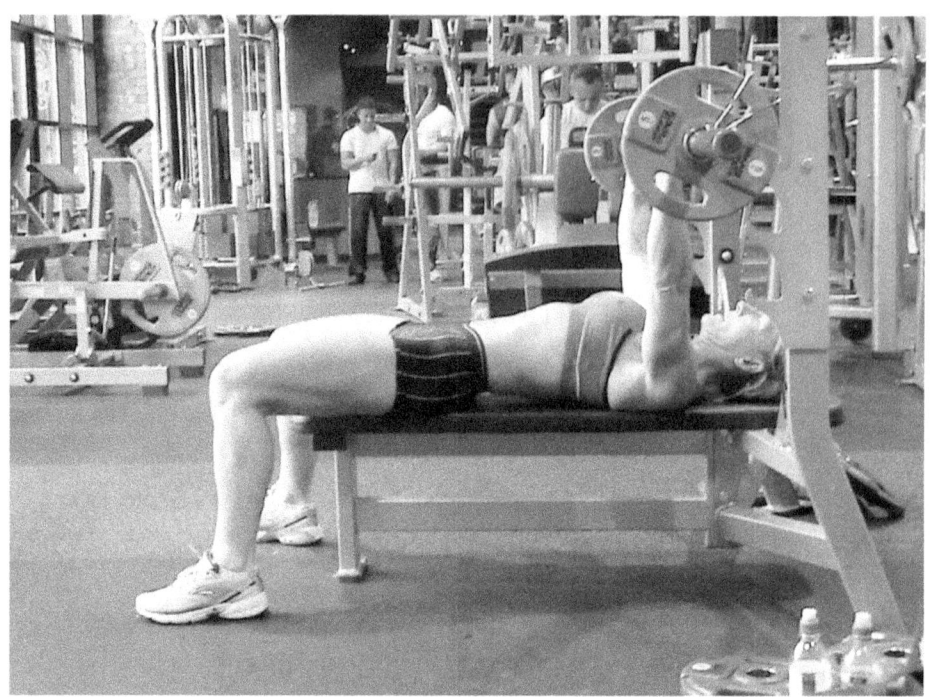

exercise we perform very often, we are in the minority, most trainers love it as they can build up to impressive poundage's very quickly. I guess it is great for the ego. We feel that for chest development there are more effective options. However, this exercise is credited with many a trainers upper body muscle. Bench press would be the first exercise on most people's list, I suggest try it for yourself and see if you get good results. There will be no shortage of exponents willing to give you advice on this one. Make sure you stay strict though, Shoulder injury is common with poor form.

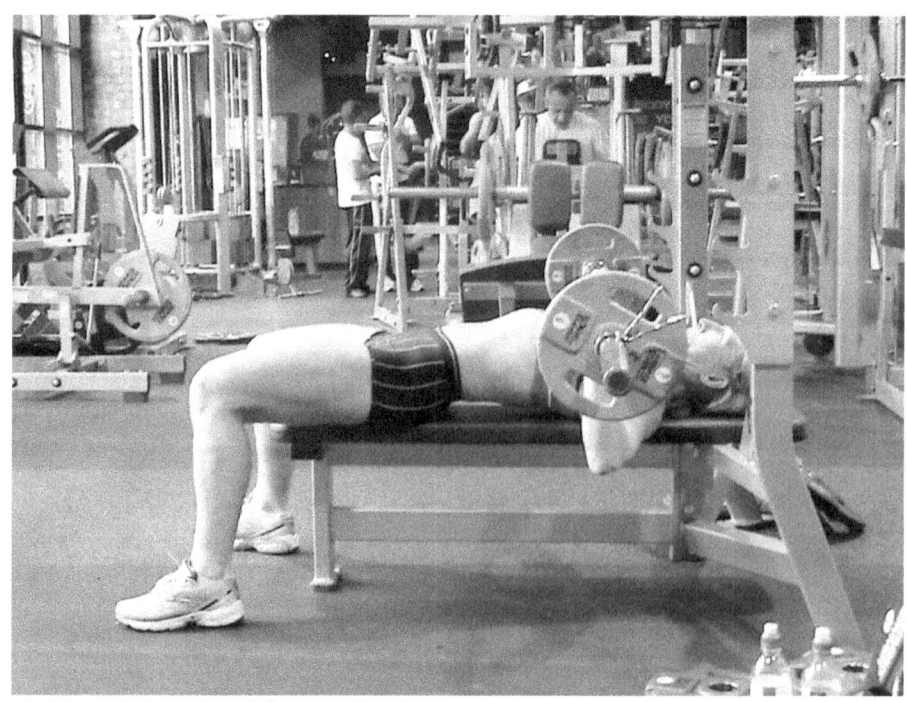

Inclined Dumbbell Fly

Set the bench at 30/45 degrees as we did on the dumbbell presses. This time the motion is a flying or hugging motion. Make sure you control the descent and stretch only as far as is comfortable at first. The dumb-bells elbows and shoulders all need to remain in line. At the bottom of the movement you should feel a stretch in your pecs, across your chest, control this stretch. An important aspect of any flye motion is not to lose control on the downward motion as this is where you will pull a muscle. Keep the chest high and maintain the arc in your arms with your elbows slightly bent throughout the movement. Fill your chest with air at the top as you lower the weight and exhale as you hug the weight back to the top. Do not use a weight that is too heavy or this exercise will turn into a dumbbell press and defeat the object of isolating your chest.

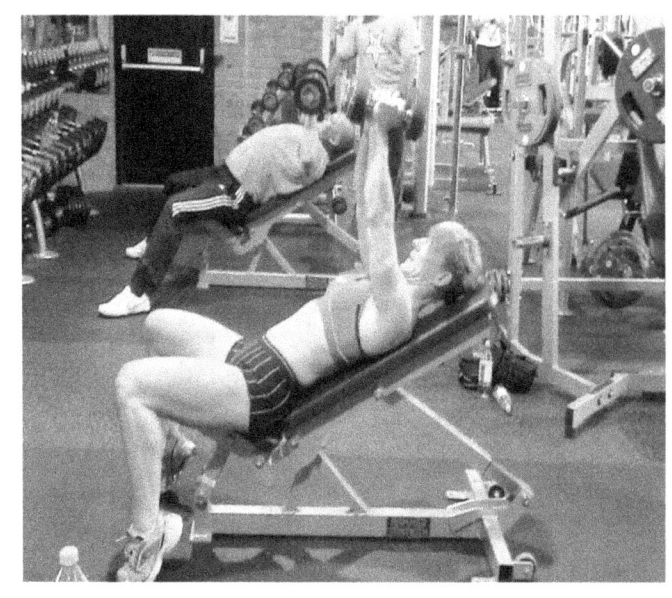

Replace the dumb-bells between sets so somebody else may use them when you are not. Always share the weights, although you will see trainers monopolising dumb-bells, don't become one of them.

Hammer Decline Press

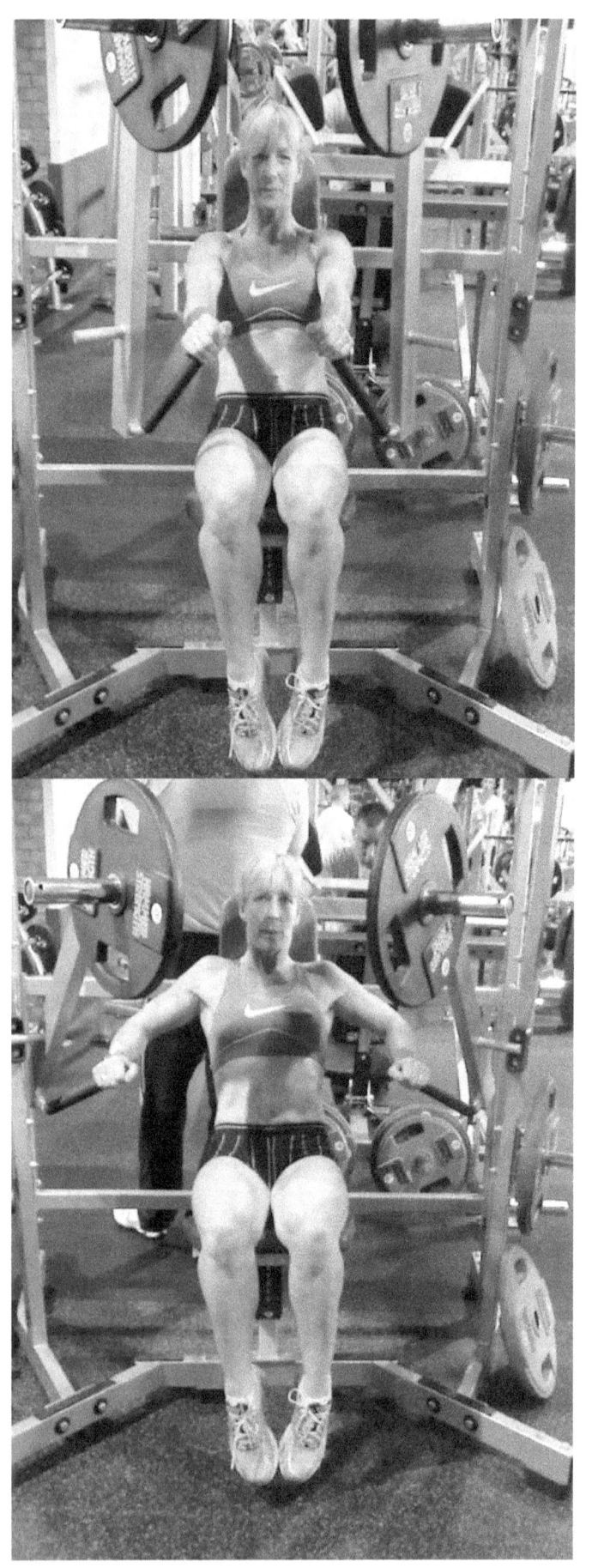

Credited with working the lower portion of your chest are decline presses and dips. Again you will be able to use quite a lot of weight with this exercise so it does tend to attract the ego trippers. The range of motion is quite small. A nice fluid motion will give great results and as added variety to an overall chest workout this will work very well. When you are picking a gym to train at, it is a good idea to keep in mind that you will need a selection of equipment for all body parts, not that you will use them all at once but it is good to change things around every now and again. A change is as good as a rest as the saying goes.

Plate Loaded Dips

Another lower chest machine that also works triceps and shoulders. A quick look at the declined chest press previously will show you the similarity in the movements. Julie

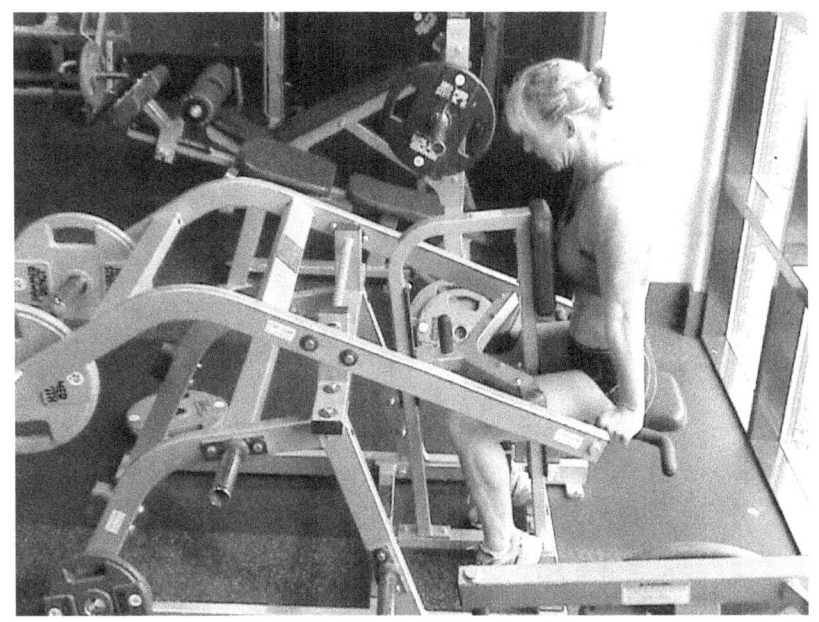

remains slightly more upright to work the outer line of her chest. The need for lower chest development on a lady is not such an issue for obvious reasons. I would favour bodyweight dips over this machine but a dip machine does add some much needed variety. I have been working out since 1975 so I appreciate the need for variety. Julie since 1980, also loves variety. Keeping it fresh, keeps you motivated.

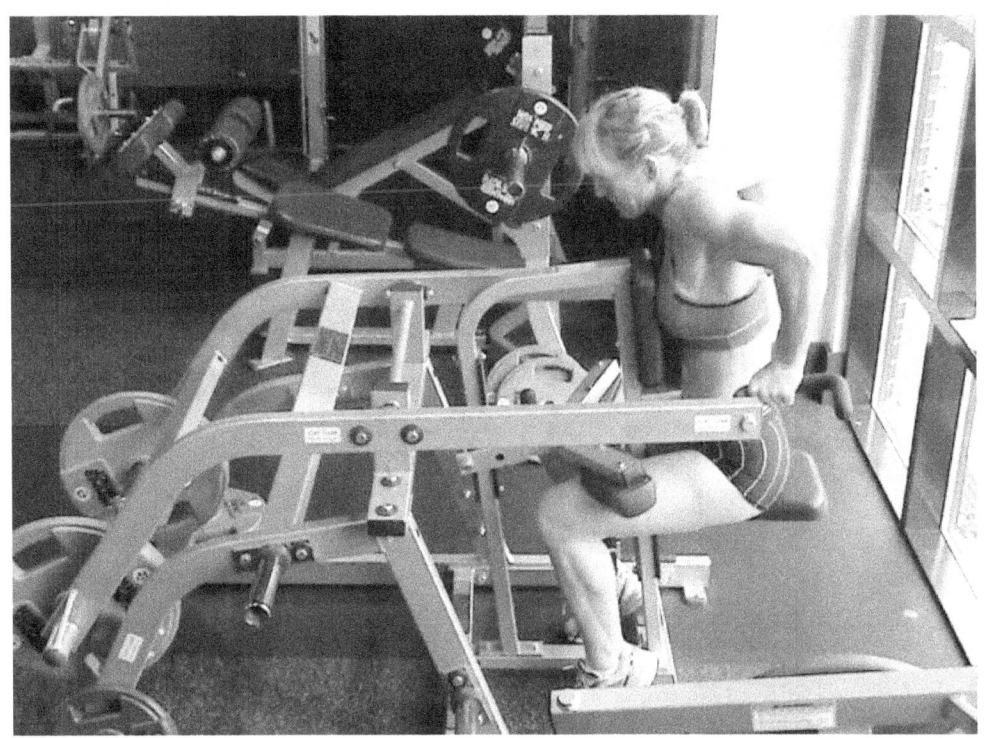

BICEPS

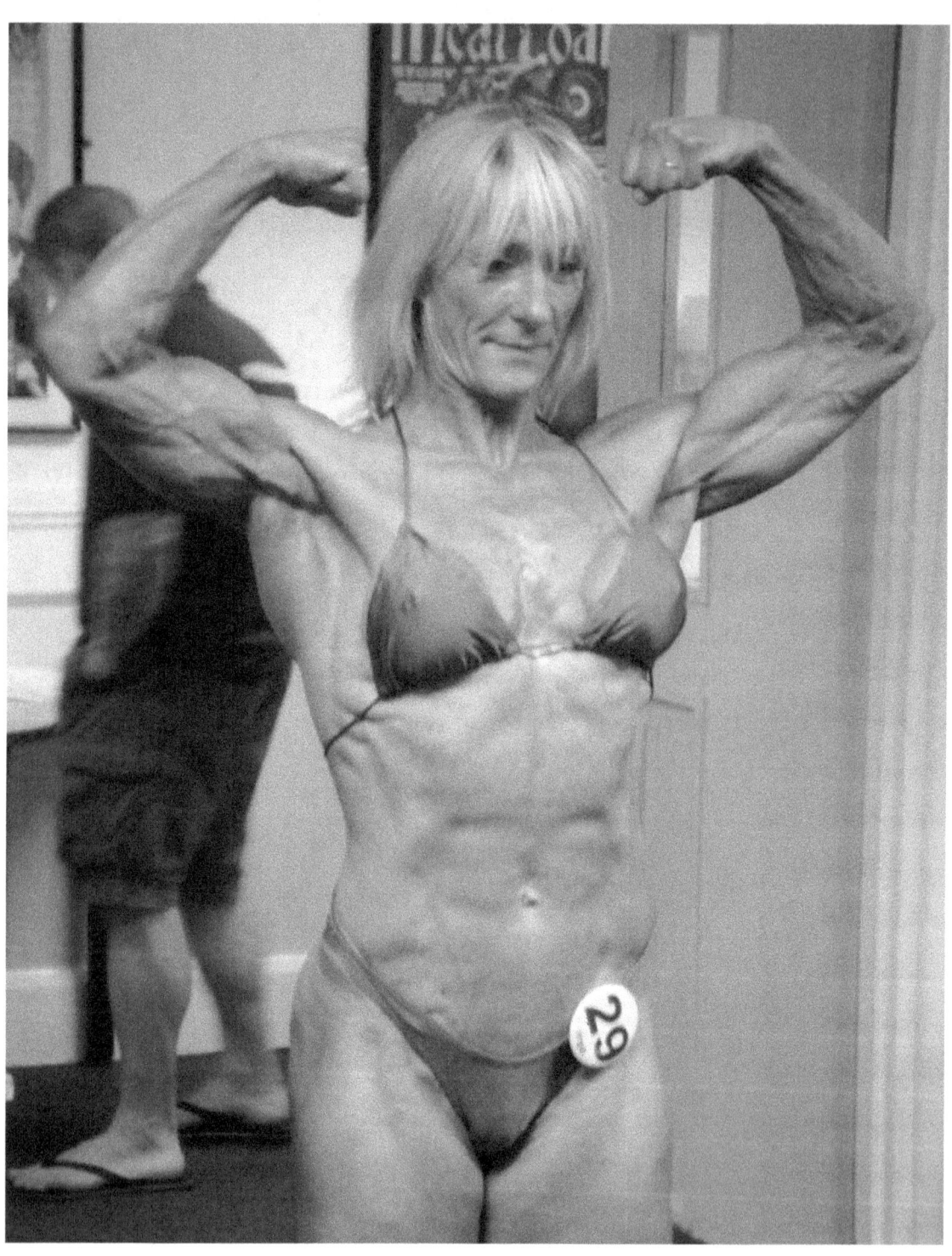

Machine Preacher Curls

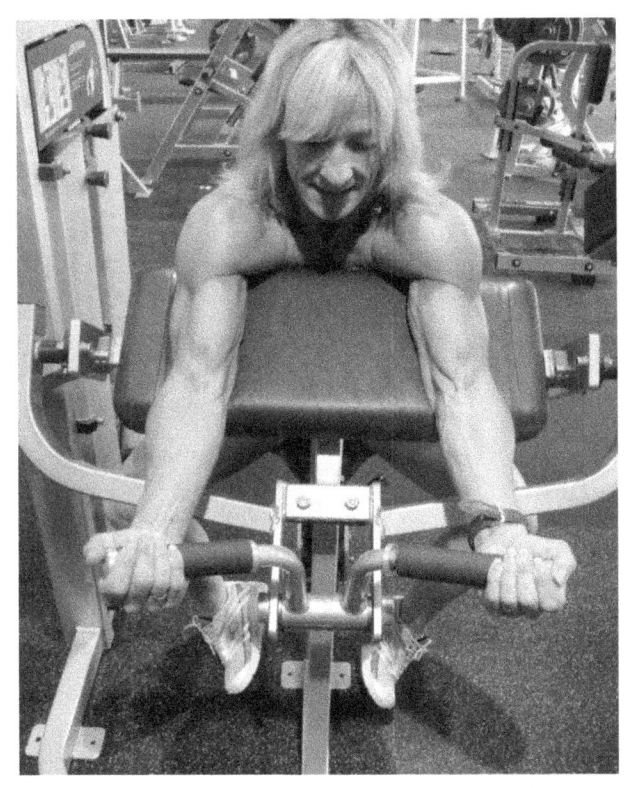

Something to keep in mind here is that biceps will always get a great deal of stimulation from any pulling work that you do. That includes most back work and some shoulder work. With this in mind you will find that you will not need an awful lot of exercises or sets to make your biceps respond. The preacher curl machine pictured is a personal favorite as you can really isolate your biceps with it. This exercise lends itself to extreme concentration. Execute the full range of motion and focus hard on the full stretch and squeeze hard with your biceps at the top. Flex like crazy and by the time you reach

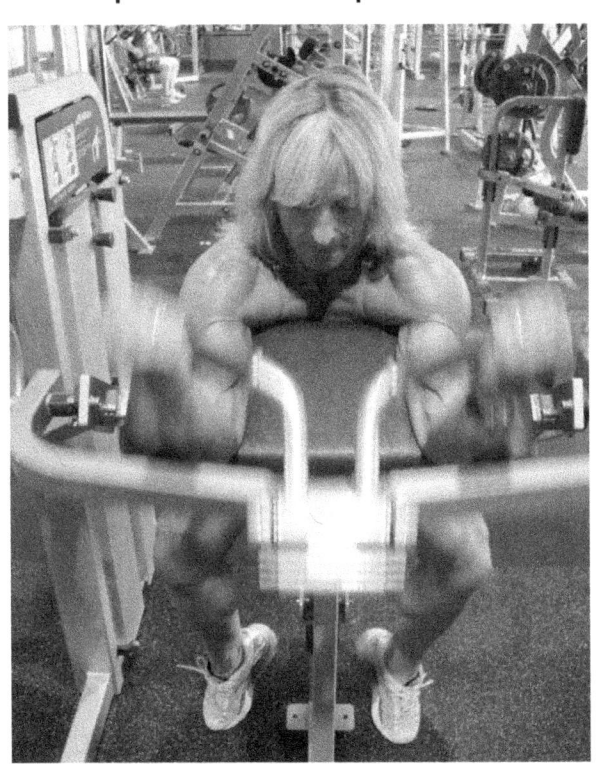

your last rep your biceps will be rather warm. Adjust the seat so the pad is tucked into your armpits. Raising the seat so you can get over the top of the weight and use heavier weights makes the designer's time a waste. Use the machine as it was designed to be used and you will reap the benefits, which is guaranteed super guns. Have fun.

Standing Barbell Curls

If you could only perform one bicep exercise for the rest of your life then standing barbell curls would probably be the wisest choice. Too much weight will result in your body rocking backward and forward to move the weight, often resulting in lower back strain for over enthusiastic or ego driven trainers.

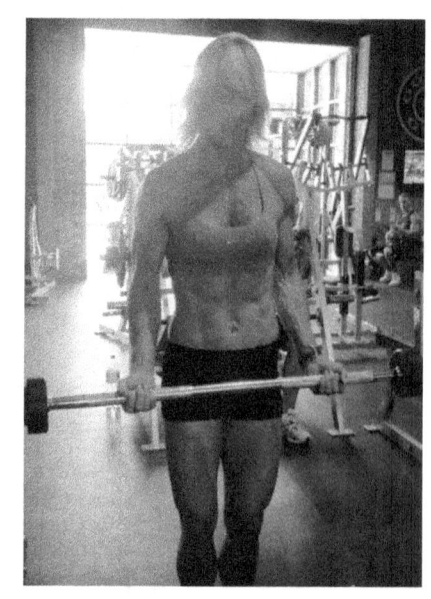

Resist the temptation and "train don't strain" Your arms should stay in line with your body as pictured and a good grip is slightly wider than shoulder width although you may experiment with different grips. It is always wise to use a light/moderate weight for your early sets as you can always increase on subsequent sets but if you start too heavy, you will hurt yourself. Never be afraid to admit to yourself that a weight is too heavy no matter who may be watching. Corny saying time: "even a journey of a thousand miles begins with a single step". Train smart and before long you will be getting noticed for all the right

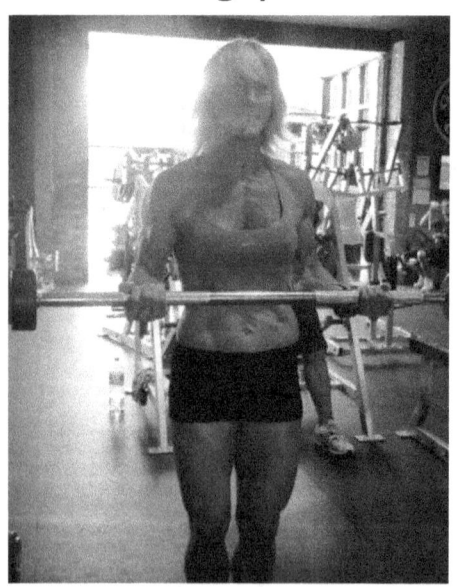

reasons. You will not need much more than 3 sets of these, any more than that will mean a drop off in intensity and would be counterproductive.

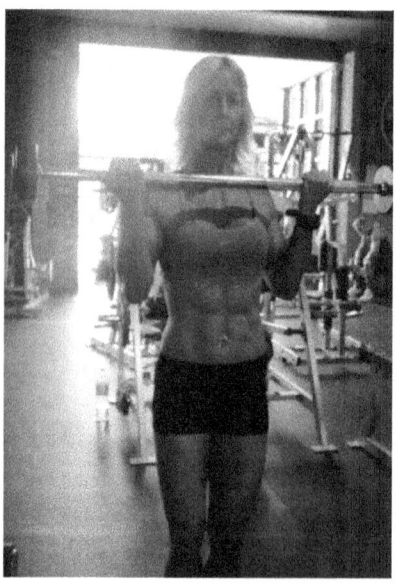

Seated Dumbbell Curls

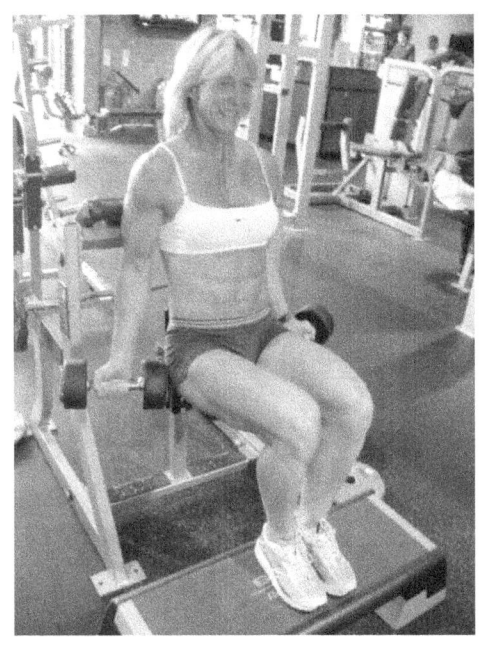

With dumbbell curls you may vary the angle of the bench down as low as maybe 45 degrees. The idea and secret, if there is one, is to keep your arms held back while you curl up. Logically you must negate any movement from the shoulder joint by the way of swinging.. You may either do both arms simultaneously of perform them alternately. We do both together, just as it seems much more time efficient. Benefits can be gained by the supination of your hand at the top of the movement. If you are unsure of what this means just turn your little pinky out towards your shoulder and you are supinating. Breathing should be exhalation on the raising and inhalation on the descent. Count your reps and breath as you count that will work. If you feel you are having problems with your breathing rhythm, just do what comes naturally and forget about it. Too much focus often causes a problem where there is none. After all you have been breathing without our advice for years now,

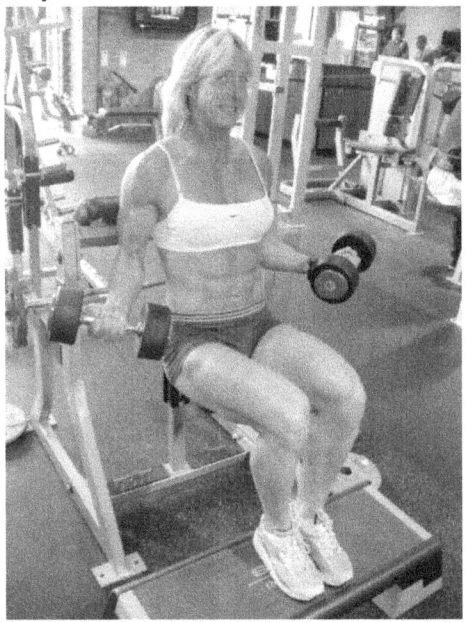

just focus on the movement of your arms breathing will carry on subconsciously and you will be OK!

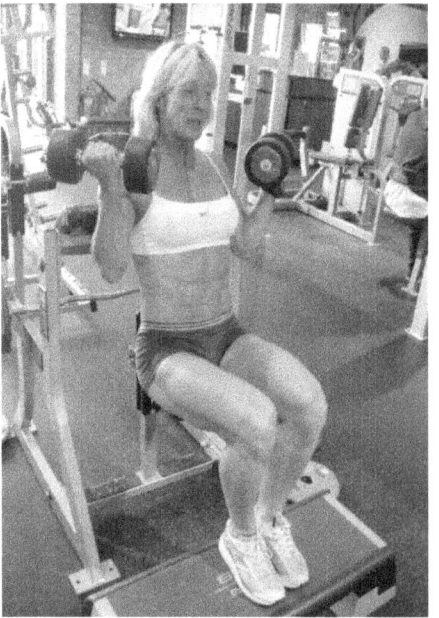

Dumbbell Hammer Curls

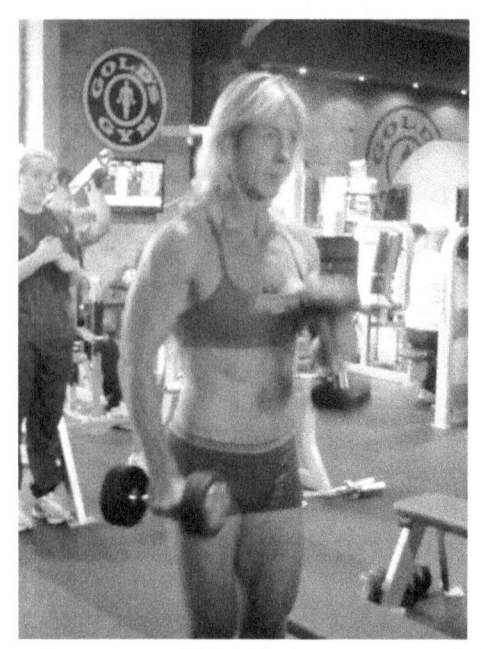

Hammer curls, Tie in your forearms and biceps brachia. They need to be performed singly as the plain of the movement would clash doing two arms together. The dumbbell is to be raised just as though you were holding a hammer in your hand. Your elbows should hardly move at all, just a slight movement across your body.

Generally these would be performed towards the end of your bicep work. We have found that higher reps work better for us, around 15 reps per set and also that they tire quite quickly so never more than 3 sets per arm. Too heavy a weight will result in splayed elbows and a rhythmic sideways swaying more like a dance than an arm workout. The result of this will pretty much be a waste of time and an increase in the chances of injury. That is, no biceps muscle to show and a pulled back or elbow, that's' right it hardly seems worth it

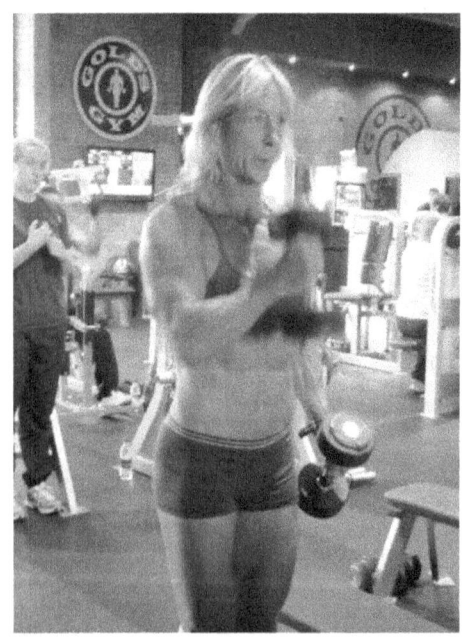

does it. It hardly ever, no make that NEVER, is worth the trade off of good form for shifting more weight.

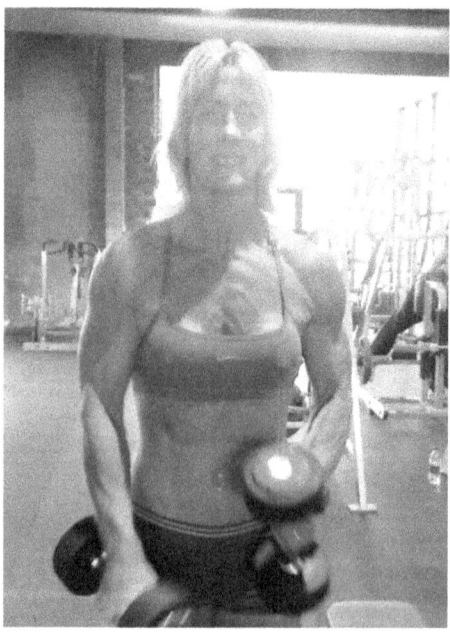

Standing Pulley Curls

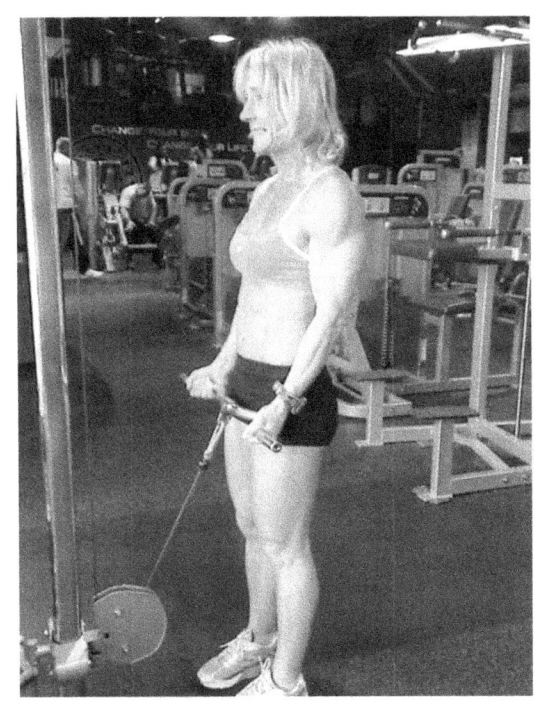

A variation on the barbell curls, that will feel totally different and the constant tension that pulleys offer are great for working biceps. Stand quite close to the pulley and again try to keep your arms by your sides throughout the move. When you upper arm moves your shoulders become activated. You will see that in the last picture Julie's arms have moved forward slightly to contract her biceps, this movement is within allowable limits but should never be extended much further. Raising the arms works your anterior deltoids. You will see many variations on biceps work using pulleys when you are working out. By all means experiment but please make sure that the movement is verified by a professional and not just a random hybrid that has evolved from trainers watching other trainers train badly and almost copying. Kind of like a

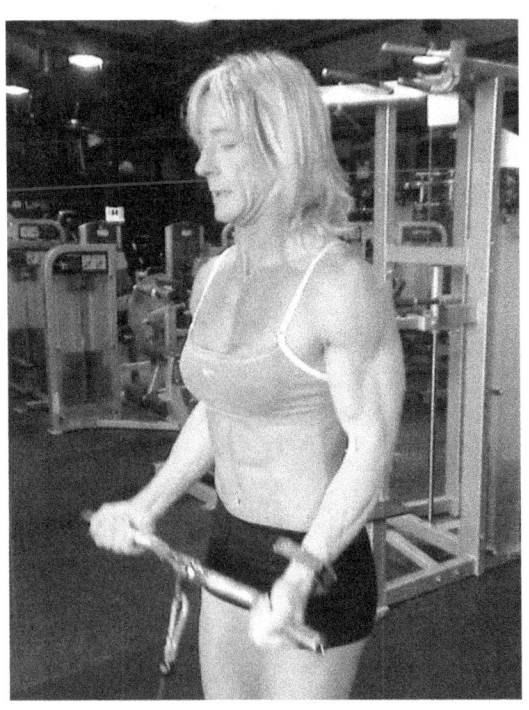

workout Chinese whispers, which everyone involved modifies to suit and then labels it "THE SECRET" exercise.

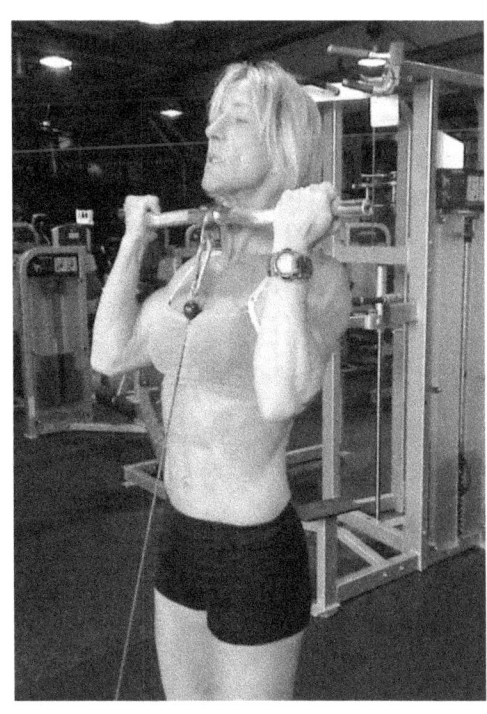

TRICEPS

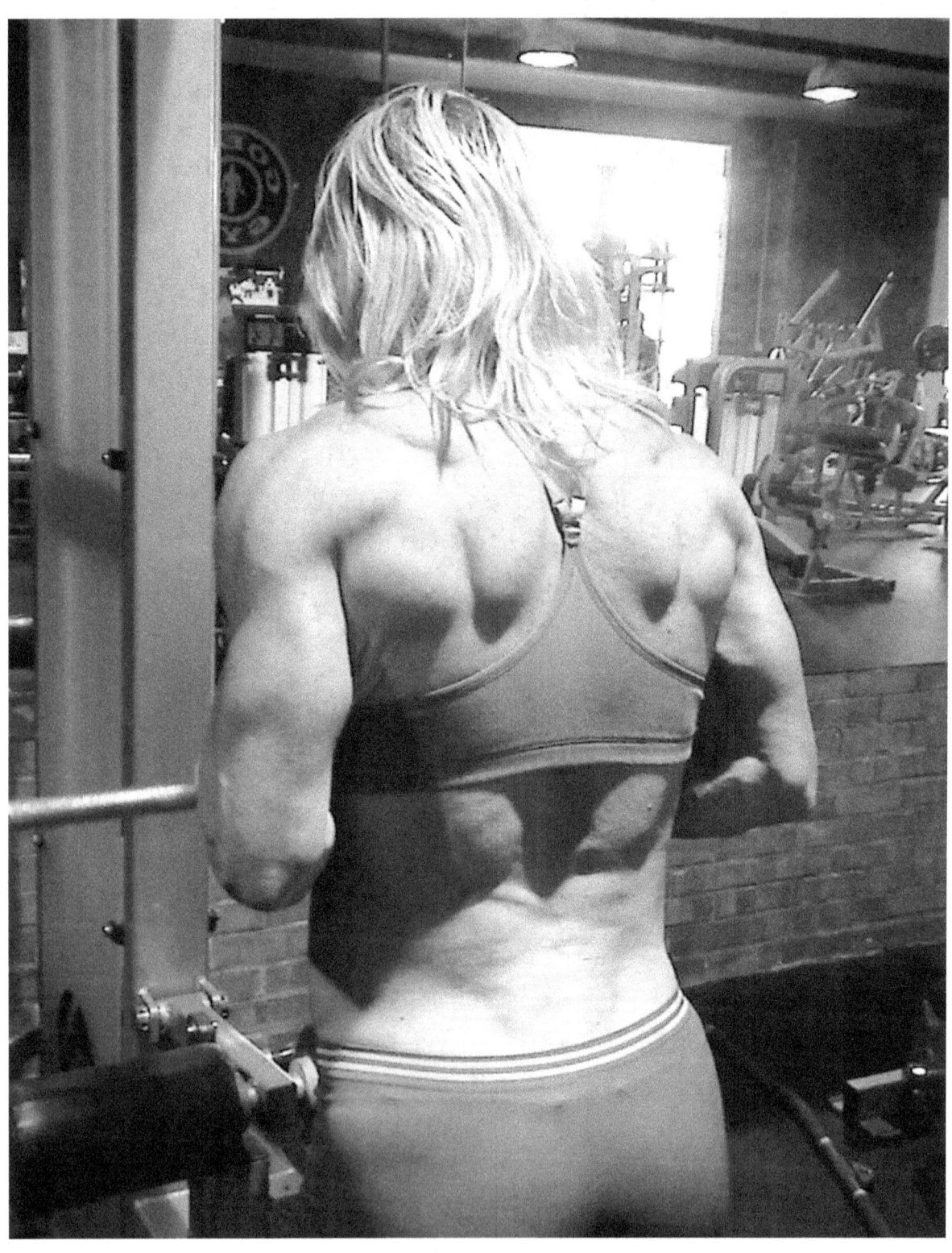

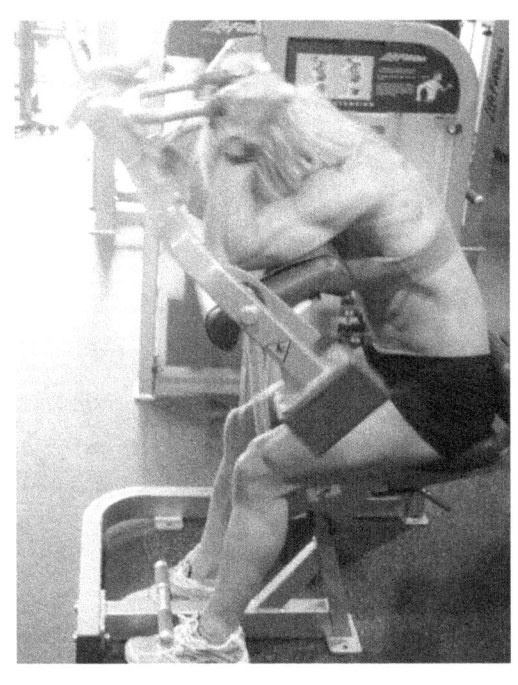

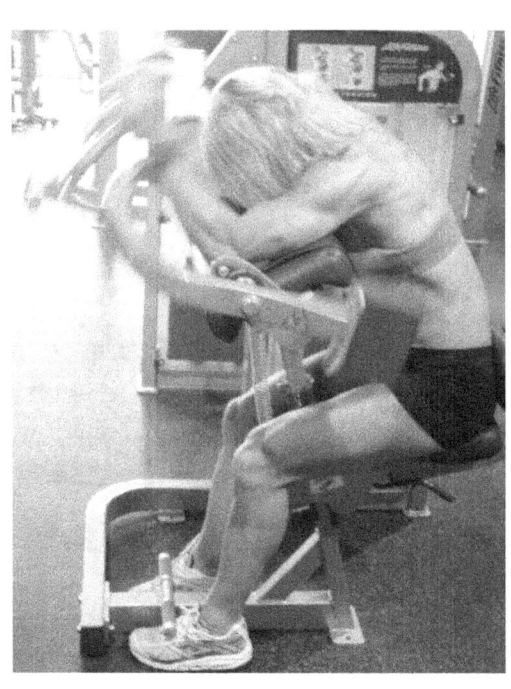

Machine Triceps Extensions

The triceps extension machine pictured is a good way of isolating the triceps muscles on the rear of the upper arm and combined with good nutrition a great way to avoid the dreaded bat wings or dinner lady arms. I always thought that was a bit unfair to dinner ladies but the term seem to have stuck. All that is needed here is to adjust the seat for your height, move the pin to the required starting weight and grasping the handles as in the pics forcibly straighten your arms before controlling them back to the start position. There are many variations on this machine in gyms across the world and all add much needed variety and ease of use to a triceps routine. With the machine there is no balance and very little coordination needed so this would not be the primary triceps exercise of choice, however this is great for finishing off your already warm and tired triceps.

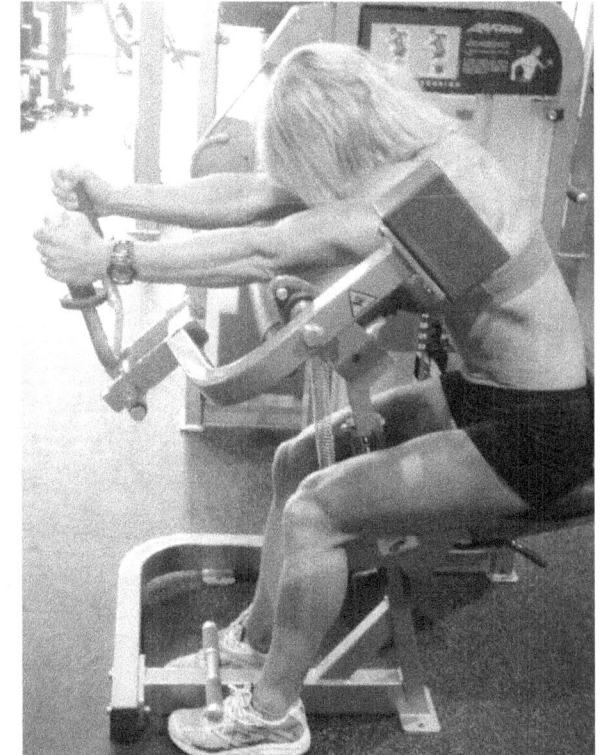

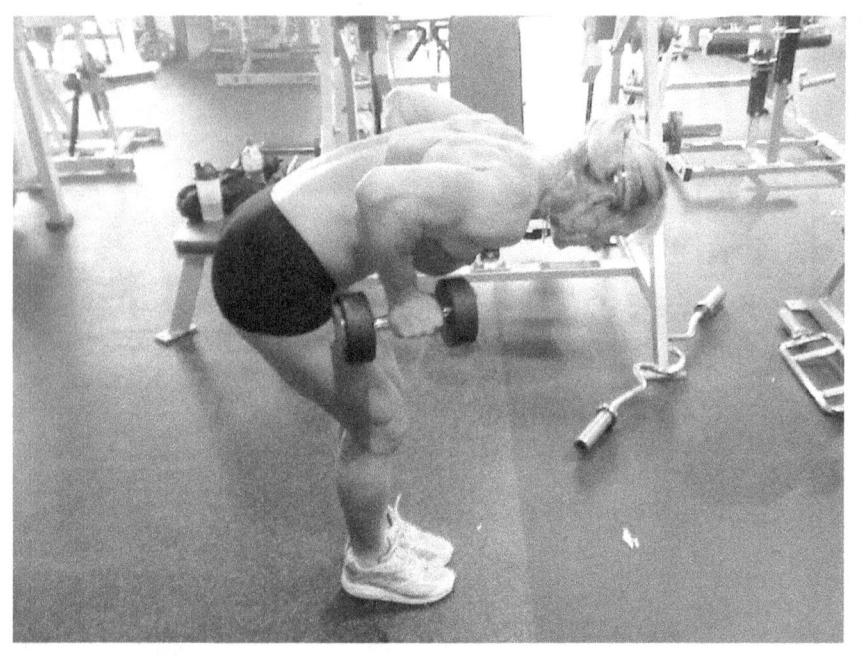

Dumbbell Kickbacks

The triceps kickback can be done with your bodyweight supported with one arm a t a time. Isolating the triceps muscles on the rear of the upper arm and combined with good nutrition a great way to avoid the dreaded bat wings or dinner lady arms. I always thought that was a bit unfair to fit dinner ladies but the term seem to have stuck. We prefer to always work both arms or legs simultaneously when we exercise, as it is quicker and your body does tend to use its limbs as a team, otherwise we may only have evolved with one of everything in the middle of our bodies. I am only kidding of course, if you wish to work one arm at a time that is perfectly ok. It is important to stand, bent over in a strong position

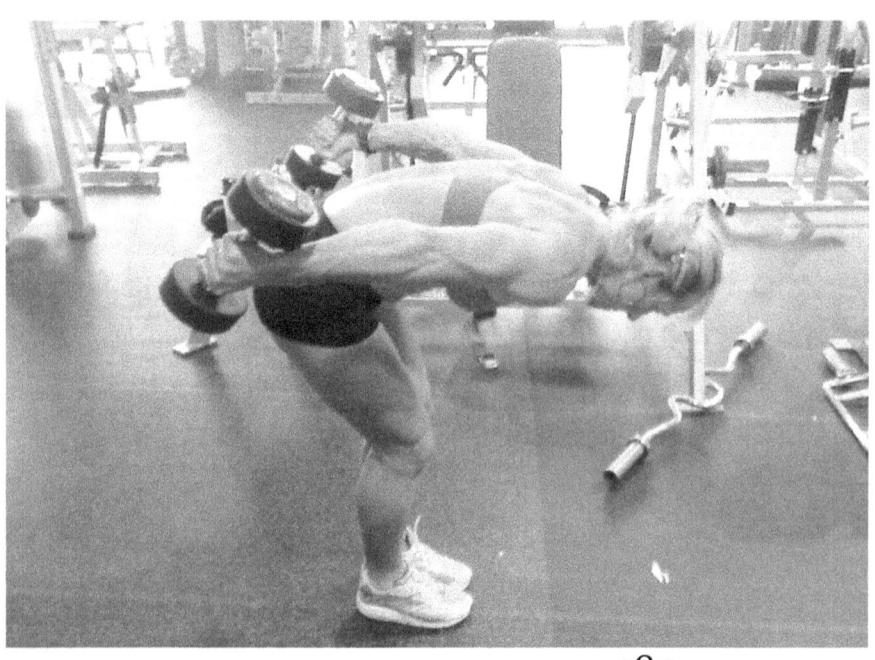

although the dumbbells do stay very close to the centre line of your body. Do not use heavy weights, you will not need them kickbacks is a exercise for light to moderate weight, good form and focused attention

Machine Dips

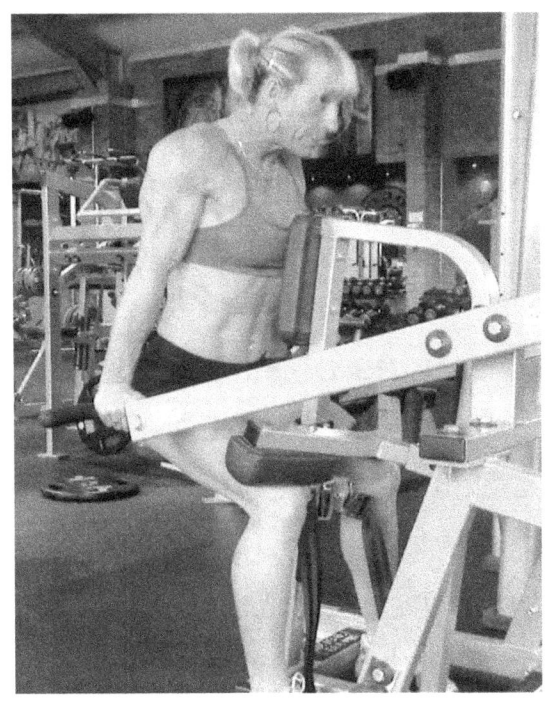

This dip machine is plate loaded and we always begin light and work up with each set letting our strength level o any given day determine our top set. Your legs are anchored under the pads to prevent you being fired across the gym with each rep. Dips work the triceps but also enlist the help of shoulder and chest muscles, Dips of any kind are a compound exercise, meaning that more than one muscle group is involved however the prime mover is the triceps as long as you keep your body as erect as possible. Any forward lean increases the chest activity.

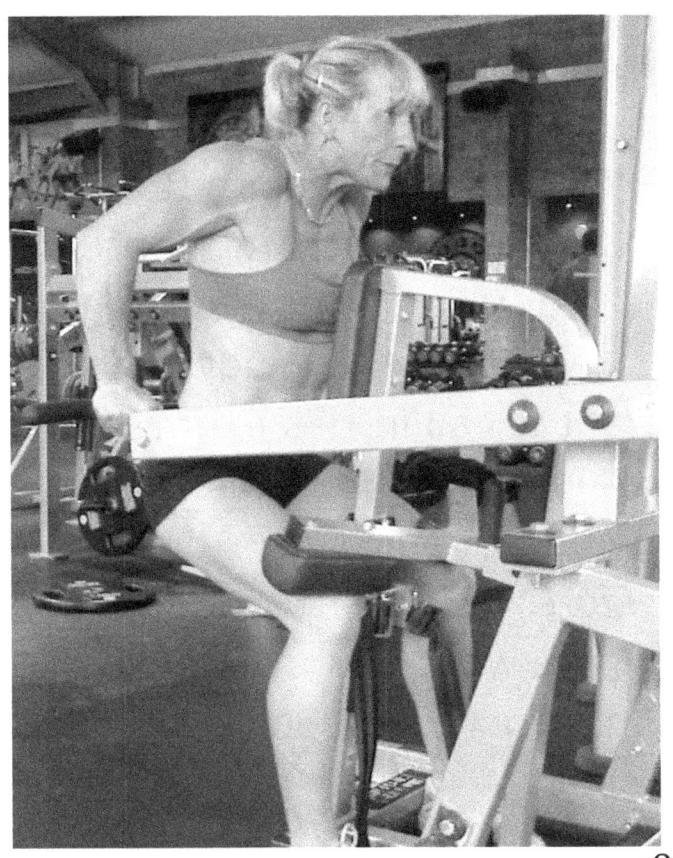
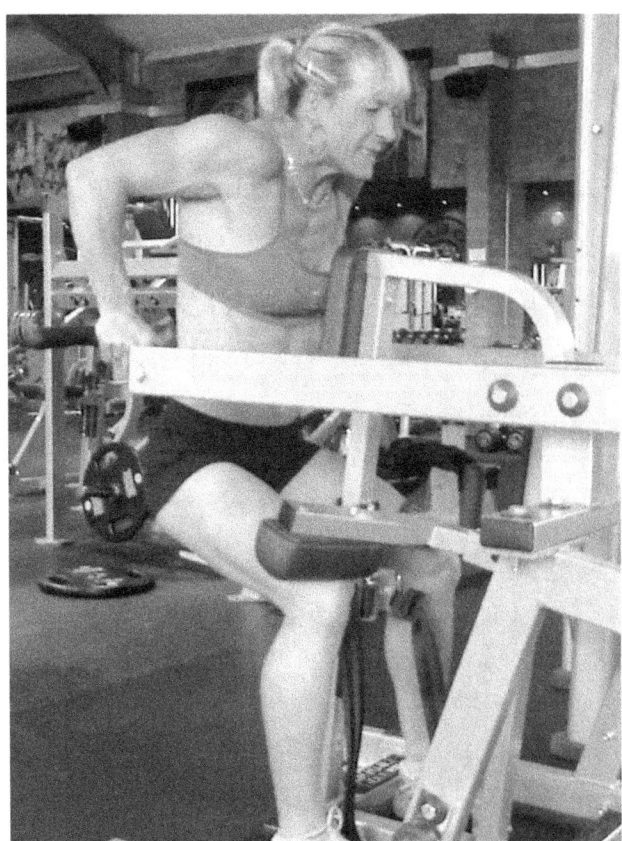

Bench Dips

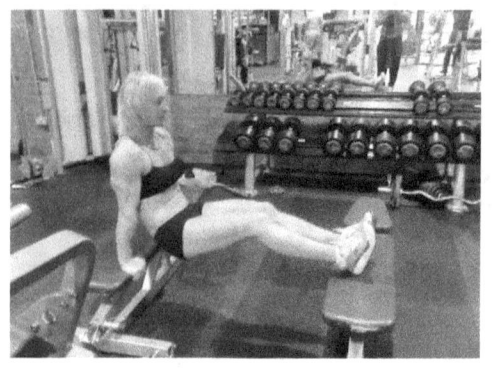

You will notice the big difference here is that your body is stretched out if front of you and your arms are bending quite far behind your body. This not only provides a great stretch for your chest and shoulders but also makes the triceps work in a unique way. Julie keeps her hands close together, this makes the exercise harder and more beneficial for you triceps. With a closer grip your supporting cast muscles have to work harder to balance your body throughout. We very

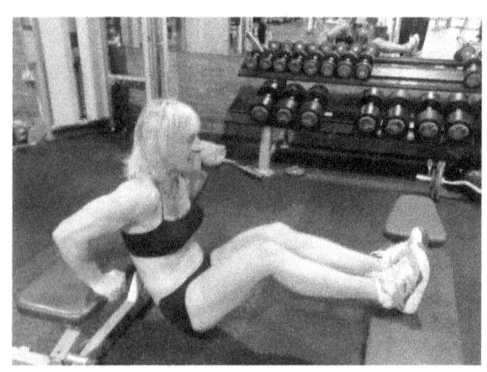

often use this exercise in a superset with kickbacks. Performing a set of kickbacks followed immediately by a set of bench dips to failure. To progress you can place a dumbbell across your lap. Julie works up to 40kilos added weight. She invariably kicks my ass on this exercise. D'Oh! Take care with the placement of the benches to ensure there are no mishaps and if you are using added weight via a dumbbell make sure the spotter places it gently and is there to take the weight back off again promptly You do not want to fail in this exercise and

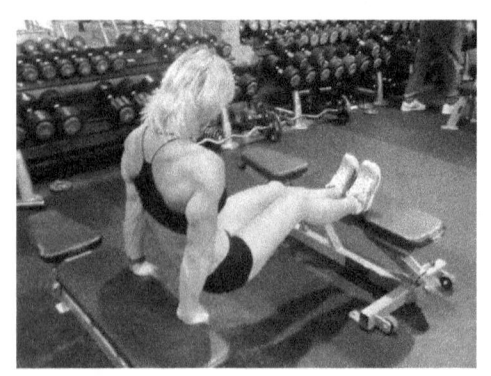

have to wait for a spotter with a gnats attention span to answer his or her mobile before your are rescued. Communicate what you expect clearly. If you don't trust the spotter don't ask them to spot

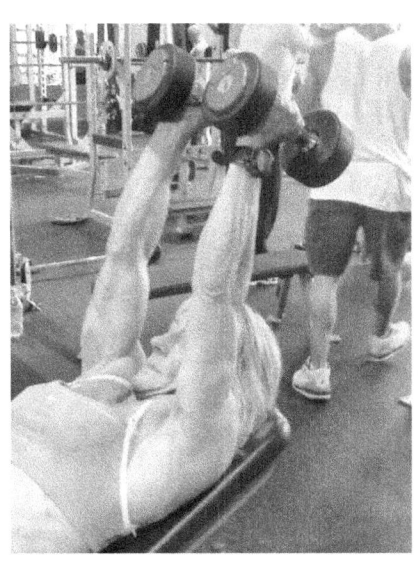

Inclined Dumbbell Triceps Extensions

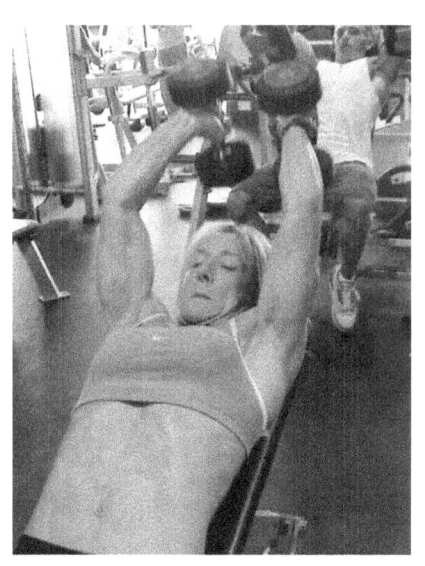

Again straightening the arm under tension but this time dumbbell triceps extensions do need both balance and coordination in order to complete the reps. This is a great primary exercise for this reason and should be one of the first exercises in your triceps routine, leaving the machine work for later in the session. Your elbow is the fulcrum in this exercise and theoretically should remain relatively stationary. your form must be slow and controlled and your elbow joints do need to be warmed up before any such triceps exercises. The concentration needed for primary exercises is obvious on Julie's face. This is not the time to mess about or adopt sloppy form or do the shopping list in your head, if you have a training partner then good communication as to your needs is also important, unless they are telepathic of course, a good partner will seem to become telepathic over time, knowing instinctively when you need help and what you need. Total concentration from start to finish is paramount. The result will be impressive triceps muscles.

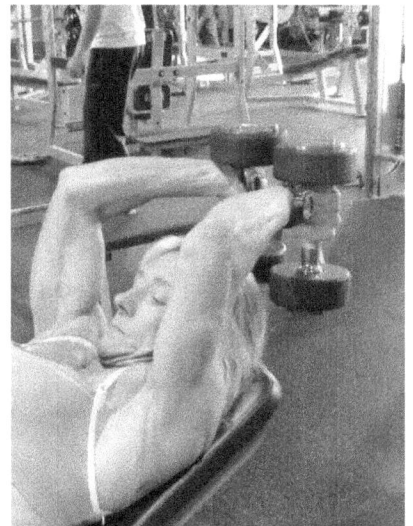

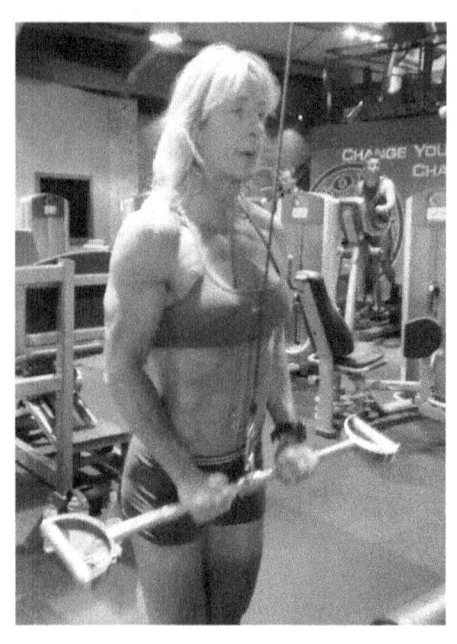

Triceps Pulley Pushdowns

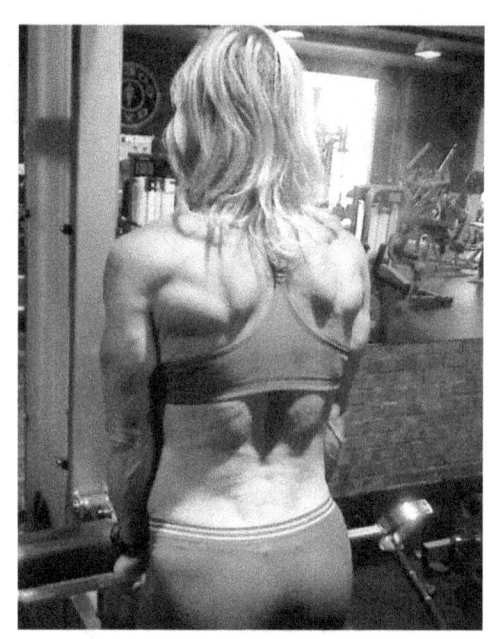

This is a body part that was once considered a weakness for Julie. She had nothing on the back of her arms at all. The impressive triceps Julie now displays are a testament to her hard work and perseverance. There is a tendency amongst trainers to work on their strong body parts and neglect weaker areas. This philosophy needs to be turned on its head and the weak parts brought into line with stronger areas in a way that makes it difficult for a observer to pick out individual areas to compliment on your body. It takes self discipline to stick to a balanced workout and not just keep doing what you are good at. We have all seen physiques that are all upper body or all arms etc, that is a result of neglecting rather than prioritizing weak body parts. Beware of this and get somebody you trust, value and respect to give you an honest appraisal at regular intervals, sometimes we are so close we don't get a realistic view.

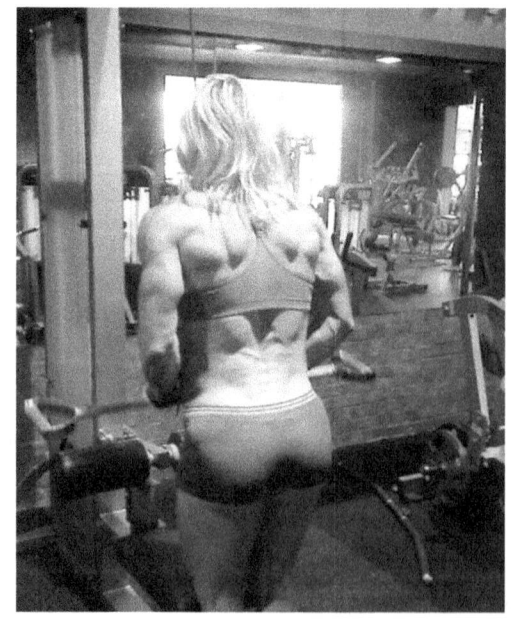

DELTS

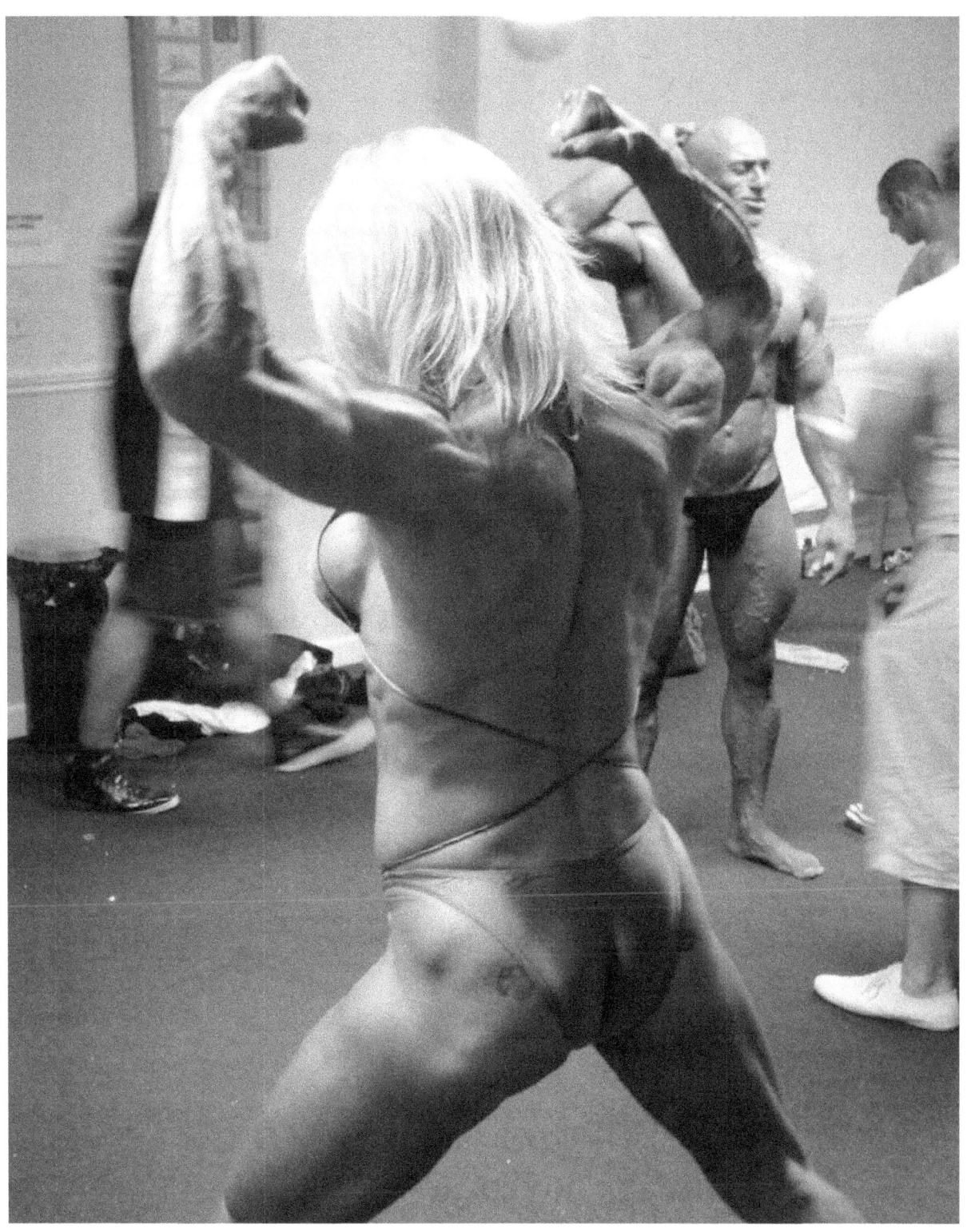

Barbell Upright Rows

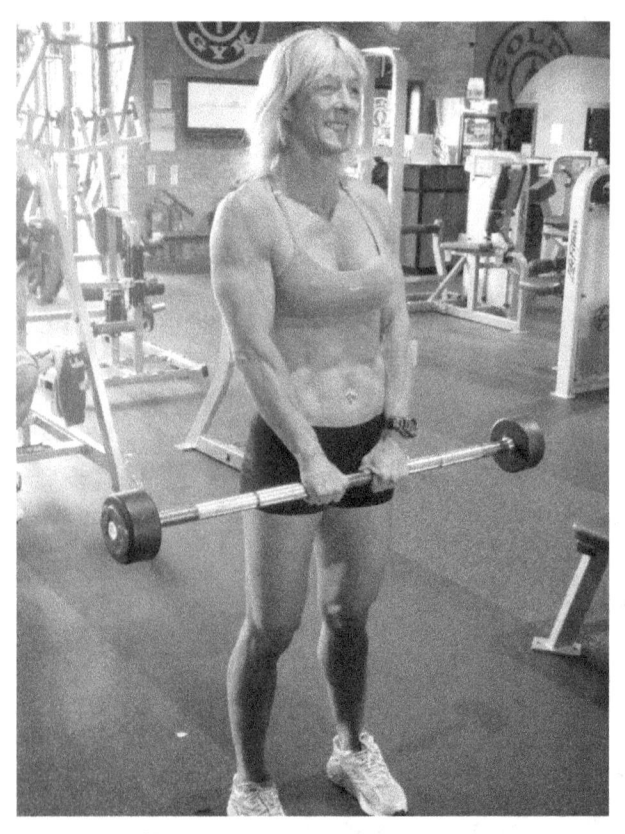

Upright rows work the Traps as well as the deltoid muscles. This is the only real trapezius work we do as we feel too much development of the traps can give the trainer a round shouldered look. Julie uses about a 6" inch grip, I like to grip the bar even closer. Find the grip that is most comfortable for you. We always try to raise the bar past the chin to illicit a more intense contraction in our shoulders. We stand with feet shoulder width apart and work to maintain good posture throughout the set. The biceps are involved quite heavily in this compound movement and if we were to pick two exercises to give a well rounded deltoid workout, we

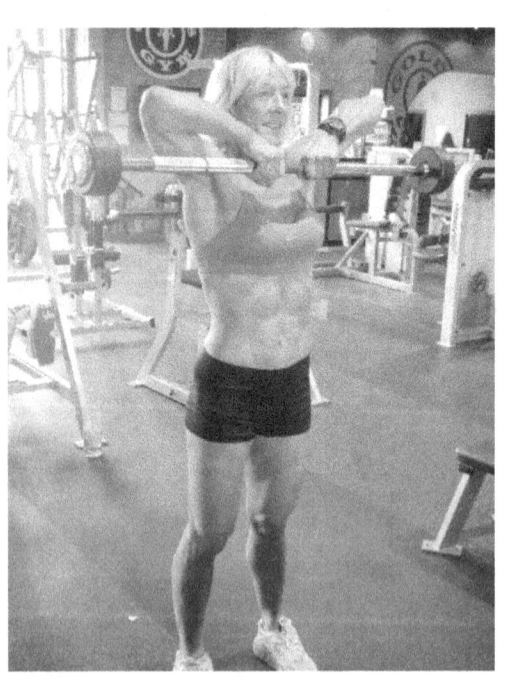

would pick upright rows and a shoulder press. That would give a push and pull balance to a deltoid session.

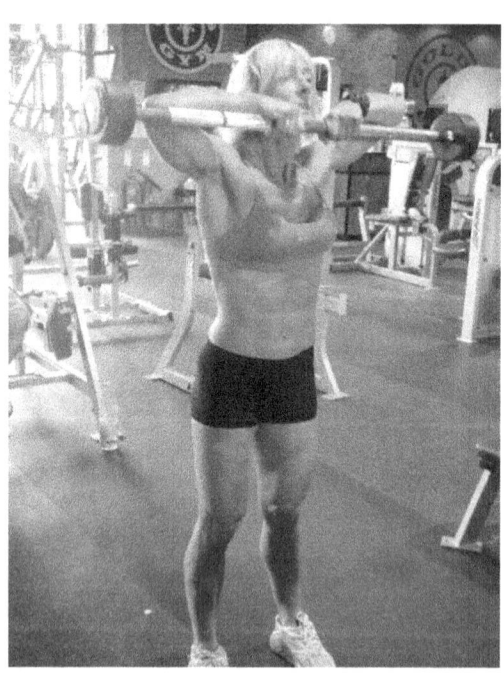

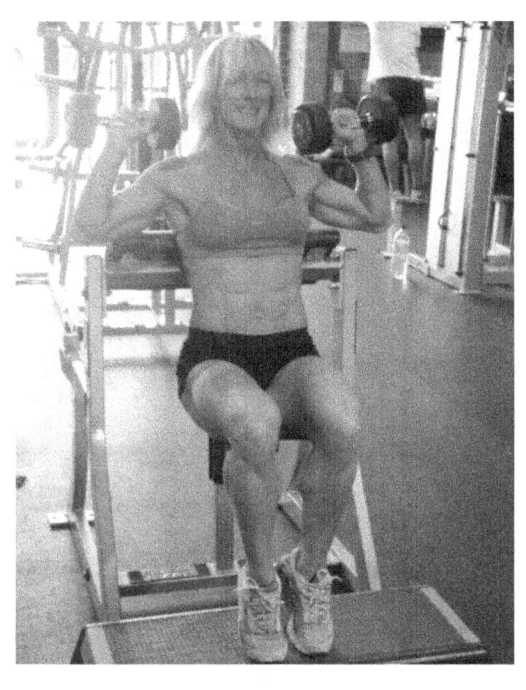

Seated Dumbbell Press

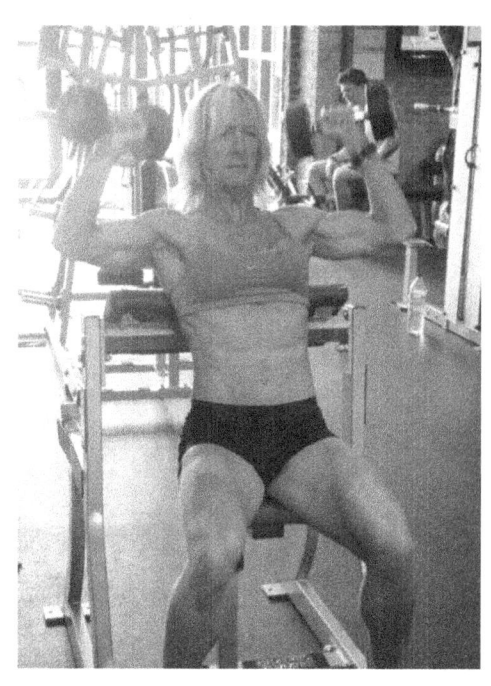

We like to perform our dumbbell presses sitting back to front on a preacher bench, as pictured with feet on a step for stability. This gives a lot of freedom while still giving some support to the back. The dumbbells are lowered until the inside bell touches the shoulders and then pressed back up to arms length. To assist when the going gets tough a partner can stand behind and help support the elbows on the press for a few assisted reps. always remember to work up in weight with each set, never start with a heavy weight, build up gradually. I would like to point out here the action of Julie's abdominals clearly visible in these pictures. The abdominals work in many exercises to support and stabilize the spine. Many trainers do very little direct work for abs because of all the indirect work they perform.

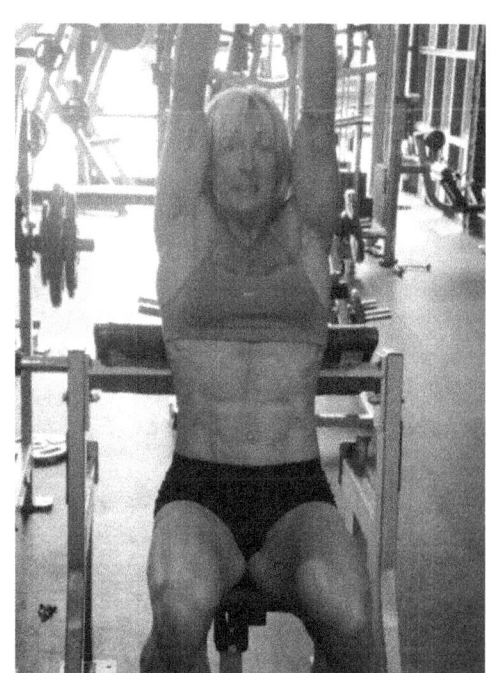

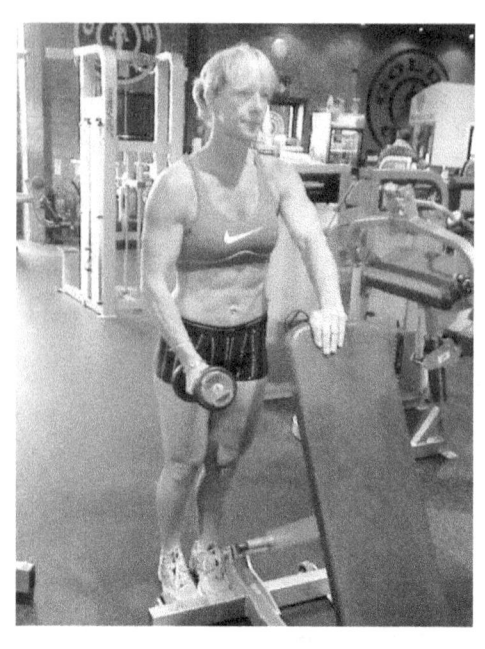

Single Arm Lateral Raise

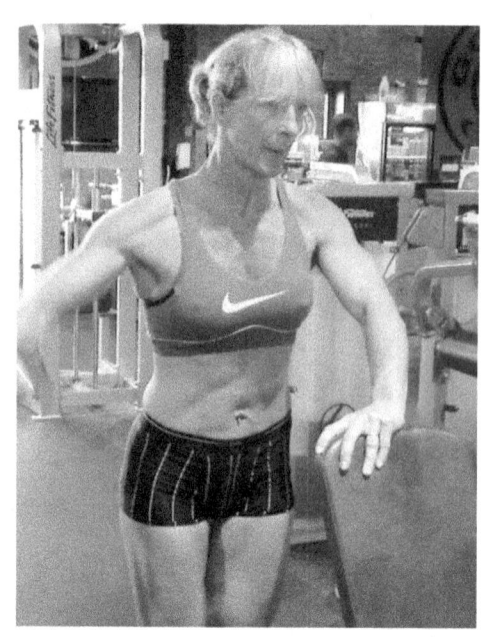

There are many variations of the lateral raise. For this particular technique, we raise a bench up to 90% and use the back to support our movement and reduce any swaying, rocking and reduce the possibility of cheating the weight up with momentum. Once a comfortable position is established Julie performs 12/15 reps with each arm and then rests before repeating the action for subsequent sets. The dumbbell only need be raised to the point where the arm is parallel to the floor or just above. Julie is demonstrating the start and finish positions perfectly. When performed correctly the shoulders start to fatigue and maybe even get a lactic acid build up in the muscle. If pain is felt anywhere else you are probably doing something wrong and need to reassess your form. Side lateral raises work the medial head of the deltoid muscle.

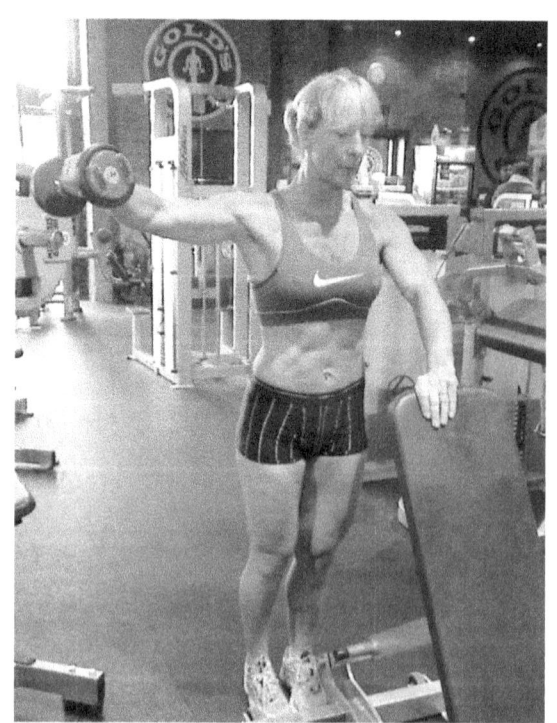

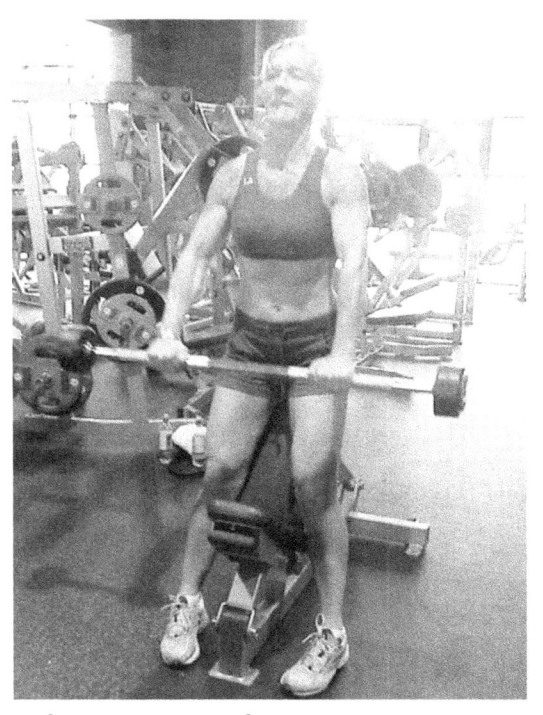

Barbell Forward Raise

Again for forward raises we raise a bench up to 90% and use the back

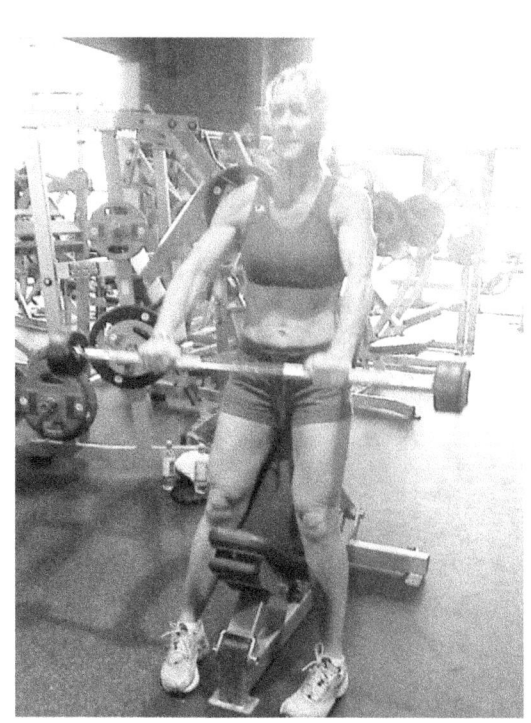

to support our movement and reduce any swaying, rocking and reduce the possibility of cheating the weight up with momentum. Once a comfortable position is established Julie performs 12/15 reps. Laterals and raises are not exercises that need heavy weights and caution should be applied.

Elbows should be slightly bent and palms are facing down. The emphasis turns to the anterior, or front head of the deltoid. When performing any raises there is always a tendency to sway and swing, you have to constantly be critical of your own form and stay strict with your movements.

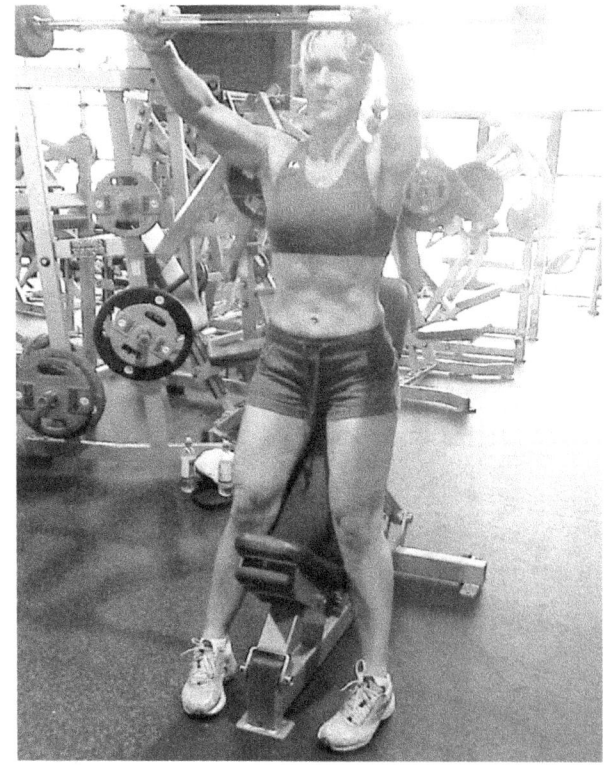

Seated Rear Deltoid Lateral Raise

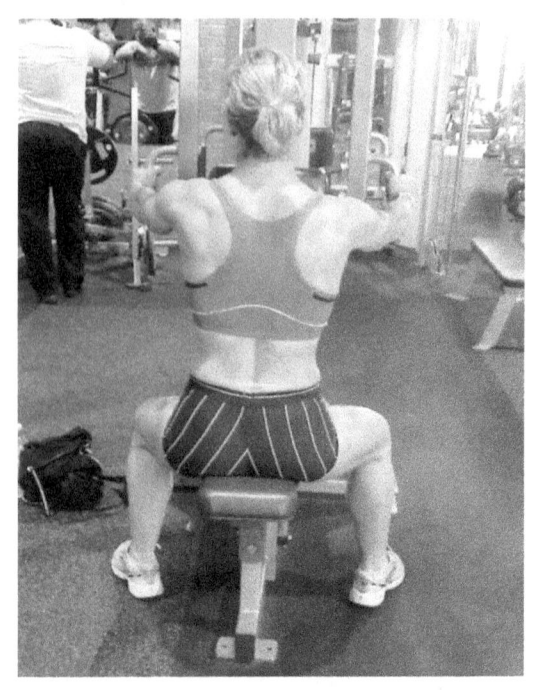

This machine has evolved to enable trainers to perform the bent over deltoid raise in a seated position. Rear raises target the posterior head of the deltoids. Once again, not much weight should be used. In the pictures we can clearly see Julie's rear delts working. Arms are parallel to the floor and posture is maintained at all times. The wonderful thing about all the latest machines is that they not only enable the exercise to be performed safely but also provide tiny differences in the exercise so as to create a whole new if very similar exercise.

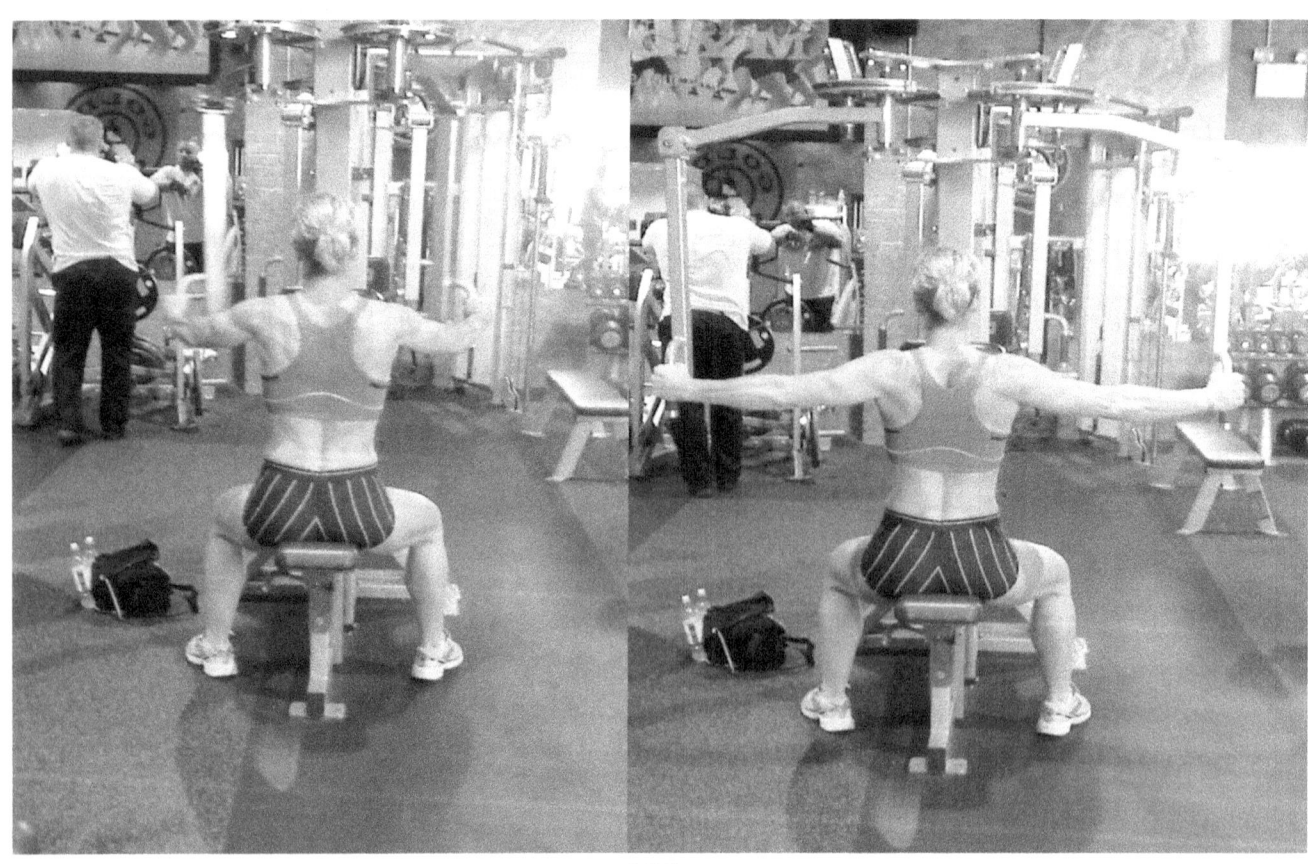

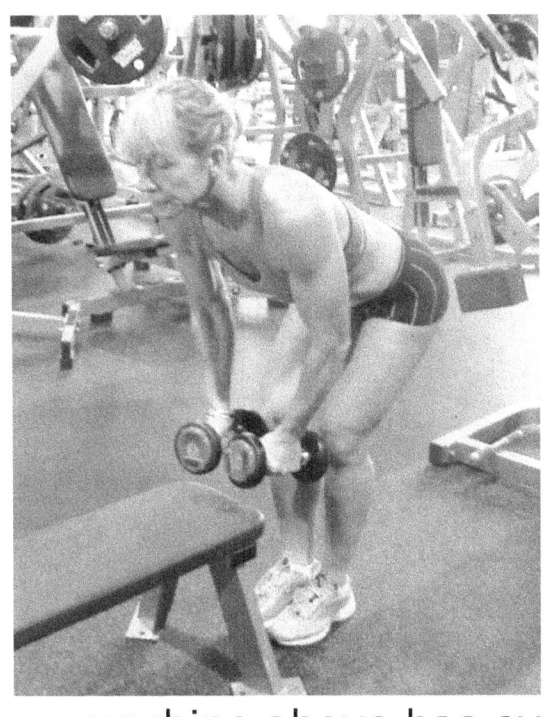

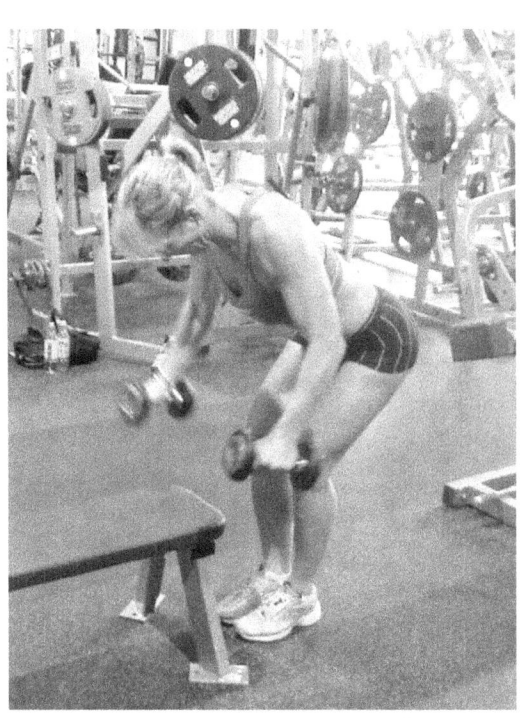

Bent Over Rear Lateral Raises

Now this is the free weight exercise that the machine above has evolved from. Rear raises target the posterior head of the deltoids. Once again, not much weight should be used. Importantly here is to maintain a strong stance throughout the exercise as you can see it is quite an awkward position. Arms are parallel to the floor and posture is maintained at all times. The wonderful thing about all the original free weight exercises is that your body has to enlist the help of many stabilising muscles not used in machine equivalents in order to perform, this is why free weight moves should be performed early in your workout before you are too fatigued to perform them safely and effectively.

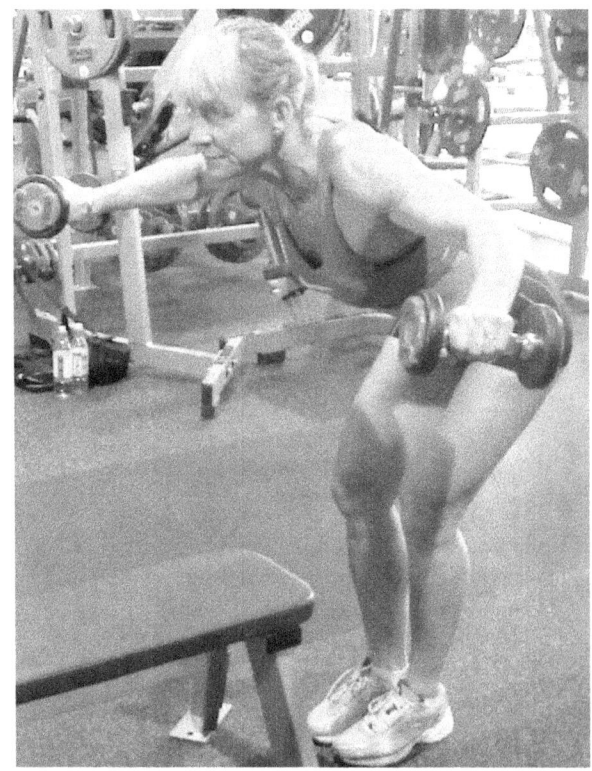

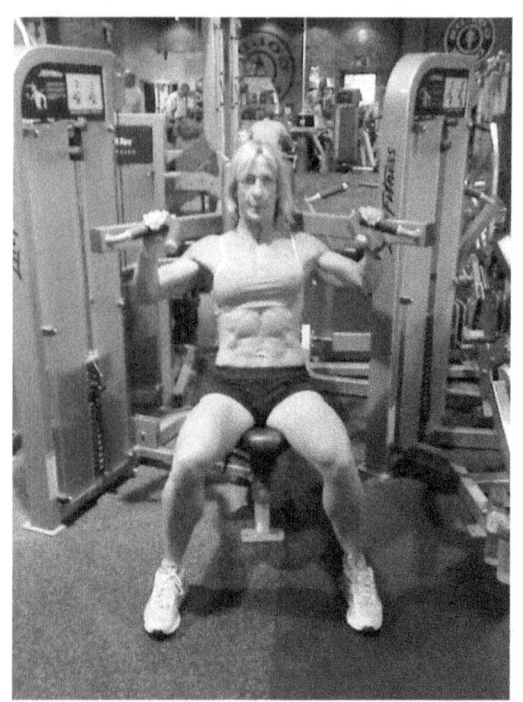

Machine Deltoid Press

Machine press is an example of an exercise that can be done later in your workouts as there is no need for balance or any technique or timing particularly. All you need to do is power the handles up in a predetermined groove and control them back down. If you compare this to dumbbells where you have to stop them going forward, backward and side to side and the groove to press out is determined by the trainer, you can see why machine and free weights are so different and how the variety and availability of both can be so beneficial.

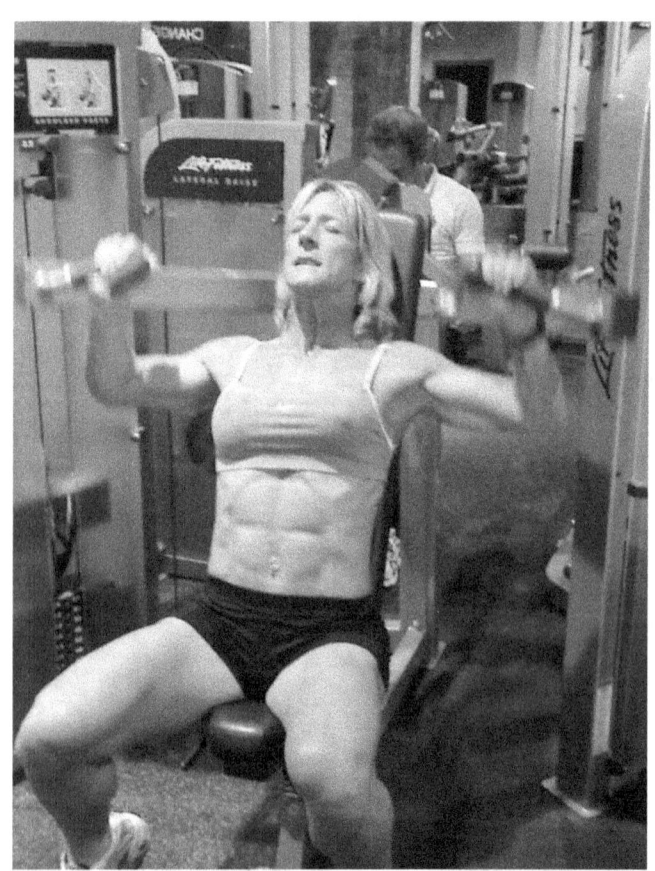

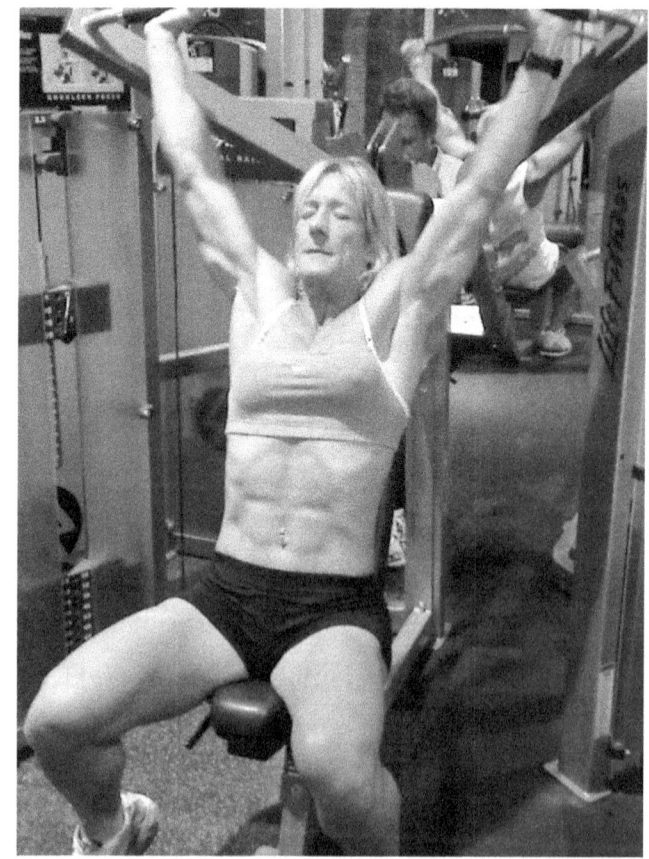

ABS

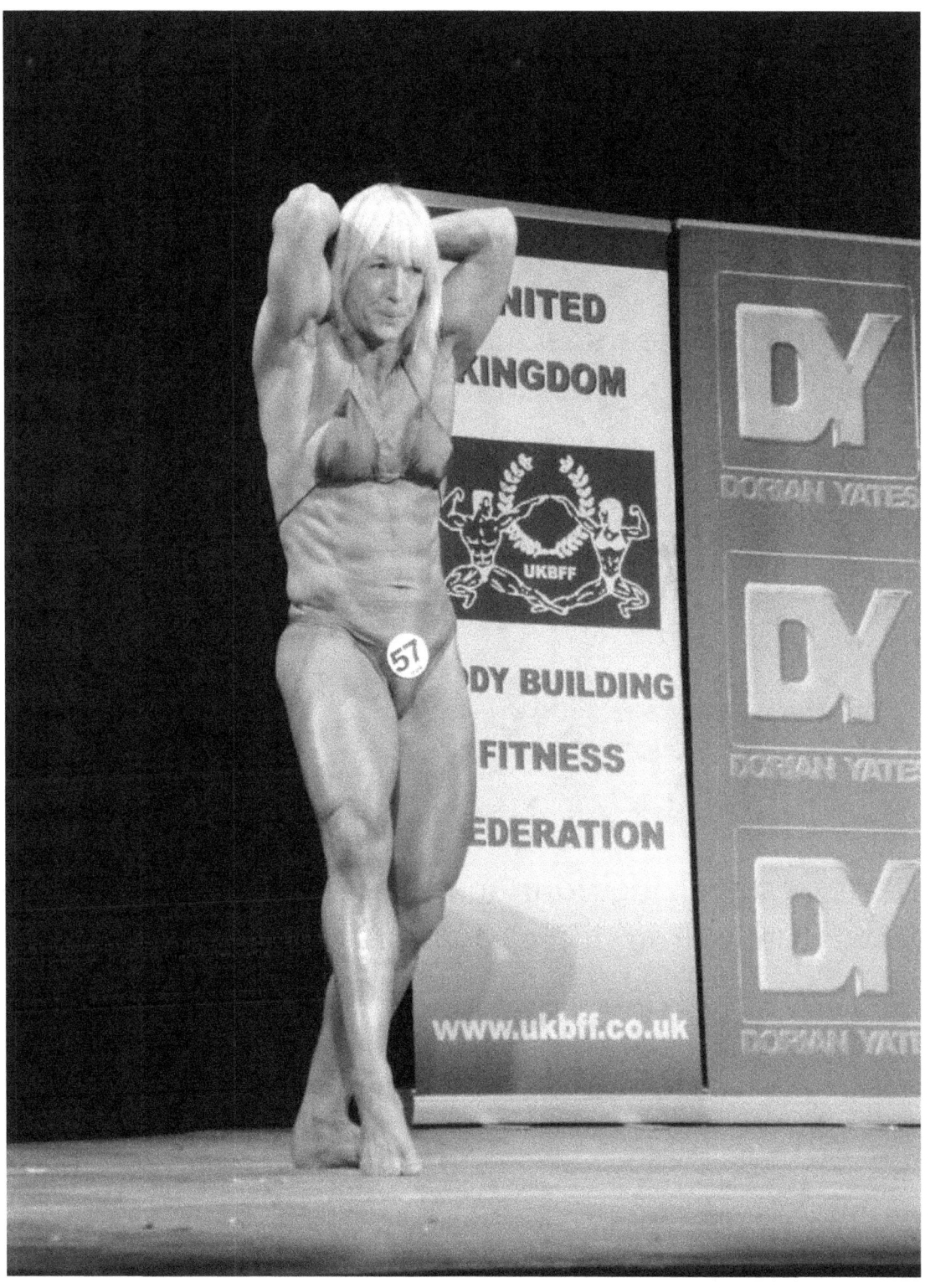

Cycle Crunches

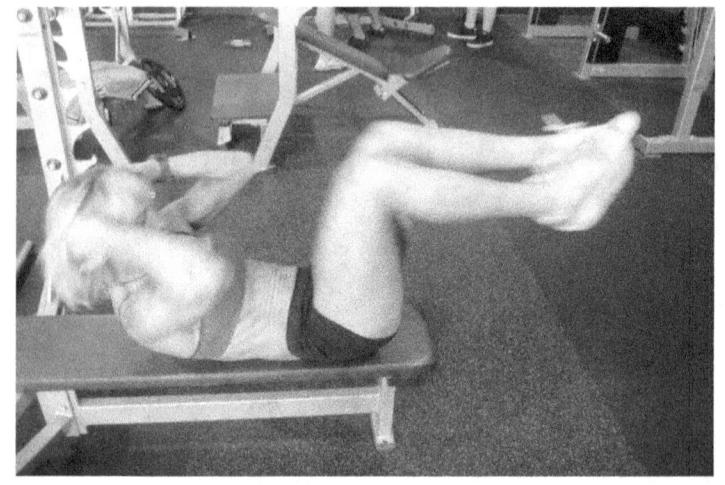

The first myth I wish to dispel in this section is spot reduction. Spot reduction is where it is believed that working an area such as your midsection hard and often will result in the loss of bodyfat in that area specifically. The order your body stores fat is unique to you and the first place you gain fat will be the last place you lose it, there is nothing you can do to change that. 1,000 sit ups ten times per day will not simply reduce your tummy, whatever the gadget manufacturers are misleading you to believe. Working the abs is still

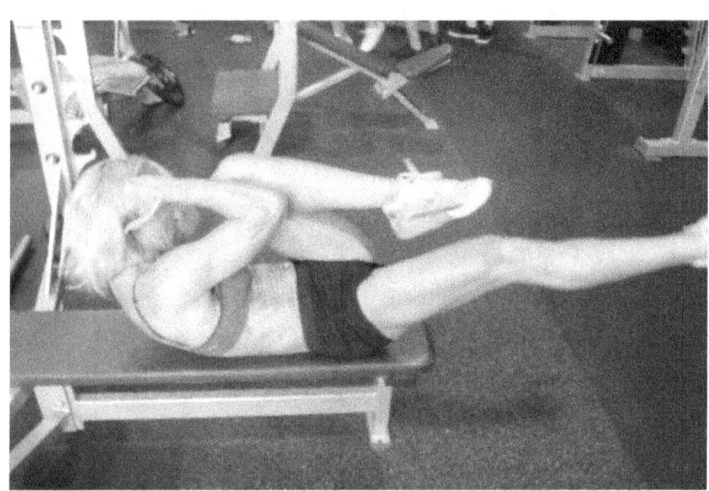

important in stabilizing your spine and when your body fat levels eventually drop due to a combination of weights, cardio and diet you will see a fine set of fat free abdominal muscles. With cycle crunches you alternate opposite elbow to knee in a slow yet rhythmic style. There are video demonstrations online.

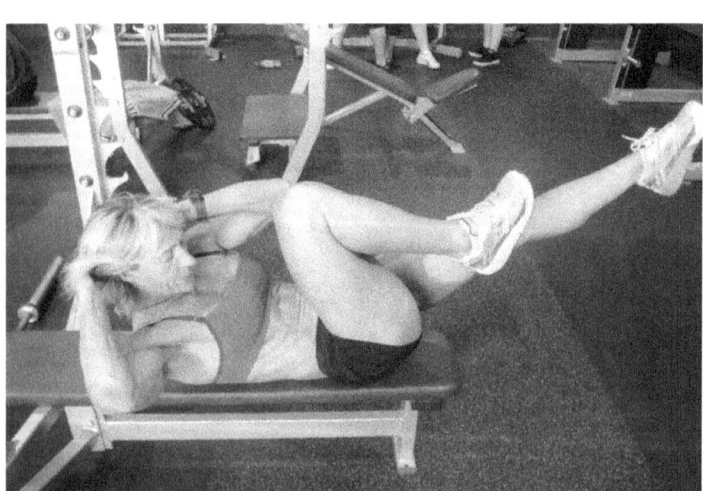

Leg Lowers

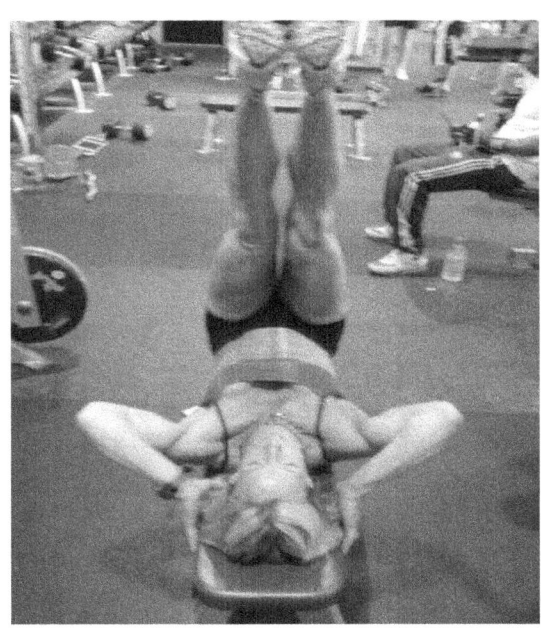

The way to perform this at first is to slowly lower your legs until you feel your low back leaving the bench and then pull your knees into your chest before straightening them and lowering again, The time to bring your knees to chest is ideally just before your back start to leave the bench. As you abdominals become stronger you will lower further and eventually be able to keep your legs straight throughout the movement as Julie is going. Eventually it is possible to have a partner push you legs down from above on each rep. We cannot stress enough the importance of not exceeding your abdominal strength levels on this movement as back strain is the inevitable result. Train smart and if in any doubt pick another exercise until your strength improves.

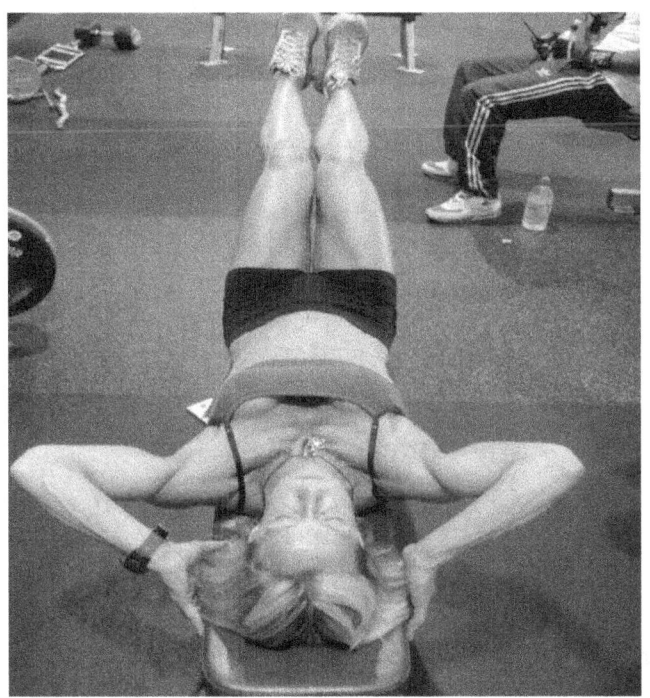

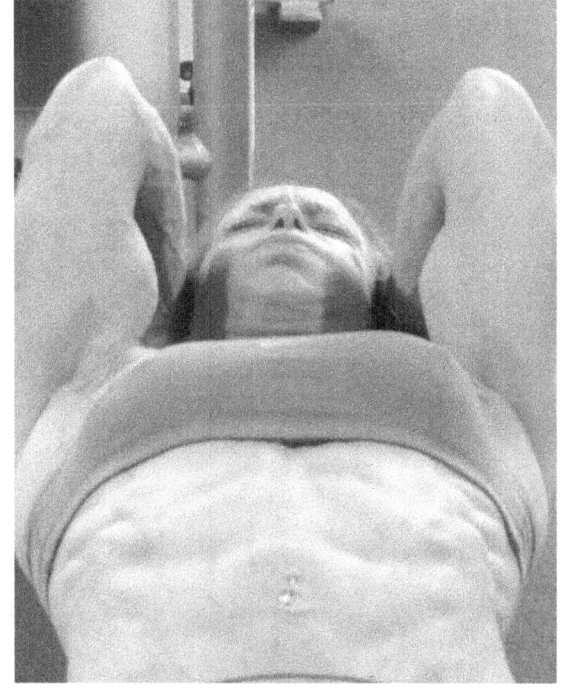

Weighted-Decline Sit Ups

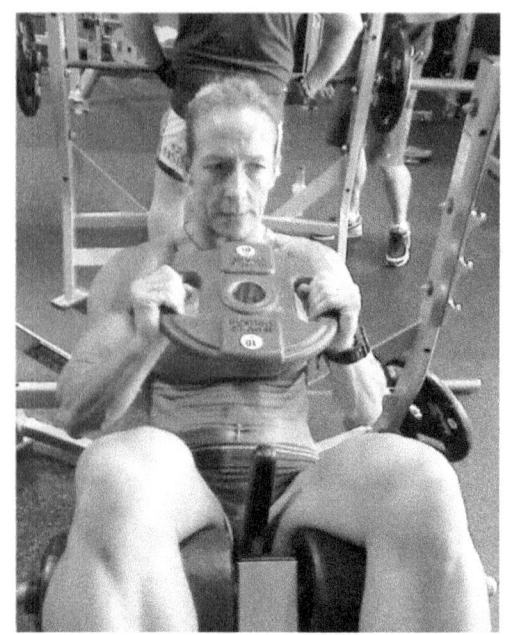

So far all three exercises shown are compound exercises for the midsection, unlike say crunches which attempt to isolate the abdominals. Compound movements enlist all of the muscles of the midsection, hip flexors abs etc working together as they do in life. It has become fashionable in the last decade or so to work muscle groups partially and in isolation whilst I do see the advantage of the addition of isolation exercises to a programme I do not see any advantage in choosing partial isolation over compound movements, Compound movements synchronize your muscles to work together as they do through life. Far better that your weights sessions compliment your life. Sit ups fell victim to the crunch revolution basically because fitness levels dropped so low nobody could do them. Well toughen up because they are back to stay. Your midsection muscles working in harmony.

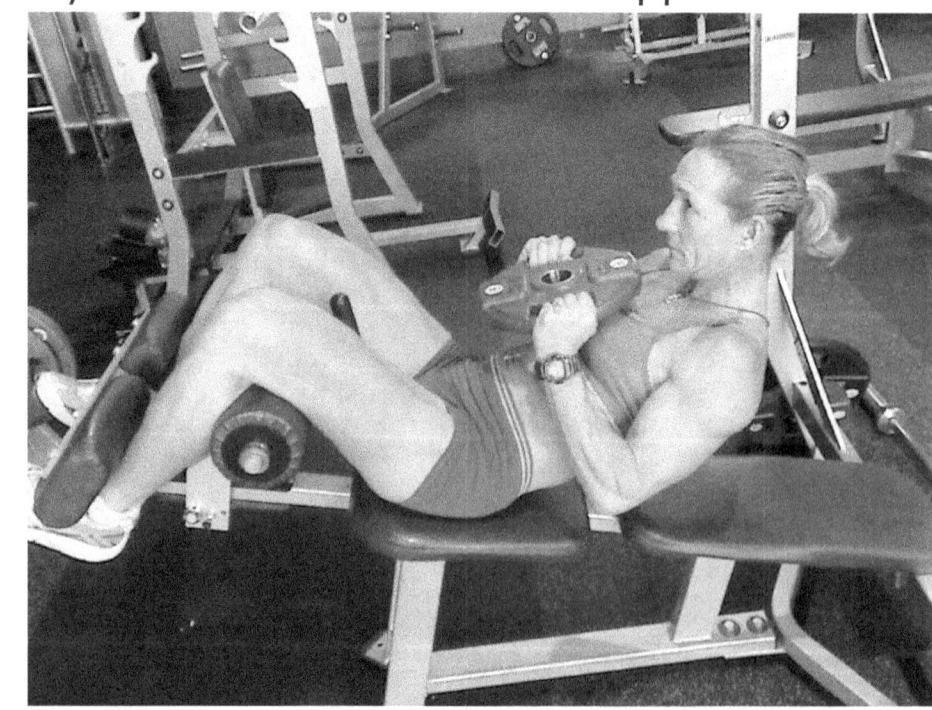

Hanging Leg Raises

If you found sit ups, cycles and leg lowers fun then you are going to love these. These are by far the most advanced of all abdominal exercises. We own a pair of abdominal slings which are available from Maxi Muscle. Pulling a bench close to the suspended slings we adopt the position Julie is in for the exercise. Important point here is to remember that as you raise your legs either bent (hard) or Straight(harder) or somewhere in between you are attempting to rotate your pelvis upward toward your body. As you progress you may wish to hold a light dumbbell between your feet. Making sure not to catapult it across the gym. Face pulling is optional but does seem to help. Demo available online.

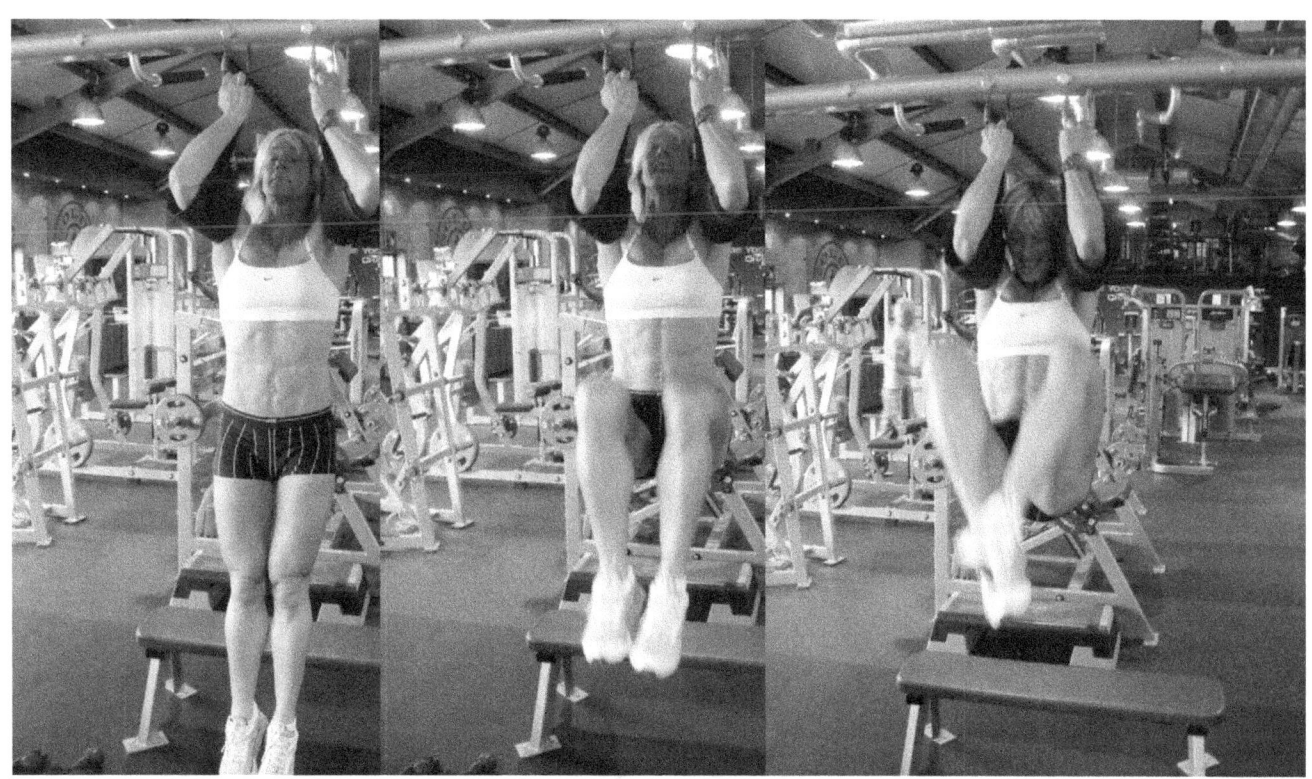

Basic Crunches

The important thing to remember here is that you are not trying to sit up. Crunches are the starting point for any newbie to training. Coaching point would be - do not pull on your head with your hands as that may strain your neck and exhale forcibly at the top of each and every rep this will ensure your abdominals are contracting on the effort. Don't rush and don't bounce up and down and keep your lower half pulled up to you as you crunch. You will see Julie pulls her legs in to meet her chest slightly.

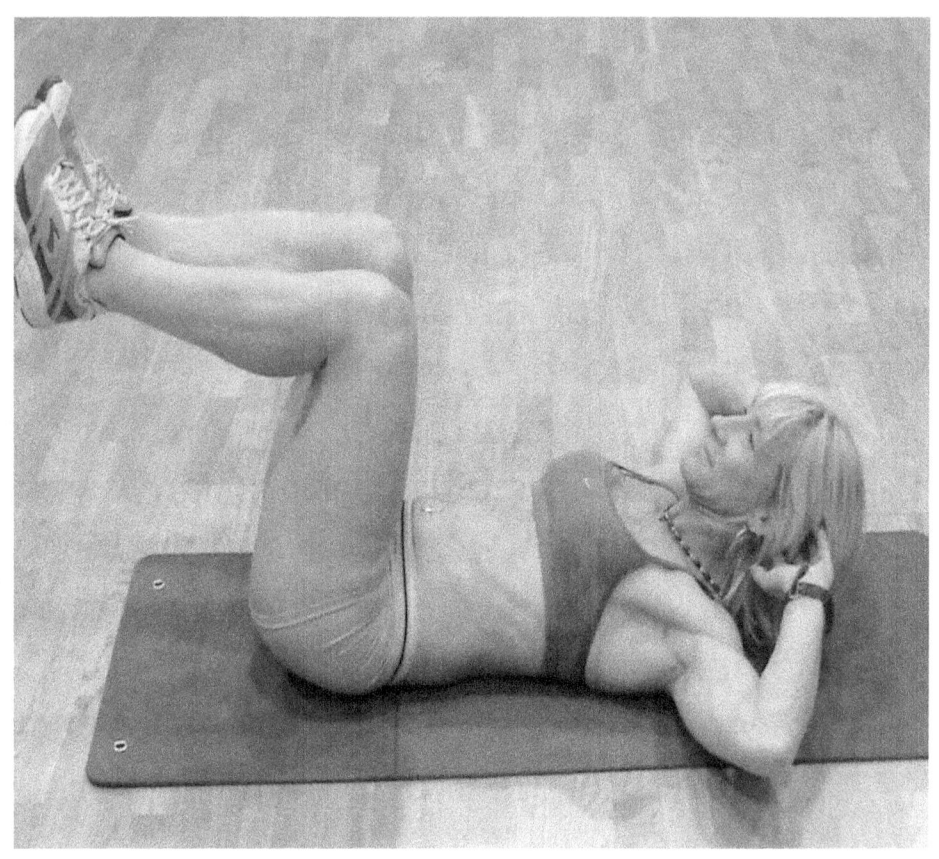

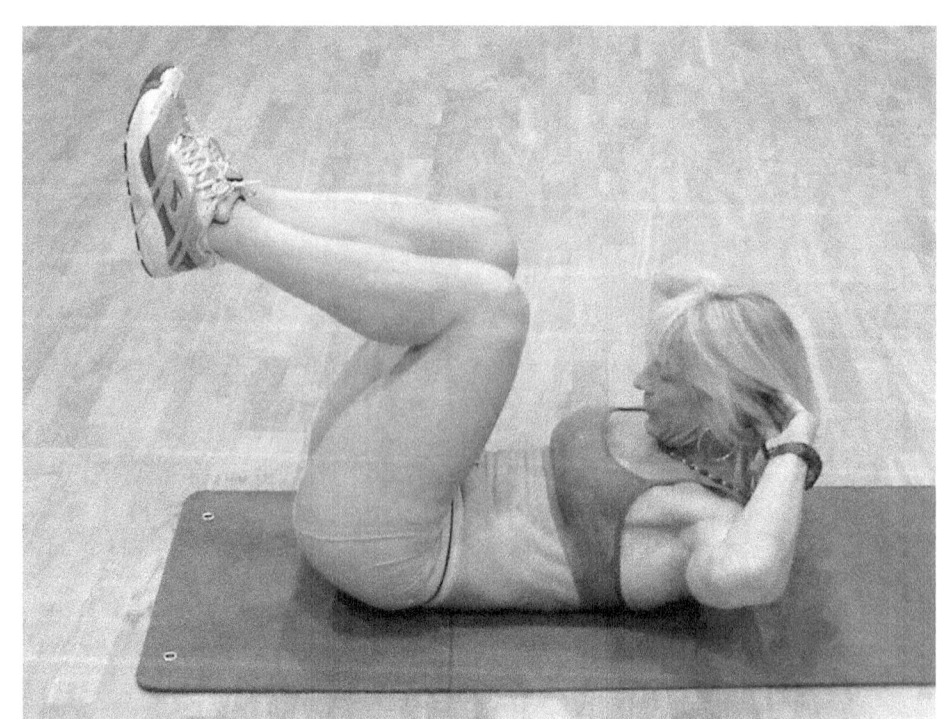

Abdominal Crunch Machine

This machine has been designed so users may perform the crunch motion in an upright position and also add weight by way of a selectorised stack. The important thing to remember here is to take the time to set the seat and chest pad to a reasonably comfortable position as you can see with Julie. Crunches are the starting point for any newbie to training. Coaching point

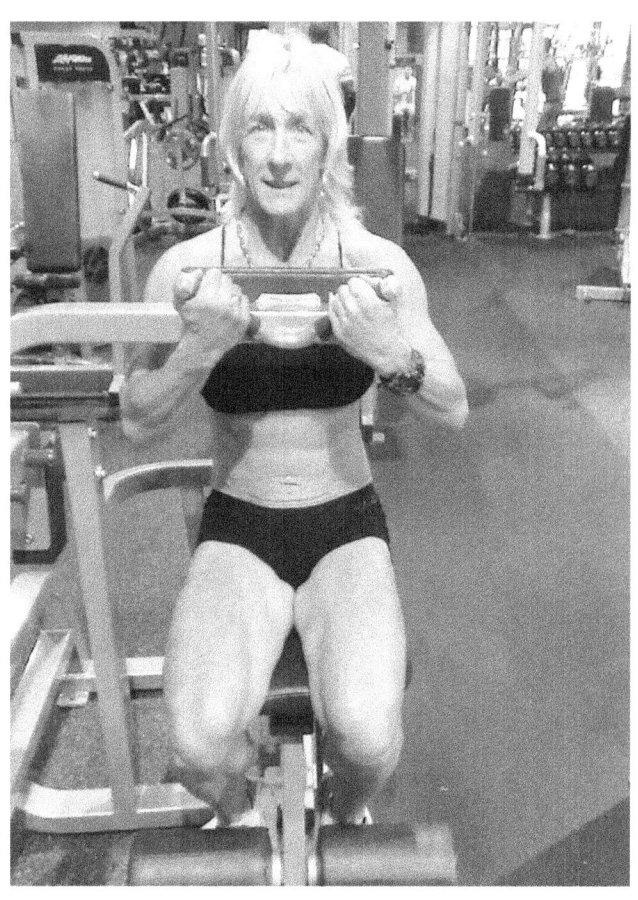

would be - keep your reps smooth and the weight moderate until you get a feel for the movement and exhale forcibly at the bottom of each and every rep this will ensure your abdominals are contracting on the effort. Don't rush and don't bounce up and down. With progressive resistance exercise momentum is always a bad thing. smooth reps and breath and count to yourself and you will not go far wrong.

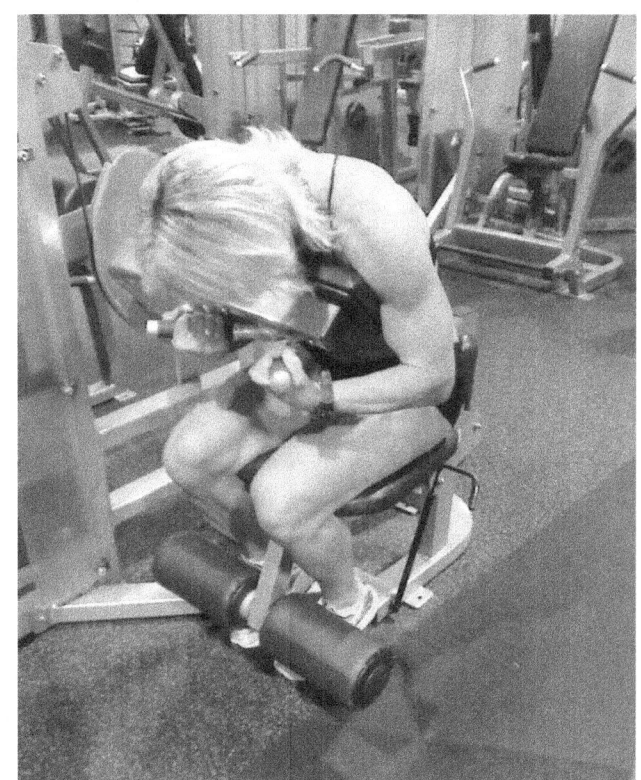

Crunch Machine

Yet another variation on the crunch. Weight can be added to the back of this machine. Again you are not trying to sit up. Crucial coaching point would be -

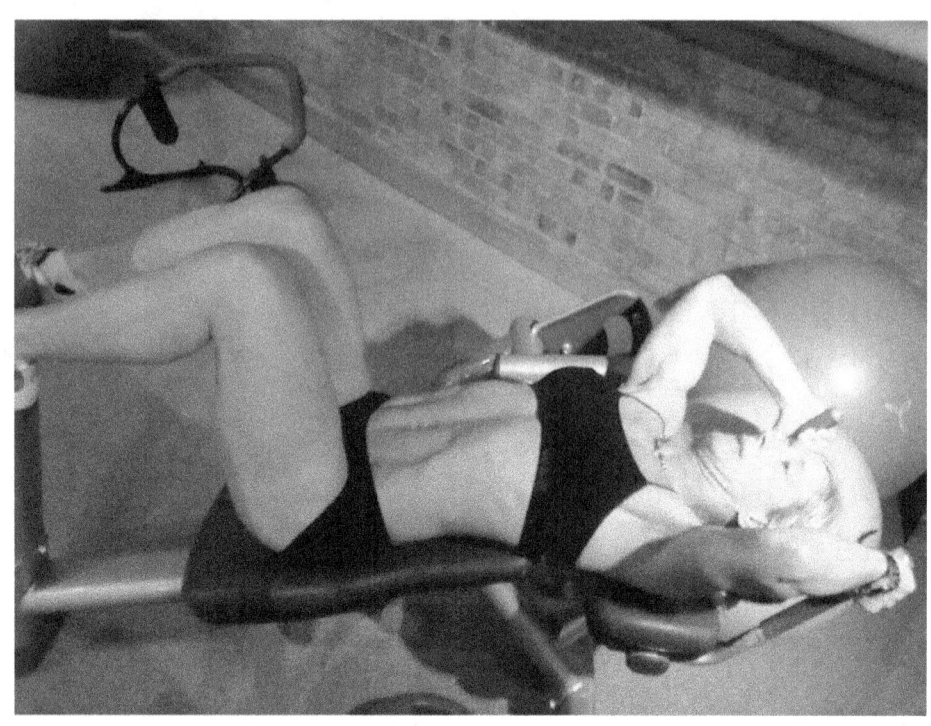

to exhale forcibly at the top of each and every rep this will ensure your abdominals are contracting on the effort. Stay smooth with your motion.

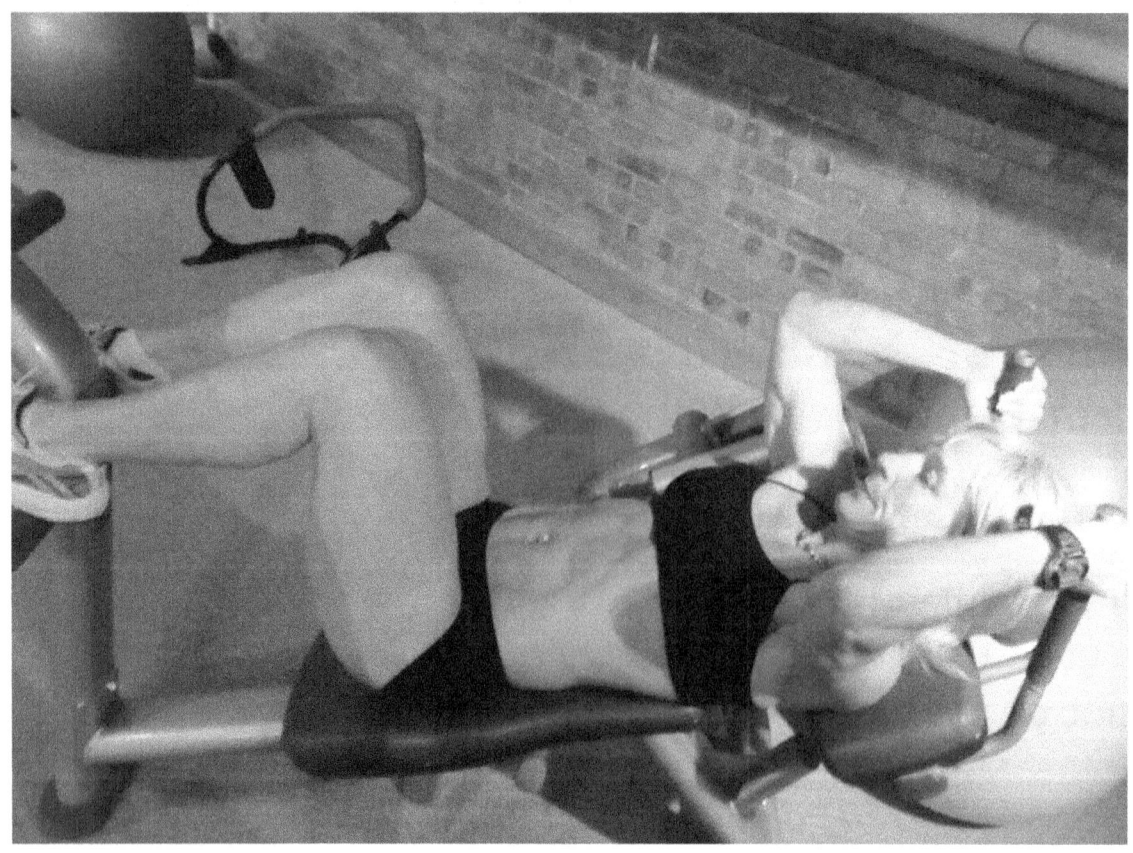

CARDIO

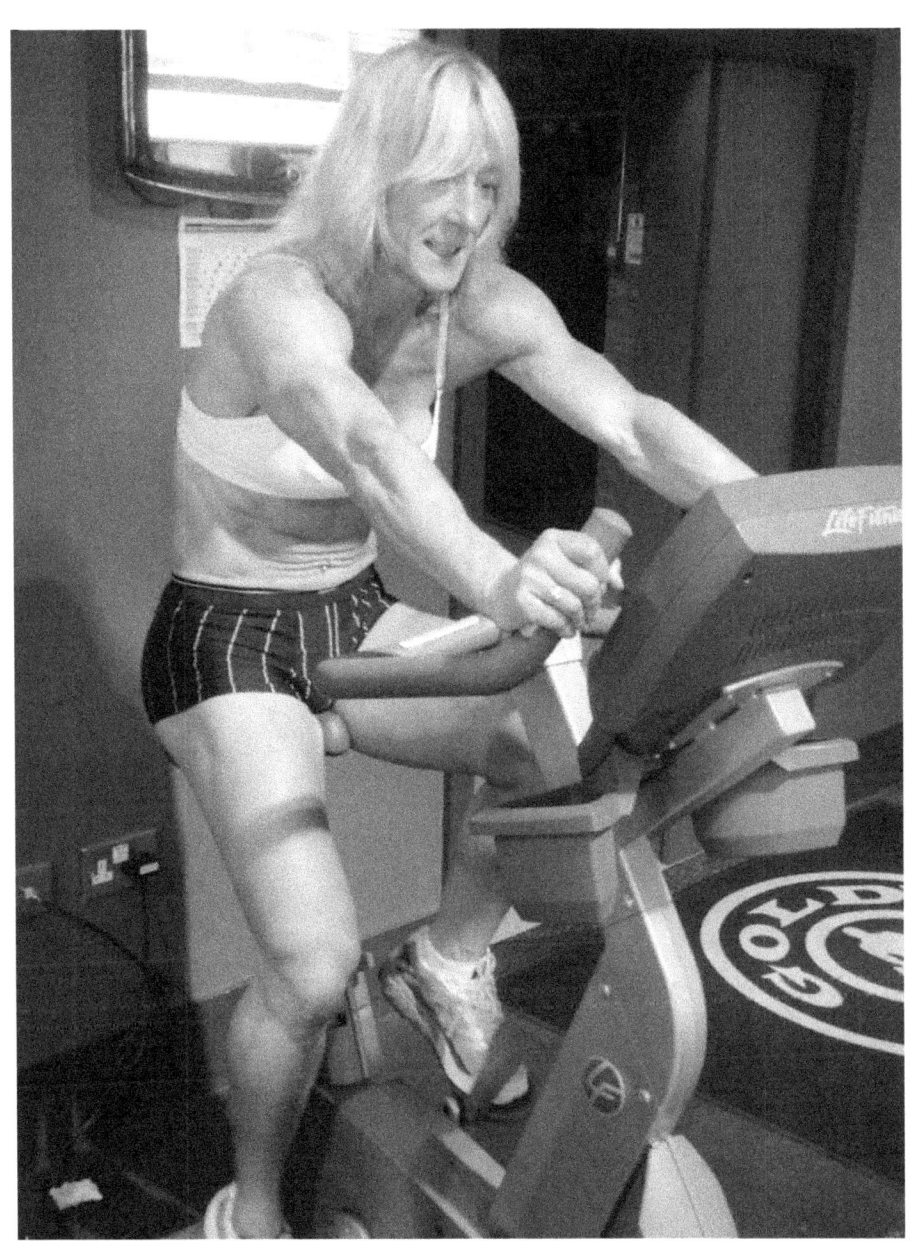

Recumberent Cycle

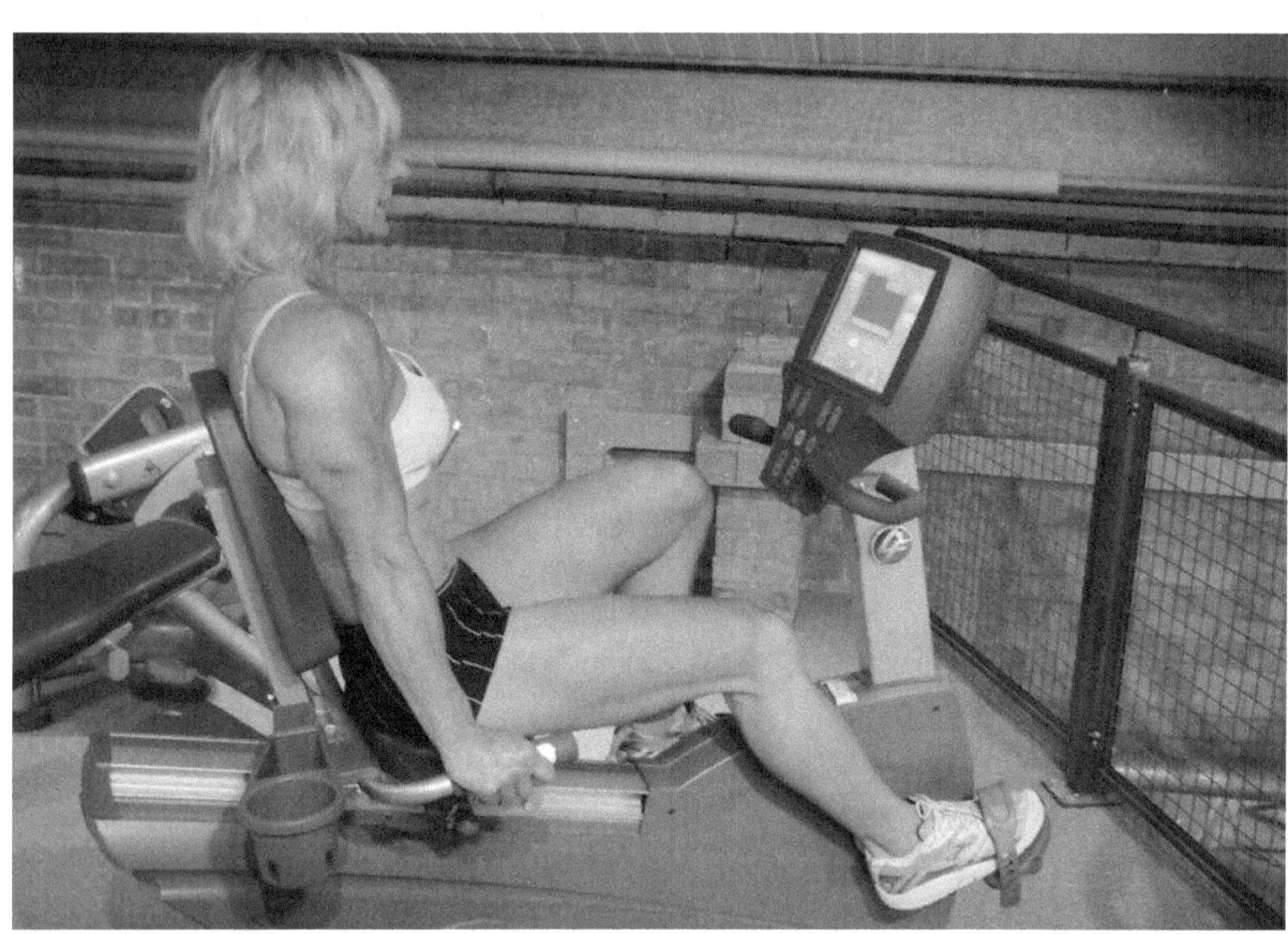

Stationary Cycle

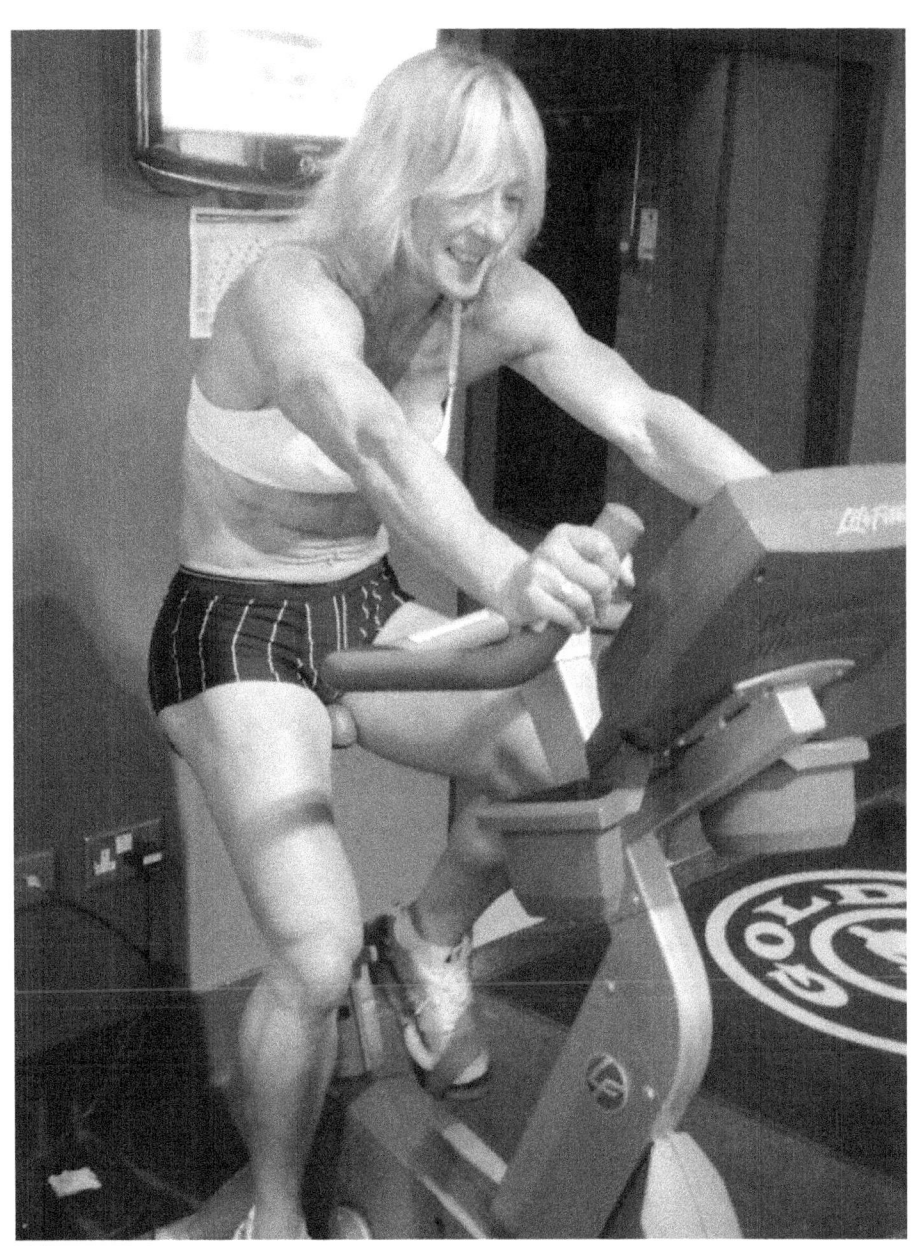

Stepper

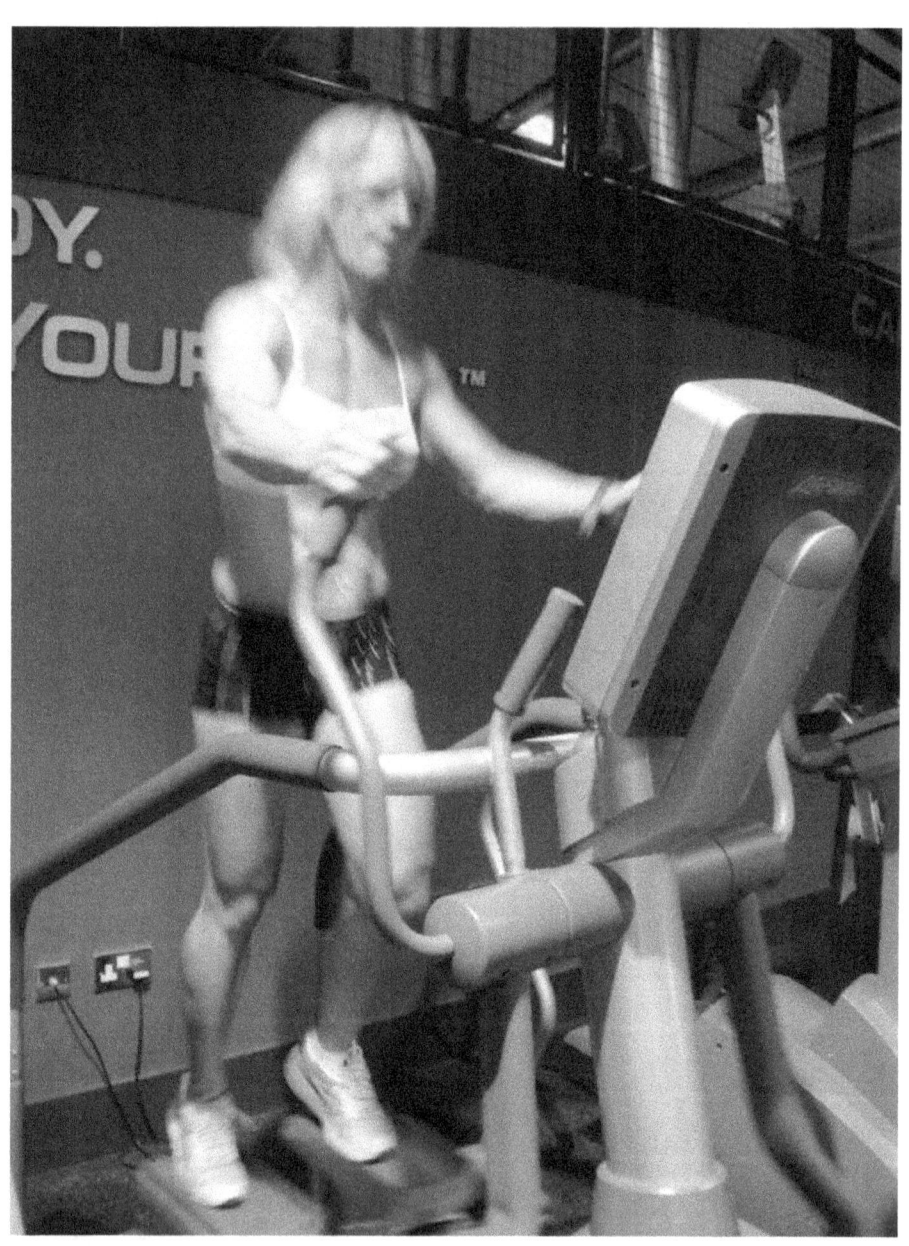

Treadmill

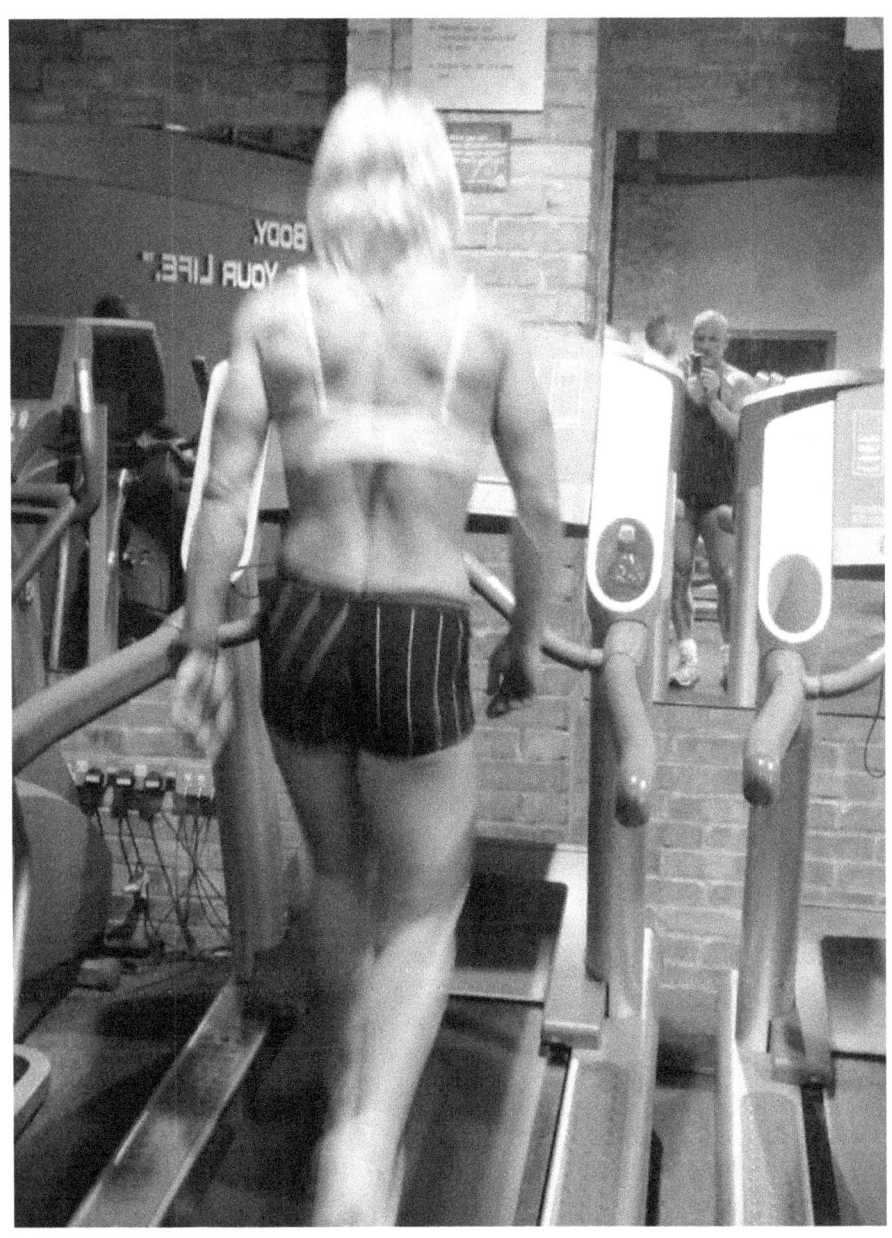

Cross Trainer

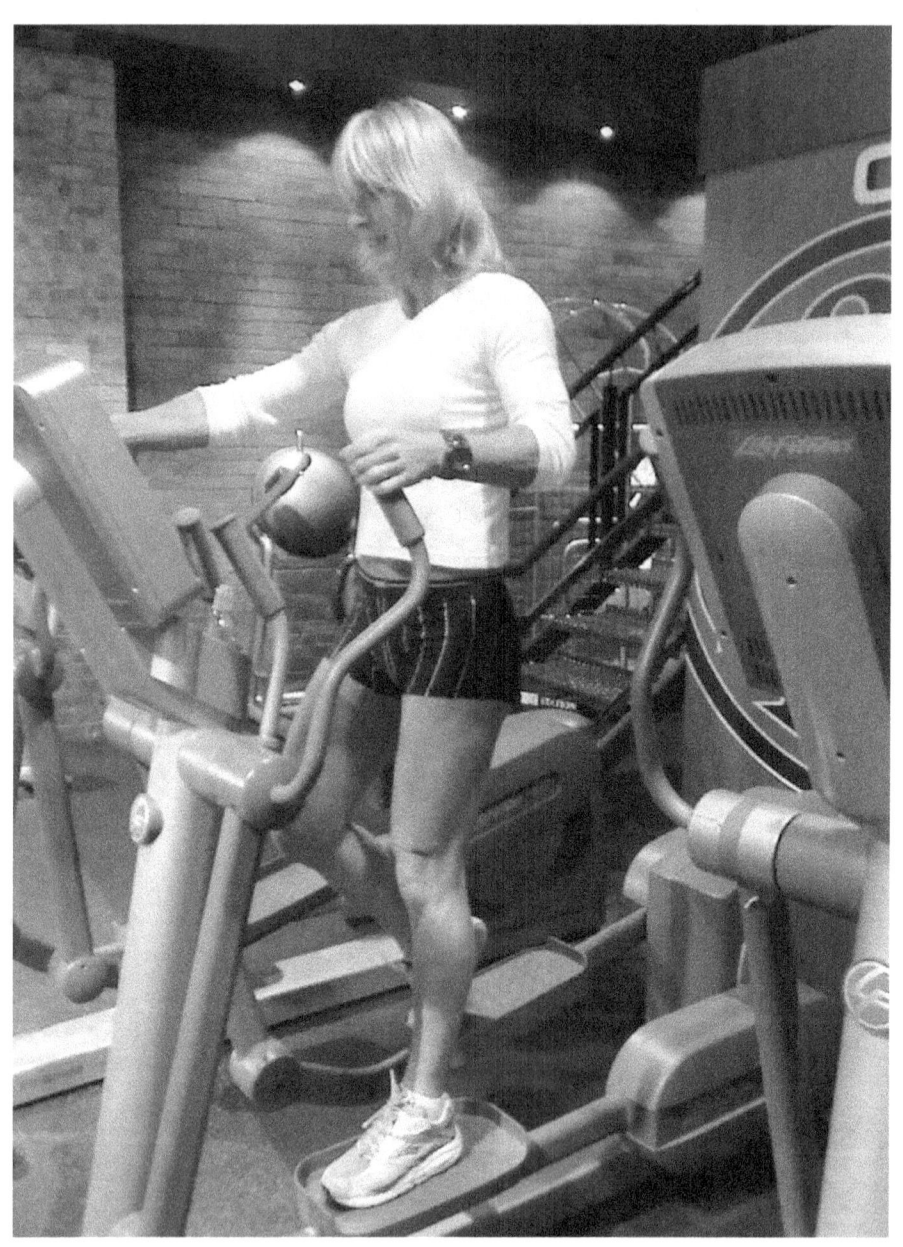

STRETCH

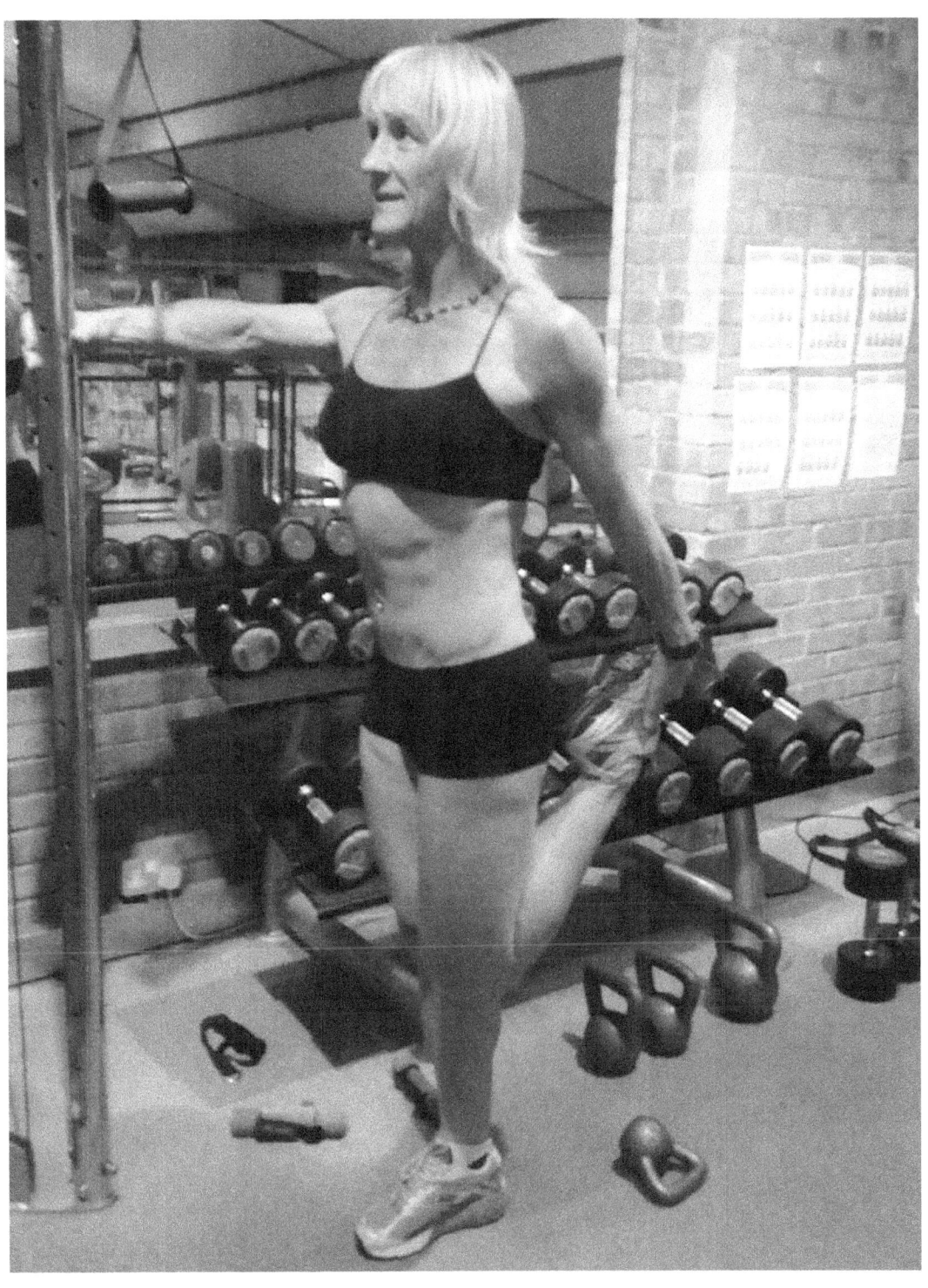

Hamstrings

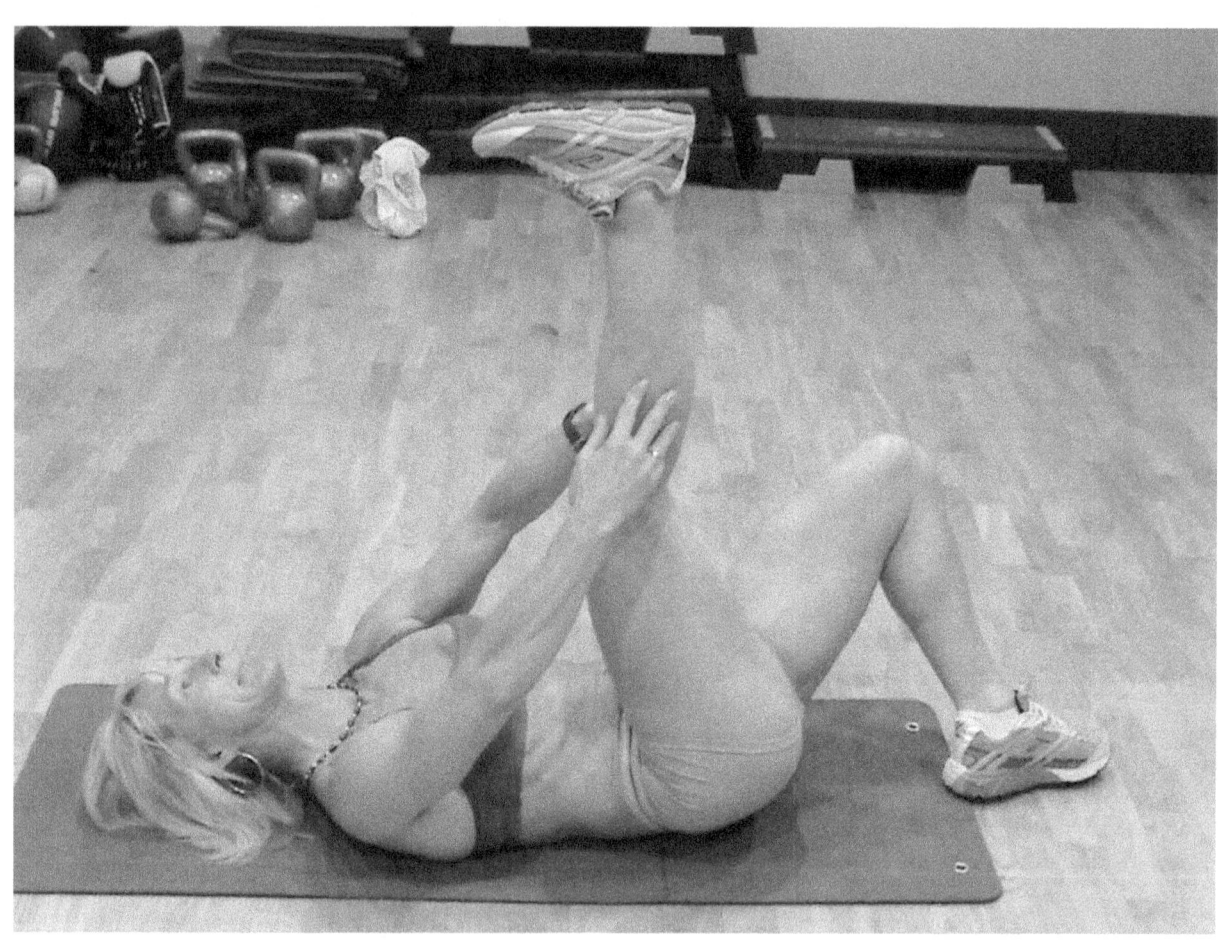

Neck

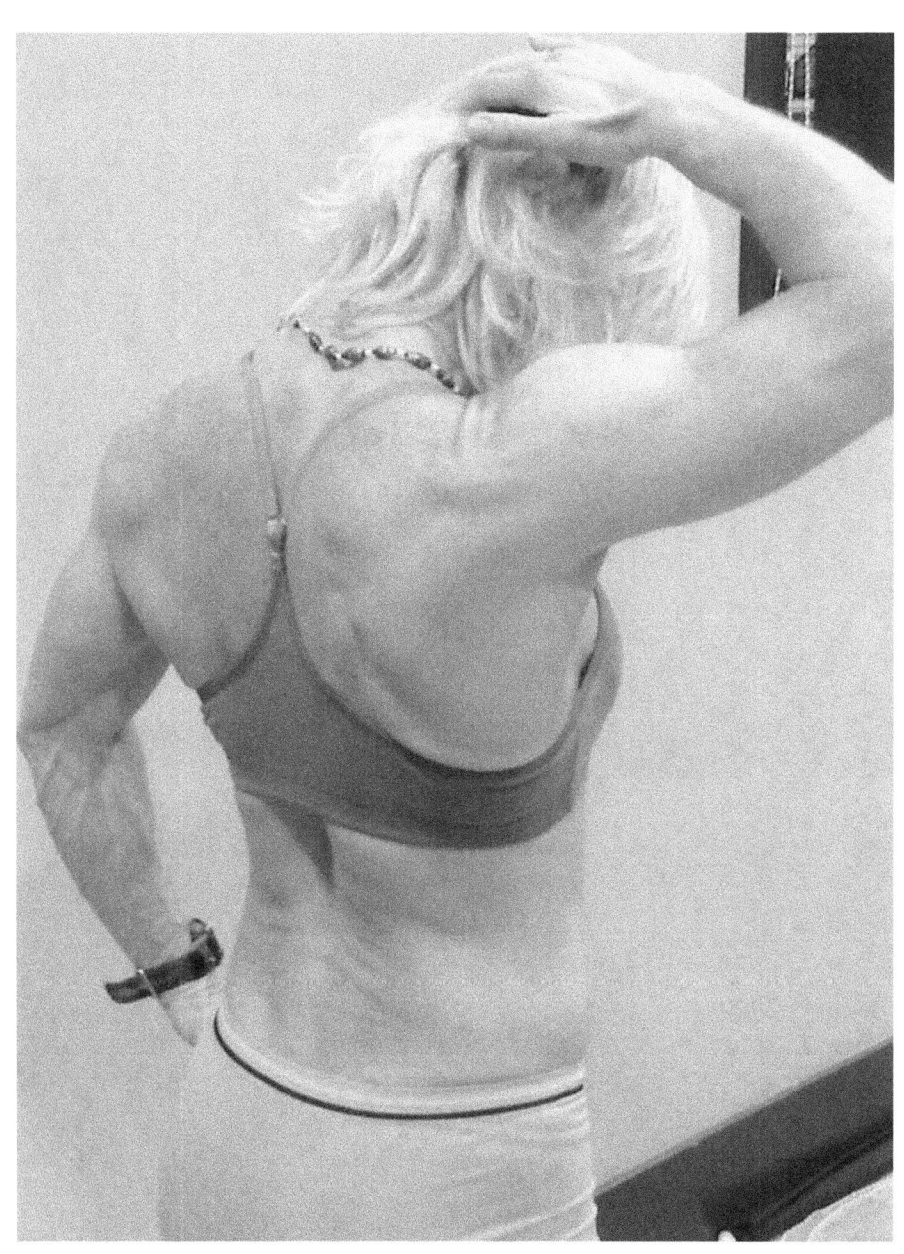

Forearms & Wrists

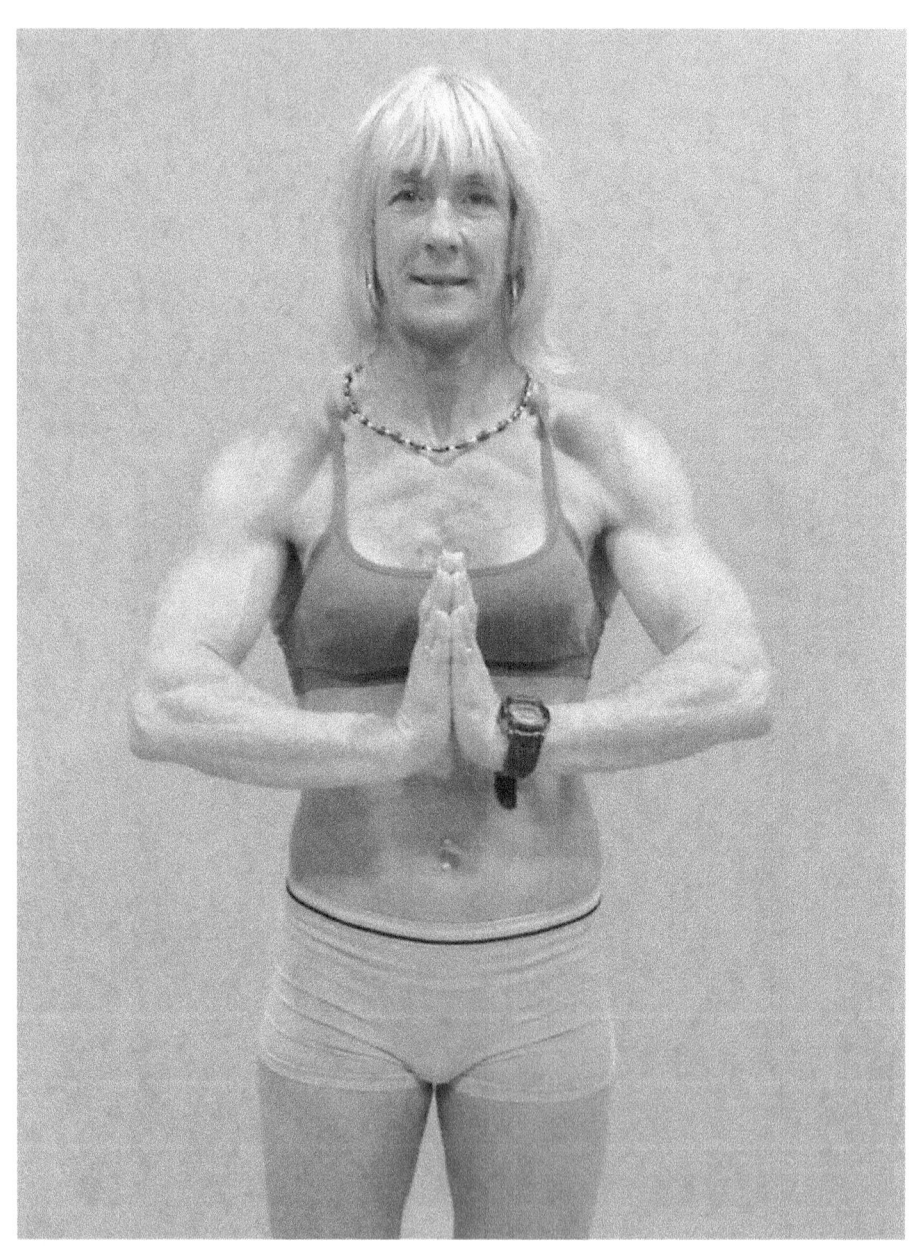

Quads

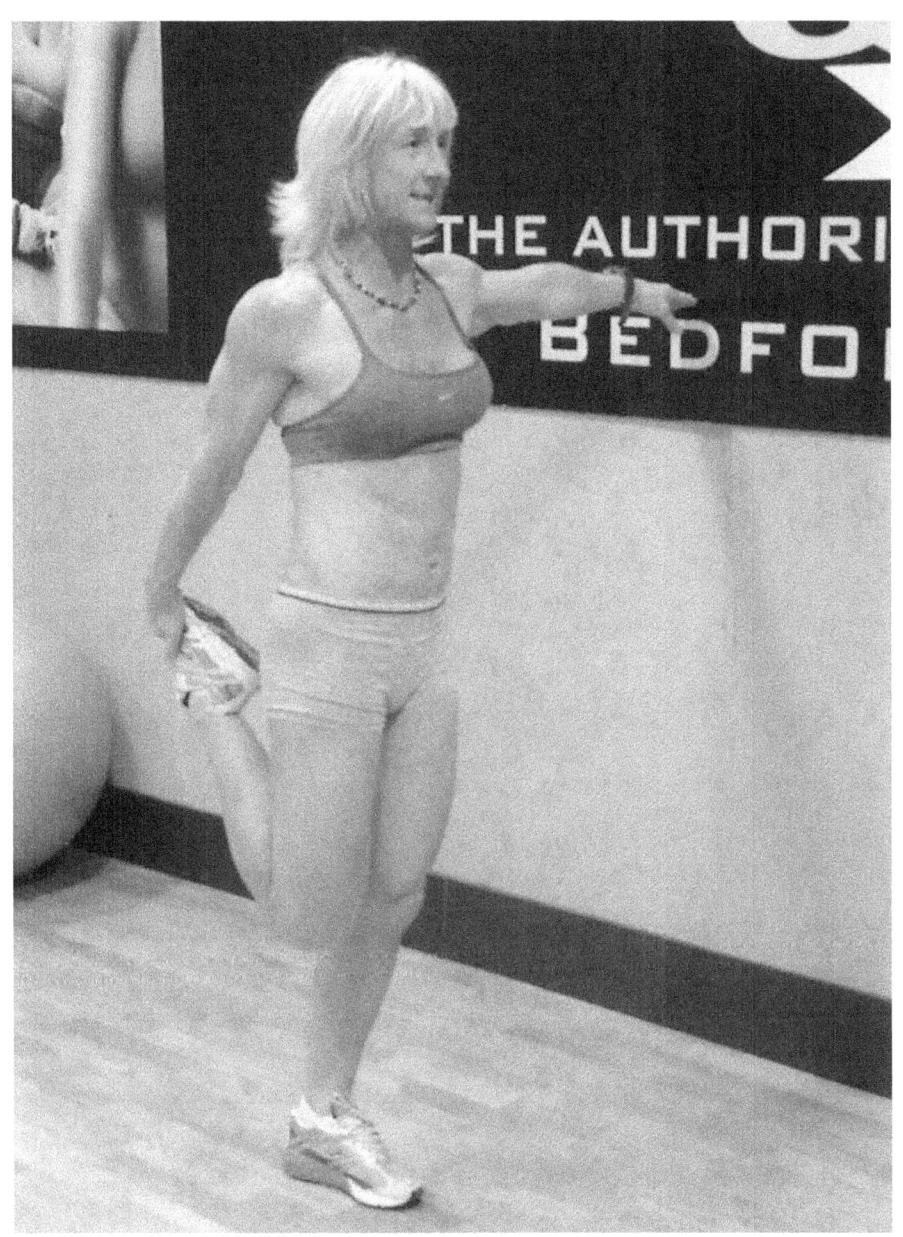

Neck

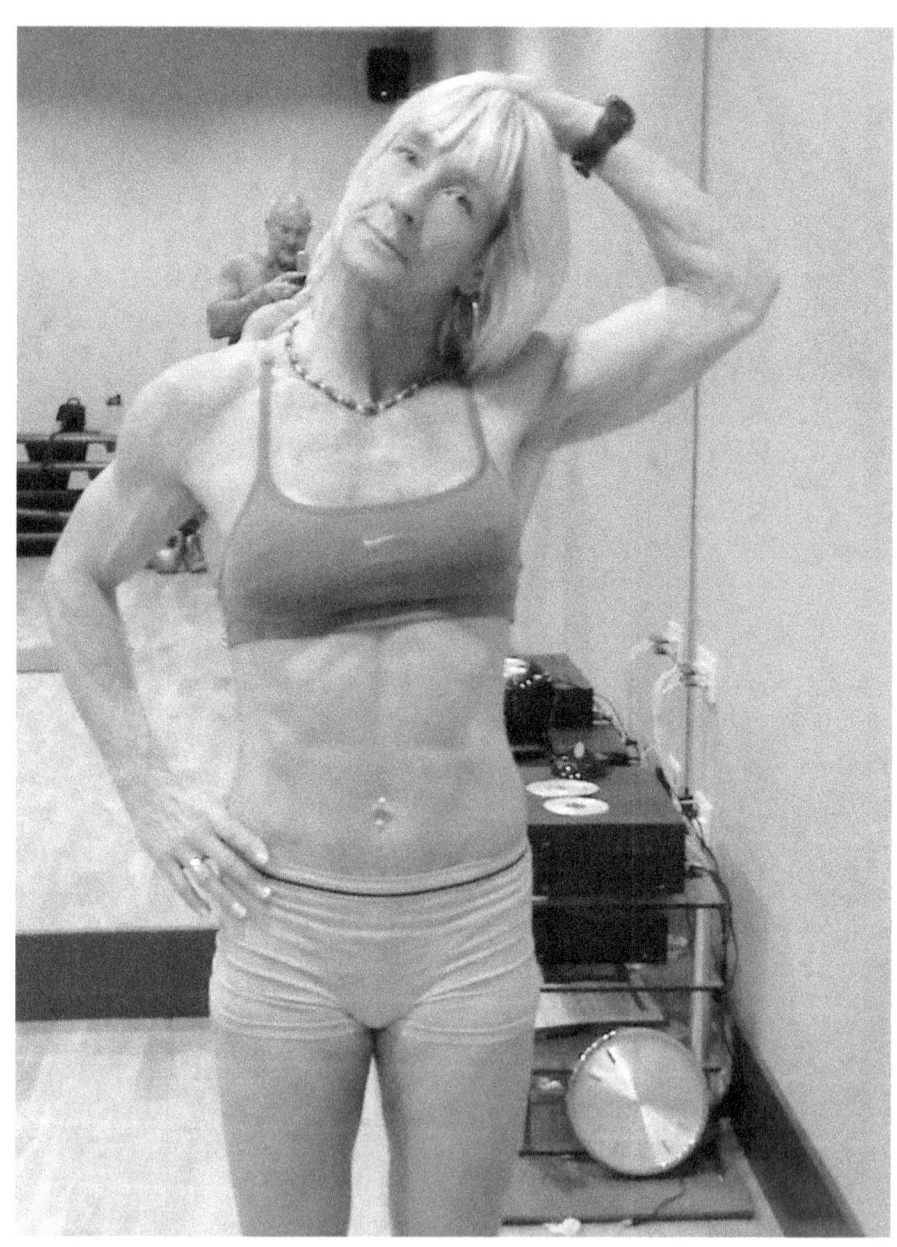

Biceps

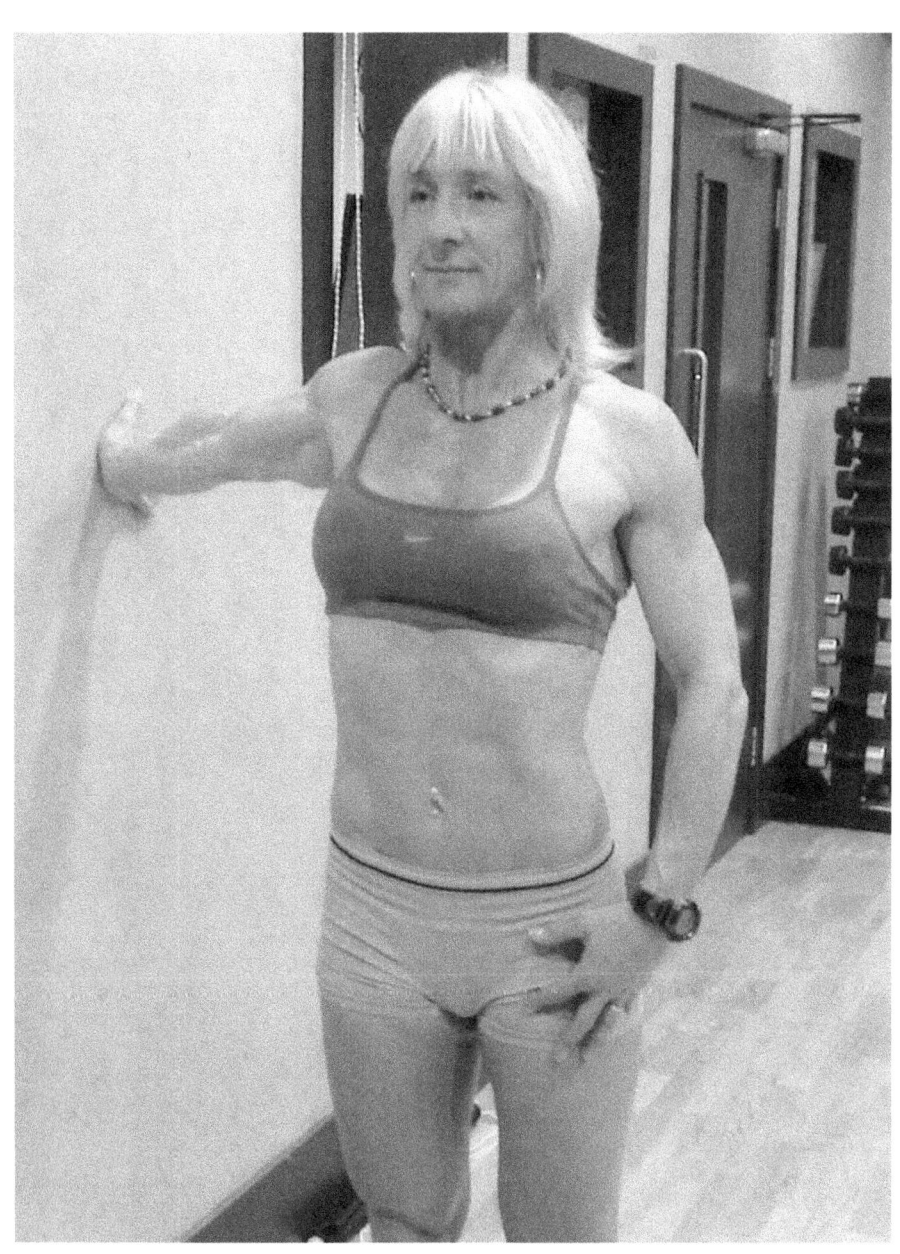

Chest & Delts

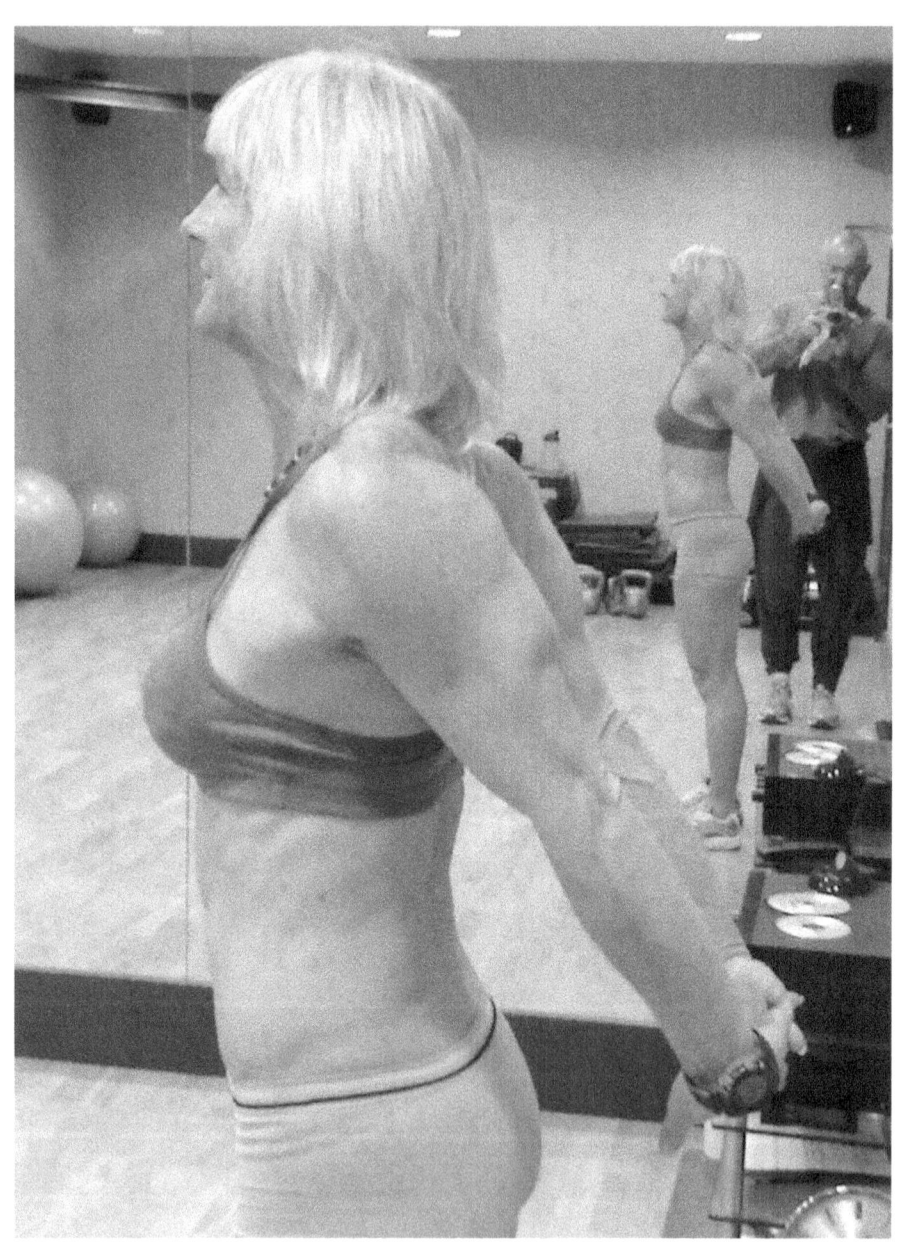

Hips & Low Back

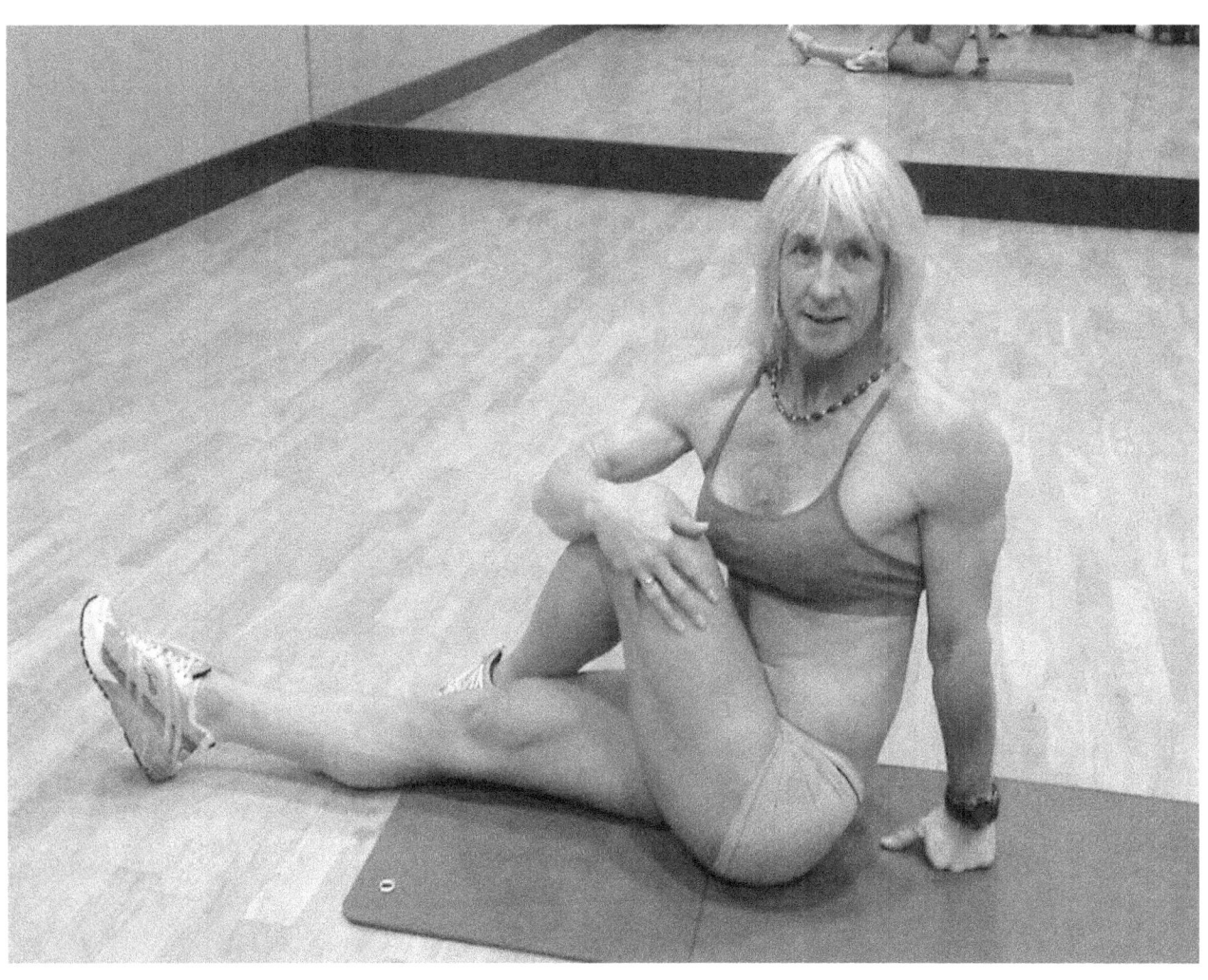

Lower Back

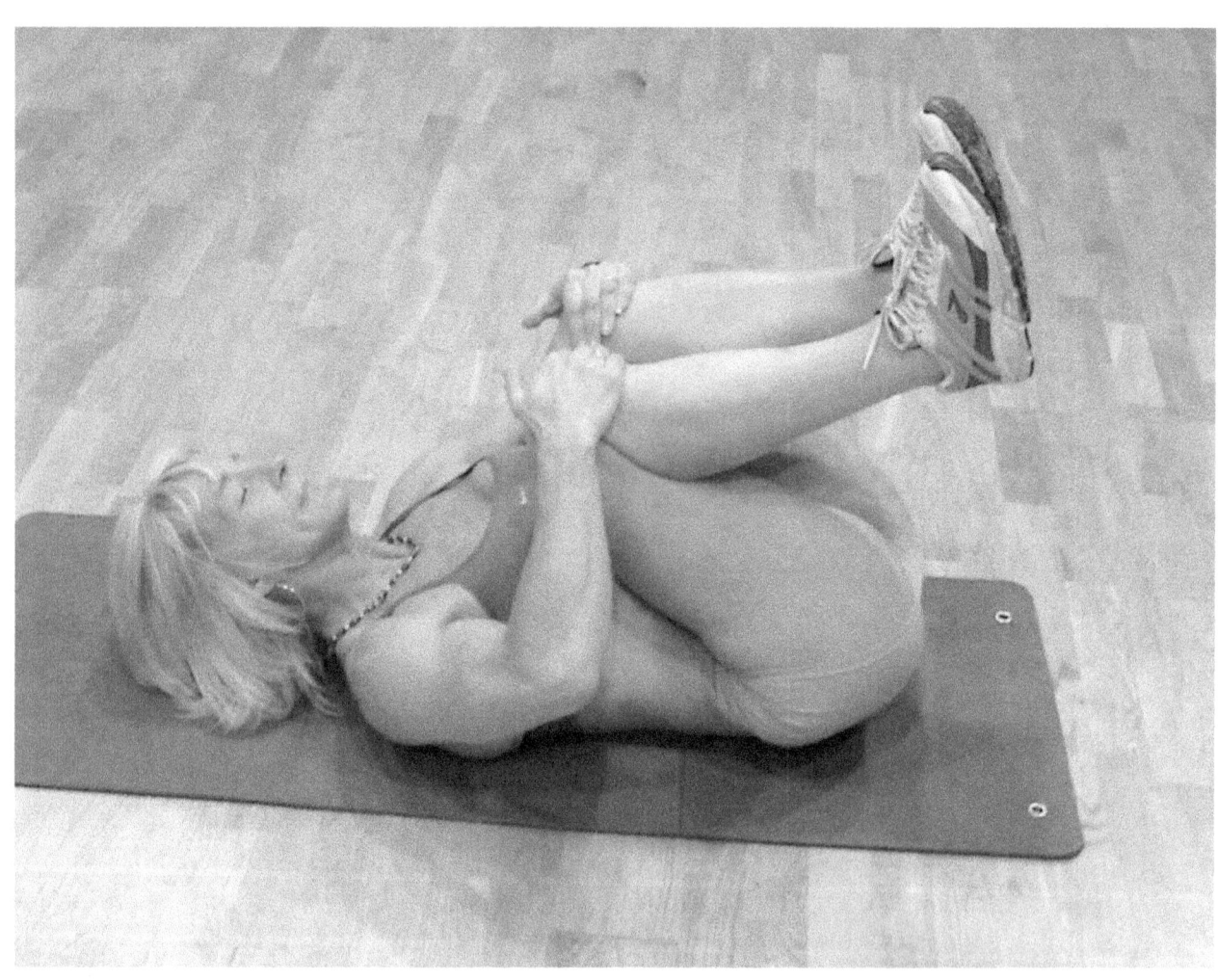

Calves

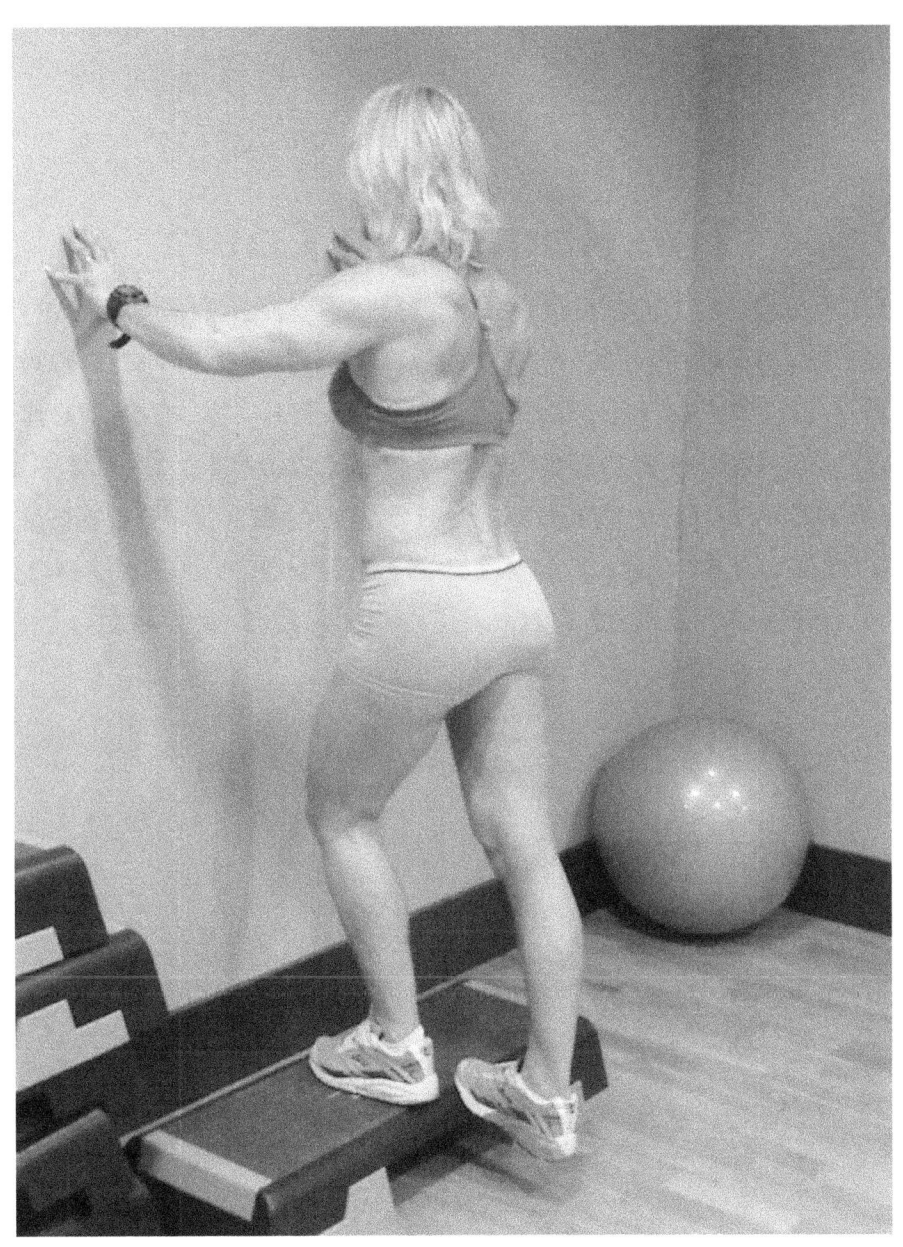

PART 5 - JUST SOME FUN??

The Kangaroo Court

Capitalist society and the mass media in particular, stand charged with reproducing and reinforcing a feminine body ideal that is unfair to women and in particular female athletes. The charge holds that this action is knowingly maintained purely for self interest and financial gain by the media, the sponsors, associated industries and sports.

"Kant's categorical imperative tells us never to use other people merely to satisfy our own ends" (Furrow, 2005, p.23).

When it comes to the sporting body are females free to choose who they are, what they do and how they think? This essay will look at whether deeply embedded myths and ideologies perpetuated by the accused are unfair to women. The first section will look at the case for the defence and how these images are positive for women. Section two for the prosecution, will examine the very real health and psychological damage that such ideologies can cause. Section three will use Bentham's utility principle to reach a verdict and then enlist the help of Ralph Waldo Emerson and Immanuel Kant to discuss solutions that we all have at our individual disposal. Finally concluding and summarising the findings.

"There can be no doubt that Western culture in the 2000's promotes unrealistic body ideals to women, and that nonconformity to these ideals leads to social disapproval" (Grogan, 2008, p. 79).

The Case for The Defence

The first point for the defence is that not all women are susceptible to body dissatisfaction upon viewing "perfect" female bodies.

Data suggests that only a specific subsection of the population - those who agree with such statements as "being physically fit is a priority in today's society (awareness of societal attitudes); "photographs of thin women make me wish I were thin" (acceptance of societal attitudes); or "my value as a person is related to my weight" (cognitive distortions related to physical appearance) - are "at risk" from such images (Grogan, 2008, p. 114).

Point two is quite straight forward and it is that they are doing nothing wrong in the eyes of the law.

Point three argues that the women are freely buying into the ideologies, as it is ultimately their money that continues to fund the ongoing processes. The women have a choice. The media & associated industries are just supplying a demand.

Point four argues that many women are motivated to lose weight and get fitter in order to reach the ideal feminine body shape due to their motivating influence.

The Defence rests its case.

The Case for The Prosecution

To begin the case for the prosecution we will briefly address the four defence points.

In response to point one that not all women are susceptible to media images, evidence will show that enough women are being affected for there to be a problem, maybe of epidemic proportions.

Point two could be answered that not everything that is morally wrong is illegal. Lying is not illegal but is often immoral.

Responding to point three, a quote from Body Image, states the case admirably:

> "The women interviewed are aware that the images presented are unrealistic and unhealthy (although they still aspire to look like fashion models in magazines) and are often angry at what they see as the media manipulating them into feeling bad about the way they look" (Grogan, 2008, p. 127).

So it would seem that even though the women seem to support the media and industry they are angry at what they feel is manipulation to an idealised body type.

On point four, there may indeed be agreement in that there are always a number of highly disciplined, motivated and self reliant individuals that will reach their personal goals. The argument would be that they would probably reach their goals without any media motivation.

The prosecutions first point is that the images are a lie and are not real in any way due to digital modification.

> "These images are teaching us how to see. Filtered, smoothed, polished, softened, sharpened, rearranged. And passing. Digital creations, visual cyborgs, teaching us what to expect from flesh and blood" (Bordo, 2003, p18).

Presenting women with an impossible goal and then selling them the needs so they may continually strive to reach the unrealistic ideal that they see in front of them at every turn.

Now we move to see the problems faced by a sport widely considered as feminine inappropriate, female bodybuilding. In could be argued that female bodybuilding amplifies the body issues faced by sporty women in general.

> "Women experienced pressures from within the body building community defining the acceptable size and appearance of their bodies. They were

engaged in a 'balancing act' where they were trying to attain a body that was muscular but not too muscular, and that maintained some aspects of traditional 'feminine' appearance. It is concluded that women who engage in Physique-level body building face complex layers of social pressure from within and outside the body building community" (Grogan et al, 2009, p. 49).

Women face health risks by trying to attain the ideal slim body revered by western society. Research was undertaken to assess bone mineral density in women.

"The main aim of this study was therefore to investigate how physical activity together with performance in selected tests in adolescence and physical characteristics in adolescence and/or adulthood are related to adult BMD in women. A second aim was to investigate whether performance in physical capacity tests for a specific body region in adolescence may be associated with adult BMD for this body region. Thus, physical performance tests were performed around the age of 16 years, coinciding with attainment of peak bone mass, and measurements of bone mass were performed at a second visit at the mean age of 36 years............ This supports earlier findings that activities started in late adolescence or young adulthood are not as effective in enhancing bone mass as activities started in earlier ages, i.e. around puberty. It also suggests that mechanical loading should be continued after puberty to maintain the increase in BMD gained from physical activity." (Barnekow-Bergkvist, Hedberg, Pettersson, Lorentzon, 2009, p.447).

This report shows that lifetime high impact and weight bearing activity started at adolescence, dramatically increases bone mineral density in later life, drastically decreasing the likelihood of osteoporosis. This is exactly the sort of exercise that women avoid in order to reach the ideal female form. Top of the list would be full body progressive resistance training, an advanced version of which, is bodybuilding. On this evidence it would appear that current ideologies could be harmful to women.

Here is another example of the damage perfect body ideologies can represent to young women athletes:

"A 15-year-old girl finishes a 1-hour dance rehearsal that prepares her for an upcoming recital. At the end of her practice, her dance instructor pulls her
aside to give her the usual critique and pointers. Instead of merely telling her to work on her positioning, the instructor tells the dancer that before she will be allowed to perform, she must lose 10 or more pounds. The instructor

tells her that this weight loss will help her look like a "real" ballerina. In a track practice across town, a 19-year-old woman talks with her teammates about the best way to drop a few pounds before the next meet. Although her coach has never openly suggested weight loss, he has made it clear that the thinner the runner is, the faster she will be. Are these examples a clear representation of what today's female athletes face in terms of sports participation and body image? Does athletic involvement by young women put them at risk for eating disorders brought on by pressures to excel at their sports? Do some sports pose a greater threat than others to a woman's body image and eating behaviour? Over the past 20 years, female athletic participation has increased dramatically, and with this growth have come questions about the impact that athletic participation has on young girls and their sense of self" (Robinson & Ferraro, 2004, p. 115-128).

Both of these research projects build a good case for ideal female body concepts and ideologies being both physically and psychologically damaging to women of all ages.
There is some evidence however to show that a gradual acceptance of female muscularity is occurring and in some cases even sought after.

"The muscular physique for women was once largely unacceptable by many; however, in the wake of the current social trend, women's muscularity is not only accepted but has also become desired. Although in the past the ideal woman's body was slender, the present standards are much more specific, with the ideal physique being not only thin, but also muscular and toned. Despite this trend, societal norms seem to have an upper limit as to what amount of muscularity is acceptable for a woman to possess, resulting in women attempting to negotiate the correct amount of muscle and an intensification of the difficulty in trying to attain this ideal. Although there is still a continuum of body ideals, it has become increasingly clear that women do aspire to muscularity goals" (Mosewich, Vangool, Kowalski & McHugh, 2009, p.99).

From this quote it would seem that although progress is being made women are still a long way from having the freedom to display a body without limitations. Where does the responsibility lay for keeping women locked into an idealised body image that is so damaging physically and psychologically? Two studies give an indication as to where the responsibility for promoting such idealised images may lay. The first quote here is based on research undertaken with young volleyball players, showing how their evaluations of body image were negative after looking at the perfect images depicted in non athletic poses, within a volleyball publication.

> "Body image is heavily influenced by the social comparison process and involves evaluations of overall physical size and specific body parts—arms, abdomen, and thighs. Although the self evaluations of physical ability are predominantly positive, evaluations of body image are frequently negative and appear to be exacerbated by photographic poses that emphasize an athlete's aesthetic beauty rather than her athletic prowess" (Thomsen, Bower & Barnes, 2004, p. 266).

The next journal examined the eating habits of young women after viewing media images of the perfect female body.

> "Among women with a discrepancy between perceptions of their actual body and the body their same-gender peers believe they ought to have, exposure to images alone and images plus congruent text led to a reduction in the amount eaten in front of female peers" (Harrison, Taylor & Marske, 2006, p. 507).

From this it would indicate that media manipulated images of how the perfect woman should look are the primary source for unrest, and the resulting lack of freedom that women experience when it comes to their physical appearance and ultimately their health.

There is no doubt that Western culture in the 21st century promotes unrealistic body ideals to women, and that nonconformity to these ideals leads to social disapproval.

The Prosecution rests it's case.

The Verdict - Utility & Individual Free Will (agency)

Jeremy Bentham (1748 - 1832) - The principle of utility will be used by this Kangaroo court to reach a verdict.

According to utilitarianism, the principle of utility is the sole source of moral rightness. No action is right or good, regardless of its source unless it conforms to the principle of utility.

> "The principle of utility is as follows: Of the courses of action available, choose the one that produces the greatest aggregate well being. In other words, we take everyone affected by a contemplated action, determine how

the action will affect them , add all these effects together, subtracting negative effects from positive effects and compare the sum with the sum of effects of alternatives" (Smart, Williams, 1973, p.48)

In order to reach a verdict this kangaroo court must adopt a model of an alternative to the current hyper-reality purveyed by the media. This court will assume that legislation is passed tomorrow that orders all forms of the media, advertising and associated industries that from now on that they have to represent the body shapes and sizes reflected in society in general. No digital enhancement, from now on all media must keep it real. Heavy penalties will result from any contravention of these new rules. Sports publications must be more true to the sport and depict serious athletes with muscles if they have them, playing their sports. Although initially the current deeply embedded ideologies would continue to drive women, it is believed that eventually women will either find comfort in themselves or else strive for a body ideal that is more realistic and achievable, closer to how they are. Models would no longer need to make themselves sick in order to conform, as they could work at any weight. Eventually body dissatisfaction would all but disappear. As the rules would be the same for all, even the accused would not suffer long term.

The verdict of this kangaroo court is that the new model would be better for all parties concerned, delivering the greatest aggregate well being. Taking away some freedom from the accused to do as they please, would give back freedom to millions of women. For the accused it would eventually be business as usual, well not as usual but with a good deal more honesty and integrity and without inflicting suffering on millions of young women worldwide. Incidentally a similar situation exists for men with muscle dysmorphia due to media pressures.

One could argue then that although the accused appear to be guilty, that the continued cooperation of the defendants makes it impossible to make a case and the changes will never happen. The victims are financing and supporting the crime as it were. The perfect crime. What then is the answer to combat the perfect crime. The answer is to be found in each and every individual. Kant would argue the perfectly autonomous female, or in Emerson's words the perfectly self reliant female.

Immanuel Kant (1724-1804) - would suggest procedural autonomy.

"A person achieves procedural autonomy if she critically evaluates her beliefs and desires, and she endorses them without excessive interference by external authority. In other words, if the beliefs and desires that generate your actions are a sincere expression of your deepest values, and you settle on these values after sufficient deliberation, then you are autonomous. This is what it means to make one's own decisions, to be a self directed person"(Furrow, 2005, p.25).

This sounds simple in theory but maybe challenging with today's media bombardment and swamped as we are in detrimental ideologies which are rarely absolute truths. Know your values, make your own decisions and direct your own life.

Ralph Waldo Emerson (1803-1882) - This gentleman may offer up a possible solution for prospective sporty women that are scared to take the plunge because of contemporary ideology, and sporty women detractors alike to consider. Both the aforementioned have lost an element of human freedom, to think what you like and to act how you like as long as it harms nobody. This is the path most of us take, happy to go along with society's program in exchange for a level of status and reasonable material circumstances, in essence to fit in. Though we all profess to be individual and breakaway from limitations, the reality is comfort in conformity. In his 30 page essay called self reliance, Emerson called his philosophy idealism and sells the virtues of resisting conformity in order to find your true self. To follow your unique calling and resist being steered through a pre - programmed predictable life. If the thoughts and actions are predictable then so too will be the results. The only proper defence against numbing conformity due to the scripting of our lives by society is to find and walk the trail of uniqueness in both thought and action. In Self Reliance there are many calls to that end.

> "We but half express ourselves, and are ashamed of that divine idea which each of us represents.........What I must do is all that concerns me, not what the people think.....It is easy in the world to live after the world's opinion.... It is easy in solitude to live after our own...Nothing can bring you peace but yourself. Nothing can bring you peace but the triumph of principles" (Emerson 1841/2007, p. 20).

If we can apply this to our thoughts and actions then maybe we will become the unique individuals we are intended to be and recognise the same in others and applaud individuality and the right to be different in all people.

Conclusion & Implications

In conclusion, it is clear to this court that immorality is indeed at work here. However the defendants are financing the whole affair. As long as human beings remain materialistic and vain, capitalist society will take advantage with any means at their disposal. With increased technology the situation will only get worse with more sports women and women in general suffering body image problems. The solution for now is with each individual acting in self reliance or autonomously. The ideal body has actually changed over the years to a marginally more muscular toned body. However as long as the word ideal can be used for any body type it will always signify a problem.

"Do not follow where the path may lead. Go instead where there is no path and leave a trail" (Emerson 1841/2007, p. 38).

That's All Folks

Have Fun

Julie & Gary

References

Arnoldi, K. (2008) *Chemical Pink*, New York; The Overlook Press.

Barrett, W. (1958) *Irrational Man - A Study in Existential Philosophy*, New York: Anchor Books.

Barnekow-Bergkvist, M. Hedberg, G. Pettersson, U. Lorentzon, R.(2006) Relationships between physical activity and physical capacity in adolescent females and bone mass in adulthood, *Scandanavian Journal of Medicine and Science in Sports 2006*: 16: 447–455. DOI: 10.1111/j.1600 0838.2005.00500.x. This article was downloaded by: [EBSCOHost EJS. Accessed On: 21 March 2010. Publisher Singapore: Blackwell Munksgaard.

Bordo, S. (2003) *Unbearable weight: Feminism, Western Culture, and the body* (10th anniversary edn), Berkeley, CA: University of California Press.
Brizendine, L. (2007) *The Female Brain*. London: Transworld Publishers.

Cox, G. (2009) *How to Be an Existentialist or to Get Real, Get a Grip and Stop Making Excuses,* London: Continuum International Publishing Group.

Cox. G. (2010) *How to Be a Philosopher*, London: Continuum International Publishing Group.

Dionigi, R. (2006) Competitive Sport as Leisure in Later Life: Negotiations, Discourse, and Aging - *Leisure Sciences, 2006, 28: 181–196.* EBSCOhost [Online]. Available at http://0-ejournals.ebsco.com.brum.luton.ac.uk/ (Accessed: 5th December 2010).

Emerson, R.W. (2007) *Self - Reliance*. Rockville, Maryland: Arc Manor Publishers.

Forbes, G.B., Adams-Curtis, L.E., Holmgren, K.M. & White, K.B.(2004) Perceptions of the Social and Personal Characteristics of Hyper muscular Women and of the Men Who Love Them - *The Journal of Social Psychology,* 2004, *144*(5), 487–506. EBSCOhost [Online]. Available at http://0ejournals.ebsco.com.brum.luton.ac.uk/ (Accessed: 10th November 2010).

Furrow, D. (2005) *Ethics: Key Concepts in Philosophy*, London: Continuum.

Gernigon, C., Thill, E. & Fleurance, P.(1999) 'Learned helplessness: A survey of cognitive, motivational and perceptual-motor consequences in motor tasks', *Journal of Sports Sciences,* 17: 5, 403 — 412. EBSCOhost [Online]. Available at http://0-ejournals.ebsco.com.brum.luton.ac.uk/ (Accessed: 1st March 2010).

Grogan, S. (2008) *Body Image: Understanding Body Dissatisfaction in Men, Women and Children.* Hove: Routledge.

Grogan, S. Evans, R. Wright, S. and Hunter, G.(2004) 'Femininity and muscularity:
accounts of seven women body builders', *Journal of Gender Studies*, 13: 1, 49 — 61
To link to this Article: DOI: 10.1080/0958923032000184970
URL: http://dx.doi.org/10.1080/0958923032000184970. This article was downloaded by: [EBSCOHost EJS. Accessed On: 21 March 2010. Publisher London: Routledge.

Jarvis, M. (2010) *Sport Psychology*. Hove: Routledge.

Hardy, L., Jones, G. & Gould, D. (1996) Understanding Psychological Preparation for Sport - Theory and Practice of Elite Performers, Chichester: John Wiley & Sons Ltd.

Hargreaves, J. (2003) *Sporting Females: Critical issues in the History and Sociology of Women's Sports.* London: Routledge.

Harrison, K. Taylor, L. D. & Marske, A. L. Women's and Men's Eating Behaviour Following Exposure to Ideal-Body Images and Text, *Communication Research;* Volume 33; Number 6, December 2006 507-529 © 2006 Sage Publications 10.1177/0093650206293247 http://crx.sagepub.com
hosted at http://online.sagepub.com
Downloaded from http://crx.sagepub.com at Ebsco Electronic Journals Service (EJS) on March 21, 2010. Published by: http://www.sagepublications.com

Harwood, J. (2010) *A Beginners Guide to the Ideas of 100 Great Thinkers*, London: Querec Publishing Plc.

Hotten, J. (2005) *Muscle - A writers trip through a sport with no boundaries*, London: Yellow Jersey Press.

Klein, A. (1993) *Little Big Men - Bodybuilding Subculture and Gender Construction*, Albany: State University of New York Press.

Malcolm, D. (2008) *The Sage Dictionary of Sports Studies*. London: Sage Publications Ltd.

Mill, J. S. (2001) *Utilitarianism and the 1868 Speech on Capital Punishment*, 2nd edn, Indianapolis: Hackett Publishing Company, Inc.

Mosewich, A. D. Vangool, A. B. Kowalski, K. C. & McHugh, TL. F. Exploring Women Track and Field Athletes' Meanings of Muscularity, *Journal of Applied Sport Psychology*, 21: 99–115, 2009. Copyright C _ Association for Applied Sport Psychology ISSN: 1041-3200 print / 1533-1571 online, DOI:

10.1080/10413200802575742 This article was downloaded by: [EBSCOHost EJS. Accessed On: 21 March 2010. Publisher London: Routledge.

Nicholl, A., R. & Polman, R., C., J. (2007) Coping in sport: A systematic review - *Journal of Sports Sciences*, January 1st 2007; 25(1): 11 – 31 EBSCOhost [Online]. Available at http://0-ejournals.ebsco.com.brum.luton.ac.uk/ (Accessed: 18th December 2010).

Nhat Hahn, T. (2008) *The Miracle of Mindfulness*, Edbury: Rider Publishing.

Nhat Hahn, T. (2009) *Happiness*, California: Parallax Press.
Pope, H.G. Phillips, K.A. & Olivardia, R. (2002) *The Adonis Complex*: *How to Identify and Prevent Body Obsession in Men and Boys*. New York: Touchstone.

Reiss, S. & Havercamp, S., M. *(2005)* Motivation in Developmental Context: A New Method for Studying Self-Actualization - *Journal of Humanistic Psychology*, Vol. 45 No. 1, Winter 2005 41-53. EBSCOhost [Online]. Available at http://0-ejournals.ebsco.com.brum.luton.ac.uk/ (Accessed: 18th December 2010).

Robinson, K. & Ferraro, R. (2004). The Relationship between the types of female athletic participation and female body type, *The Journal of Psychology*, 2004, 138(2), 115–128 URL: http://dx.doi.org/10.1080/0958923032000184970. This article was downloaded by: [EBSCOHost EJS. Accessed On: 21 March 2010. Publisher London: Routledge.

Russell, B. (1912) *The Problems of Philosophy*, Oxford: Oxford University Press.

Seligman, M. (2006) *Learned Optimism*. New York: Free Press

Smart, J.J.B. & Williams, B. (1973), *Utilitarianism: For and Against*, Cambridge: Cambridge University Press.

Thomsen, S. R. Bower, D. W. & Barnes, M. D. Photographic Images in Women's Health, Fitness, and Sports Magazines and the Physical self-concept of a Group of Adolescent Female Volleyball Players, *Journal of Sport and Social Issues* 2004; 28; 266 DOI: 10.1177/0193723504266991 Downloaded from http://jss.sagepub.com at Ebsco Electronic Journals Service (EJS) on March 28, 2010. Published by: http://www.sagepublications.com

Treagus, M. (2005) Playing like Ladies: Basketball, Netball and Feminine Restraint, *International Journal of the History of Sport*, 22: 1, 88-105. EBSCOhost [online]. Available at: http://dx.doi.org/10.1080/0952336052000314593 (Accessed: 20 January 2010).

Weitlauf, J.C., Cervone, D., Smith, R.E., & Wright, P.M. (2001) Assessing Generalization in Perceived Self-Efficacy: Multidomain and Global Assessments of the Effects of Self-Defense Training for Women - *Personality and Social Psychology Bulletin 2001*, 27: 1683. EBSCOhost [Online]. Available at http://0ejournals.ebsco.com.brum.luton.ac.uk/ (Accessed: 13th December 2010).

Woodman, T. & Hardy, L. (2003) The relative impact of cognitive anxiety and self-confidence upon sport performance: a meta-analysis, *Journal of Sports Sciences,* 21: 6, 443 — 457.   EBSCOhost [Online]. Available at http://0ejournals.ebsco.com.brum.luton.ac.uk/ (Accessed: 13th December 2010).